Cocaine Users

Cocaine Users
A Representative Case Approach

James V. Spotts
Franklin C. Shontz

 THE FREE PRESS
A Division of Macmillan Publishing Co., Inc.
New York

Collier Macmillan Publishers
London

The Free Press
A Division of Macmillan Publishing Co., Inc.
866 Third Avenue, New York, N.Y. 10022

Collier Macmillan Canada, Ltd.

Library of Congress Catalog Card Number: 79-7631

Printed in the United States of America

printing number
1 2 3 4 5 6 7 8 9 10

Library of Congress Cataloging in Publication Data

Spotts, James V
    Cocaine users.

    Includes bibliographical references and index.
    1. Cocaine habit--United States--Case studies.
2. Cocaine. I. Shontz, Franklin C., joint author.
II. Title. [DNLM: 1. Cocaine--Case studies.
2. Drug abuse--Case studies. WM280 S765c]
HV5810.S65   362.2'93   79-7631
ISBN 0-02-930560-8

Contents

PART 3: INTERPRETATION

Acknowledgments

We wish to express our gratitude to Charles B. Wilkinson, M.D., Executive Director of the Greater Kansas City Mental Health Foundation, and to Daniel J. Lettieri, Ph.D., Project Officer of the National Institute on Drug Abuse, whose patience, encouragement, and support throughout our research were essential to its completion.

We also wish to express appreciation to the many people who assisted us in this endeavor. We appreciate the assistance and advice received from William McNalley, M.D., Director of the University of Kansas Medical Center Methadone Maintenance Program, and Mr. Harold Brooks, R.N., of the Western Missouri Mental Health Center. We are also grateful to Gordon Halliday, Ph.D., Daniel Elash, Ph.D., and Robert Becker, M.A. for their invaluable assistance in data collection and analysis.

Finally, our heartfelt thanks go to Ms. Connie Morgan, who typed the manuscript again and again with skill and persistence.

We wish also to express our sincere appreciation to that large group of people who cannot be named but who assisted us in our participant search and served in a more direct role as intermediaries. Without the assistance, support, and tolerance which these people openly provided for two curious investigators some of these studies would never have been completed.

Finally, and most important, we wish to express our gratitude to the nine anonymous men whom we have called Arky L., Bill F., Tom P., George B., Al G., John B., Willie M., Fred S., and Rufus B.; they are what these studies are all about. They shared their lives, hopes, dreams, fears, and expert knowledge of cocaine with two investigators. We have tried to report the many things we learned from them as honestly and as accurately as we can.

This book is based on data collected in research conducted under the auspices of the Greater Kansas City Mental Health Foundation (600 East 22d Street, Kansas City, Mo.) in conjunction with Contract No. ADM-45-74-149 with the National Institute on Drug Abuse (NIDA), the Alcohol, Drug Abuse, and Mental Health Administration of the United States Department of Health, Education, and Welfare. The opinions expressed herein are those of the authors and do not necessarily reflect those of the National Institute on Drug Abuse, the Department of Health, Education, and Welfare, or the Greater Kansas City Mental Health Foundation.

James V. Spotts
Franklin C. Shontz

_____ Part 1

Background and Orientation

Background

THE SUBSTANCE

The substance, cocaine—known in the drug culture by such names as *snow, flake, girl, coke, gold dust, heaven dust, happy dust, happy trails, Bernice, the star-spangled powder, the rich man's* (or *pimp's*) *drug, her, Corrine, heaven leaf,* and *lady,* is an alkaloid derived from the leaves of the *Erythroxylon coca,* a shrub that is cultivated on the mountainous slopes of Peru, Chile, and Bolivia, in Java, and to a lesser extent in Mexico, the West Indies, and India (Clark, 1973; Froede, 1972). The shrub produces the active alkaloid cocaine within eighteen months and continues to produce it for its whole life, almost forty years. The plant can grow as high as twelve feet, but plants cultivated for harvest are kept pruned to a height of three to six feet for convenience in picking. Since *Erythroxylon coca* is an evergreen, the elliptical leaves which vary from one to four inches in length can be harvested several times a year (Hawks, 1977). The plant grows best on the eastern slopes of the Andes in Bolivia and Peru between 1,500 and 6,000 feet above sea level in a cool, humid, frost-free evergreen zone with a mean annual temperature of sixty-five to sixty-eight degrees Fahrenheit (Sabbag, 1976, p. 70).

Typically coca leaves are harvested in March, June, and November. The harvested leaves are soaked in gasoline drums with kerosene and other solvents. The fluid is then drained off and the soggy leaves are removed. The residue, a thick coffee-like paste, is ladled into smaller containers and sold to "laboratory agents" or "traffickers" for $200 to $300 per pound. These agents transport the paste to laboratories where the alkaloid is refined and shipped (Gay, Sheppard, Inaba, and Newmeyer, 1973b).

Both Carroll (1977) and Sabbag report that, in its natural form, coca is rather nourishing. It contains vitamin C, riboflavin, and many B vitamins. "It cures altitude sickness, tones the entire digestive tract, and promotes the health of the oral cavity and teeth, properties which result from the synergy between cocaine and the associate compounds in the leaf" (Sabbag, p. 71).

Cocaine is reportedly the only naturally occurring anesthetic. Froede described cocaine as a benzoic acid ester, outlining the following laboratory process for extracting cocaine:

1. The coffee-like coca paste is distilled from the leaves;
2. the paste is converted into cocaine hydrochloride through
   a. extraction of the alkaloids,
   b. hydrolization to ecgonine,
   c. methylation, and
   d. distillation into a white powder.

A cocaine yield of .65 to 1.2 percent by weight is achieved from the leaves (Buck, Sasaki, Hewitt and Mccrae, 1968). A yield of 1 percent from mature plants is considered good (Adriani, 1962).

Pure cocaine is a colorless to white crystal or crystalline powder, is odorless, decomposes on standing in air, and has a melting point of 98° C. Cocaine hydrochloride, U.S.P., dissolves in one-half its weight in water. Its saturated solution is alkaline (Clark).

Erythroxylon coca is thought to be indigenous only to Central and South America. One variety, *Erythroxylum (Erythroxylon monogynum),* is indigenous to India (Madras), but it does not contain cocaine or related alkaloids. *Erythroxylon coca* was brought to Ceylon in 1870 from the botanical gardens at Kew, London. From there it was introduced to India in 1883-85; apparently, these efforts to introduce the shrub failed, except in the hilly Nilgiri area (Chopra and Chopra, 1958). *Erythroxylon coca* was then introduced to Java and Jamaica to meet the rising demand for the drug in the United States. Clark reports that today Java is the world's largest producer of coca leaves. However, Carroll (1977) asserts that most legally produced coca now comes from Peru and Bolivia.

History

In South America coca leaves have been used for at least 1,200 years. The emblem of the coca leaf appears on ancient pottery shards, and coca leaves have been found in Indian graves dating back to the ninth century A.D. (Gay et al., 1973b). Indians chewed coca leaves mixed with an alkali (lime) and a binding agent (cornstarch or guano). Chewing coca leaves is thought to have been widespread during the pre-Inca period, but during the Inca era its use was reserved for the nobility and priesthood. The plant was declared divine, a gift bestowed by Manco Capac, royal Son of the Sun God. The Inca or Imperical Ruler dispensed coca leaves as a token of noblesse oblige during religious ceremonies or to warriors, diplomats, and other state officials as rewards for outstanding service (Martin, 1970; Mortimer, 1901/1974).

Another myth of the origin of coca asserts that a beautiful woman was executed for adultery, cut in half, and buried; from her grave the coca plant grew and blossomed to be consumed by men in her memory (Petersen and Stillman, 1977). It is reported that Inca surgeons used the coca leaves as a local anesthetic in brain surgery or trephining (Hrdlicka, 1939).

With the coming of Pizarro and the destruction of the Inca Empire in the sixteenth century, the church restricted the use of coca leaves. At this time cultivation and chewing of coca leaves was widespread. Chewing the leaves alleviated fatigue, relieved hunger, and made the arduous daily life of the Indians more bearable. Eiswirth, Smith, and Wesson (1972) report that because coca leaves suppressed appetite and fatigue and increased productivity, the practice of chewing them had survival value. When the Spanish discovered that the Indians could not perform heavy labor if they were forbidden to use coca, the ban was dropped. Thus, during the post-Inca period, mine workers and slaves were paid in coca leaves to increase productivity. This custom persists today. Later, the church recognized the economic value of coca and initiated and maintained coca plantations of its own (Carroll, 1977). Coca leaves are still chewed by Andean Indians as part of social ritual and for mild stimulant effects.

Carroll points out that *"mamita kukita"* ("little mother coca") is still used by the Andean Indians to reduce muscular exhaustion, alleviate hunger and thirst, reduce the pain of rheumatism and external sores, reduce swelling of wounds and strengthen broken bones, alleviate asthmatic symptoms, stem nosebleeds, treat diseases of the teeth and gums, treat sore eyes, alleviate headache, and ease uterine contractions in childbirth.

Coca leaves were brought to Spain as botanical oddities by Nicolas Monardes in 1569 and to England somewhat later, in 1596. Monardes published an essay extolling the virtues of the plant in combating hunger and fatigue. In 1859, Paolo Mantegazza, who had lived in South America, described the physiologic and therapeutic effects of the coca leaves. That he was a champion of the drug is illustrated by the following: "Borne on the wings of two coca leaves, I flew about in the spaces of 77,438 worlds, one more splendid than another. I prefer a life of ten years with coca to one of a hundred thousand without it. It seemed to me that I was separated from the whole world, and I beheld the strangest images most beautiful in color and in form than can be imagined" (quoted in Gay et al., 1973b, p. 423).

In 1859 Dr. Scherzer, a member of the South American expedition on the Austrian frigate *Novara,* brought coca leaves to Vienna. In 1860, the Viennese biochemist Alfred Nieman isolated the cocaine alkaloid from the leaves of the plant (Byck, 1974).

In his paper *Über Coca* Sigmund Freud (1884/1974) reported that there was active human and animal research with cocaine in Austria, England, France, and Russia during the 1860s and 1870s. Findings were discouraging, however, and there was doubt that practical applications could be found for cocaine. Freud attributed these findings to deficiencies in the preparation of the leaves.

The eminent German pharmacologist and toxicologist Louis Lewin reported that when cocaine was introduced to medical science in 1885 all that was known about its effect was that ". . . the drinking of an infusion of 12 g. of coca leaves occasioned, besides a greater frequency of the pulse, palpitation of the heart, faintness, seeing of sparks and *tinnitus aurium,* a feeling of augmented power, and a greater desire for activity. An infusion of 16 g. of the leaves produced first a strange feeling of isolation from the exterior world and an irresistible urge to use one's strength; then in full consciousness appeared a kind of rigidity with a feeling of the most intense well-being, accompanied by the desire not to make the least movement for the whole day. Finally, sleep supervened" (1924, quoted in Byck, 243-244).

Between 1884 and 1887, Freud wrote a series of papers praising cocaine (Bernfield, 1953). He experimented upon himself with moderate dosages and became an advocate of its use as a euphoriant (Byck).

Freud enthusiastically prescribed cocaine. He gave it to his sisters and even to his future wife, Martha. As Ernest Jones (1953) stated, Freud was rapidly becoming a public menace (p. 81). Perhaps as a result of the optimistic reports he read concerning the value of cocaine in treating morphine and opium addiction in America (Bentley, 1880/1974; Erythroxylon coca as an antidote to the opium habit, 1880; Hammond, 1886; 1974), Freud recommended cocaine to a friend, Dr. Ernst Von Fleischl-Marxow, in the hope that it would relieve Fleischl's addiction to morphine. Fleischl administered the drug to himself in the form of subcutaneous injections. It appeared at first that the treatments were succeeding, but over time it became necessary for Fleischl to increase the dosage until he developed chronic intoxication and full-fledged cocaine psychosis.

At this point, Von Fleischl was using a subcutaneous dosage of a gram of cocaine per day. His symptomatology included tactile hallucinations, fainting (often with convulsions), severe insomnia, and an inability to control what were described as certain eccentric behaviors. He continued to abuse cocaine until his death six years later. This caused a much needed pause in Freud's efforts to proselytize in behalf of the drug (Lewis, 1968).

Freud's open advocacy of cocaine use brought criticism upon him from the medical profession and ultimately caused him to abandon his personal use of and scientific work with the drug. The eminent German psychiatrist, Albrecht Erlenmyer, was one of the first to sound the alarm. He described cocaine not only as dangerous and poisonous, but as most certainly addictive. Indirectly he accused Freud of contributing to the unleashing of the third scourge of humanity (after alcohol and morphine) onto the Continent. Louis Lewin, who later wrote *Phantastica* (1931), also contended that cocaine could not be a cure for the morphine habit. His comments, made in 1884, have a distinctly modern ring: "I want to state explicitly that according to all evidence coca is no substitute for morphine and that a morphine addiction cannot be cured by the use of coca . . . since the real morphine addict wants the specific morphine effect and since he can very well distinguish the euphoria of other substances. Such an exchange does not suit his special needs" (quoted in Byck, p. xxxii). Lewin added that if one treated a morphine addict with cocaine the only outcome would be double addiction.

In 1887, Freud published *Craving for and Fear of Cocaine* (1887/1974) to defend himself. He noted the positive findings in America and stated that all reports of cocaine addiction and the deterioration that resulted had occurred among individuals already addicted to morphine. He further stated that cocaine was not habit-forming and could be given up at will. Freud did note one important fact concerning cocaine, namely, the variability of its effects on different individuals.

However, Freud discontinued his work with cocaine in 1887. He later eliminated this period from his autobiography.

An acquaintance and colleague of Freud, Dr. Carl Koller (1928; Becker, 1963) achieved the fame Freud had sought in his studies with cocaine. Freud had discussed with Koller the possibilities of using cocaine as a topical anesthetic. After a period of experimentation, Koller delivered a paper in 1884 on the local anesthetic effects of cocaine used topically in ophthalmic surgery—and thus became famous as the discoverer of local anesthesia (Byck).

While Freud was attempting to treat morphine addiction with cocaine, Dr. William S. Halsted in America—a leading surgeon at Johns Hopkins School of Medicine who discovered cocaine's nerve-blocking anesthetic effect—was treating his own addiction to cocaine with morphine. The story of this physician's long struggle has been described by Brecher and the editors of Consumer Reports (1972) and Penfield (1969).

In America a number of reports during the 1880s concerned the use of cocaine in the treatment of a variety of medical conditions in addition to morphine and opium addiction, including stomach irritability, vomiting, cerebral hyperemia, mental depression, neuritis of the radial nerve, sciatica, vaginismus, rectal disease, conjunctivitis, and in nasal surgery (Bentley, 1880; Hammond, 1886/1974, 1887/1974). In 1877, Dr. G. Archie Stockwell optimistically asserted that Americans would be able to begin their second century of independence with the convenient and vigorous effects of cocaine, which never depresses, has no recoil, and eliminates fatigue without adverse effects.

Dr. William A. Hammond, Surgeon General under Lincoln and one of the most successful neurologists in New York, presented a paper at the annual session of the Virginia Medical Society (1886/1974), in which, like Freud, he denied that there was any such thing as a cocaine habit. He said that he had had a chemist prepare a drink of wine with pure cocaine (two grains to the pint), which was helpful in the treatment of dyspepsia and other stomach conditions. During the questioning period one physician reported a patient whom he thought exemplified cocaine addiction, but Hammond stoutly denied that it could occur.

Hammond did make a significant contribution: He used himself as his experimental subject and published one of the few descriptions in the literature of a dose-effect curve for cocaine (1887/1974).

From 1890 to 1910, additional cases of what was thought to be cocaine addiction began appearing all over the world. The fictional detective Sherlock Holmes was portrayed as a cocaine user (Musto, 1968/1974). Robert Louis Stevenson was treated for tuberculosis with cocaine in 1885 (Perry, 1972; M. G. Schultz, 1971). It is said that during this period he wrote the first draft of *Dr. Jekyll and Mr. Hyde* in three days.

In America from 1880 to 1914 cocaine was used in all kinds of quack nostrums. One well-known pharmaceutical company produced a variety of products containing cocaine, including coca leaf cigarettes and cigars, a liqueur-like coca cordial, and cocaine in tablets, hypodermic injections, ointments and syrups (Parke, Davis and Co., 1885/1974). The consumption of wine infused with coca leaves was popular, as were a plethora of patent medicines, home remedies, and beverages containing cocaine.

In 1885 this company published a promotional brochure describing the medical uses of cocaine. The introduction stated it [cocaine] is ... "a drug which, through its stimulant properties, can supply the place of food, make the coward brave, the silent eloquent, free the victims of alcohol and opium habits from their bondage, and, as an anesthetic, render the sufferer insensitive to pain, and make attainable to the surgeon heights of what may be termed 'aesthetic surgery' never reached before" (1885/1974, p. 128).

"The 1890s to 1914 was *the Age of the Cocainized Nostrum.* Foremost of these was Coca-Cola, introduced by Asa G. Chandler (and an instant hit) in 1888, which was advertized to 'cure your headache' and 'relieve fatigue for only 5¢.' As late as 1912, Koca-nole, Cafe-Coca, Kos-Cola, Kola-Ade, Celery Cola, and Dr. Don's Kola flourished. Catarrh (an early catch-all phrase for all that might ail you, from runny nose to tuberculosis) compounds glutted the corner drug store: Agnew's Powder, Anglo-American Catarrh Powder, and Ryno's Hay Fever and Catarrh Remedy, to name but a few" (Gay et al., 1973b, pp. 415–419). However, physicians began reporting growing numbers of cases of cocaine intoxication and psychosis. By 1890 the failure of cocaine to cure alcohol or morphine addiction had become apparent. In 1898 Scheppegrell described a variety of adverse and fatal reactions associated with cocaine in medicine and dentistry. By 1903 cocaine had been dropped as an ingredient in Coca Cola.

Shortly after the turn of the century cocaine snuff became popular for its euphoric effects. It is said that blacks in particular used this form of snuff (Chopra and Chopra, 1958; Lewis, 1968). Williams (1914) reported that use of cocaine snuff among blacks in the South had developed into a epidemic. He attributed increased crime and wholesale killings to these "cocaine fiends." In many towns and cities "the bootblacks and newsboys act as common vendors —retailers, so to speak, who loyally refuse to reveal the sources of their supply even under the most extreme pressure. They sell the commodity in the form of 'snuff,' a vile concoction composed of a small proportion of cocaine mixed with some white powder (such as Epsom salts) to give it bulk. 'Ten cents a sniff' is the usual price for an individual dose. But the more affluent purchaser who can raise the sum of twenty-five cents may get a good day's supply for that price, which is dispensed in small paper pill boxes" (p. 247).

According to Dale (1903), the drug was widely used in all sectors of society, frequently with morphine. "The ease with which morphine and cocaine can be purchased from a druggist without a physician's prescription is appalling. Some druggists rely on these sales to keep up their volume of business, and some have even said they could not exist if it were not for the sale of cocaine" (p. 1216). A survey in 1902 reported that only 3 to 8 percent of the cocaine sold in New York, Boston, and other metropolitan cities went into the practice of medicine or dentistry (Gay et al., 1973b).

In 1905, Mills described several cases of cocainism and coca-mania. Later, Gordon (1908) provided a detailed description of the symptomatology and treatment of fifteen cases of acute cocaine intoxication, some involving use of cocaine alone and others involving mixtures of cocaine and morphine. Both Mills and Gordon noted that heavy use of cocaine was rarely an isolated habit; most commonly, morphine and cocaine were used together. Mills and Gordon, as well as others, were pessimistic about the prognosis for cocaine users. They felt treatment could only be successful if users were willing to undergo separation from their homes and usual surroundings for up to a year (Lewin, 1931); but even under optimal conditions they would probably resume the habit upon returning to their accustomed surroundings.

Action was taken in 1906 to control the misuse of cocaine when the United States enacted the Pure Food and Drug Act. This act required accurate labeling of the contents of all over-the-counter preparations, forbade interstate shipments of food and soda water containing cocaine or opium, and put the first restrictions on the import of coca leaves (McLaughlin, 1973). In 1914, the Harrison Narcotic Tax Act specified that anyone handling opiates or cocaine must register with the government, pay a special tax, and keep records of all transactions. Unregistered persons could buy the drugs only on prescription from a physician. In 1922 Congress prohibited most importation of coca leaves and officially defined cocaine as a narcotic (Grinspoon and Bakalar, 1976). We know now, however, that cocaine is not a narcotic but a stimulant (Eiswirth et al., 1972; Kaplan, 1970).

Petersen and Stillman (1977b) point out that the emergence of state and federal legislation to control cocaine and the opiates was due to the confluence of a variety of factors. One factor was the reaction against the excesses of the patent medicine era. Some journalists focused attention upon the patent medicine manufacturers who sold "potent drugs to anyone who had the money to pay" (Ashley, 1975), and made the public aware of the hazards of some patent medicines and tonics. At the same time, "American medicine, characterized by relatively lenient professional standards until that time, was coming of age. Prior to the twentieth century, a medical degree was easily obtained, even in the best medical schools. While still in its infancy, the American Medical Association became increasingly concerned with establishing and maintaining higher standards of medical training and practice" (Petersen, 1977b, p. 29). As Ashley has noted, both pharmacists and physicians recognized as well that patent medicines claimed many customers who would otherwise be using their services. Another important factor, cited as influencing legal restrictions on the use of cocaine, was sheer racism (see Ashley; Petersen, 1977b). Between 1900 and 1920 the mass media raised the specter of cocaine-crazed blacks committing heinous crimes. Cocaine was made to seem responsible for mass murders by crazed (black) cocaine users (whose marksmanship was supposedly improved by the drug), and was accused of driving the humbler blacks all over the country to abnormal crimes.

By the time the Harrison Narcotic Act of 1914 was passed, forty-six of the forty-eight states had passed legislation limiting the use of cocaine. Ashley notes that people apparently felt more threatened by cocaine than by opiates, for at the time of the passage of the Harrison Act only twenty-nine states had laws regulating opiates.

"All the elements needed to insure cocaine's outlaw status were present by the first years of the twentieth century: it had become widely used as a pleasure drug, and doctors warned of the dangers attendant on indiscriminate sale and use; it had become identified with despised or poorly regarded groups—blacks, lower-class whites, and criminals; it had not been long enough established in the culture to insure its survival; and it had not, though used by them, become identified with the elite, thus losing what little chance it had of weathering the storm of criticism" (Ashley, p. 89).

During the early 1920s cocaine drifted into relative obscurity. Its medical use declined as a result of the development of longer lasting and less toxic analogues in anesthesia. Before passage of the Harrison Act there had been quite a few pure cocaine addicts in the U.S. However, by 1924 almost all cocaine addicts were also addicted to opium, morphine, or heroin (Kolb, 1924). In the United States by the mid-1920s cocaine had gone underground and become limited largely to members of the Bohemian jazz culture and to the more affluent ghetto dwellers (Eiswirth et al., 1972).

America was not the only country having problems with cocaine. The popularity of the drug in Europe increased gradually until World War I. With the war, the practice of snuffing cocaine broke out in France, in the Russian army, and later in central Europe. Wolff (1932) reported that following World War I cocaine became increasingly popular in Germany. In Wolff's opinion, the physicians' casual practice of prescribing cocaine was largely responsible for the spread of its use from 1918 to 1925. When the government instituted control over prescriptions, there was a decline from 400–450 kilograms per year in the country from 1925 to 1930, to less than half that amount in 1931.

Louis Lewin (1924/1974) provided a description of cocaine use in Germany.

"Already in 1901 there were many cocainistic men and women in England, doctors, politicians, and writers. At present, the situation is evidently much worse, although morphinism has not been dethroned. In Germany, mainly in the large towns, there are many cocainists in every profession, down to prostitutes and their protectors. In certain bars and restaurants, in the street, etc., cocaine is clandestinely sold, very frequently stolen or adulterated merchandize for which huge prices up to 30 marks are asked and paid. In Berlin there are cocaine dens, both disreputable and dirty and also fashionable and up-to-date establishments. One of these was raided by the police at the beginning of the present year. About one hundred habitues, men and women, from all classes of society, even university and literary men, had gathered there, to lead for a few hours an existence of somnolence and unreality" (p. 244). One of Lewin's patients provided a picture of the effect of cocaine in capsule form. In a letter to Lewin he stated, "Time is necessary to bring my conception of the world to a point which is founded on the sentence: God is a substance!" (quoted in Byck, 1974, p. 247).

During the 1920s and early 1930s reports from Europe and Asia asserted that with heavy cocaine use persons with a previously heterosexual orientation became homosexual. One interpretation of these cases was that in heterosexual men a loss of potency—without, however, any diminution of libido—together with the craving for new sensations was the cause for the inversion (Anonymous, 1925). Chopra and Chopra (1930-1931) attributed it to the loss of control of the "higher centers" which occurs in cocaine intoxication. Wolff (1932) did not feel the shifts in sexual orientation were due directly to cocaine. He stated, "It may be that sexual impotence which occurs in men as a result of cocaine addiction brings to the surface a hitherto latent component of inversion, the degree of which is dependent upon the extent to which the individual is bisexual. . . . after a 'withdrawal cure' or, better said, 'disintoxication,' a certain number of these persons recover complete heterosexuality, while others remain homosexual or bisexual" (p. 218). In 1961 Bell and Trethowan asserted the now generally accepted view that cocaine does not cause changes in sexual orientation and that sexual behavior while using cocaine is a function of sexual orientation prior to use.

During the 1920s and early 1930s problems associated with the abuse of cocaine were reported in Austria (Anonymous, 1924); Egypt (Biggam, Arafa, and Ragab, 1932); India (Chopra and Chopra, 1930-1931); and other parts of Europe and Asia. For example, while the normal medical consumption of cocaine in Austria did not exceed 60 kilograms per year, licensed sellers of narcotics there had received and disposed of 210 kilograms in one year. During that year a single dealer had sold 73 kilograms of cocaine hydrochloride, more than the medical requirements for the entire nation.

Physicians were thought to be responsible for the widespread use of cocaine in Europe during the 1920s. The spread of cocaine in India, however, was started, according to Chopra and Chopra, by a rich landowner in a provincial town who had become addicted to cocaine when he used it for a toothache. The habit then spread along the two main railway lines toward northern India, through proselytism by commercial travelers and others. Towns on railroad sidelines and the larger part of the country remained relatively free from the problem. The use of cocaine in India spread among the educated classes and the well-to-do people in towns. The high incidence of cocaine abuse was not due to snuffing the drug—in India it is chewed with betel leaf.

During the early 1930s Lindemann (1933-1934) and Lindemann and Malamud (1933-1934) studied the physiological and psychological effects of cocaine, sodium amytal, mescaline, and cannabis indica with various clinical groups. Cocaine seemed to increase schizophrenics' interest in and contact with the outside world, but effects varied markedly from subject to subject. Aside from this investigation, interest in cocaine seemed to wane. Usage of the drug was thought to have declined from 1930 to 1965 in both Europe and the United States. However, *The Gourmet Cokebook* (1972) reported that cocaine was popular among some Nazi officials up until and during World War II.

In the late 1960s cocaine became increasingly popular among U.S. heroin addicts both on the streets and in methadone maintenance programs. This use of cocaine by addicts in methadone programs was presumably to obtain euphoric feelings they could not get with orally administered methadone. Self-reports by 180 randomly selected narcotic addicts, certified during 1969-70 by the New York State Narcotic Control Commission, revealed that 82 percent used or abused cocaine. Some 73 percent of the 1,096 narcotic addicts evaluated at the NIMH Clinical Research Center in Lexington, Kentucky between May 1968 and June 1969 reported use or abuse of cocaine (Chambers, Taylor, and Moffett, 1972). In a study of 101 former methadone maintenance patients who had been admitted to the Lexington Center under civil commitment procedures from September 20, 1971 to February 5, 1972, Stephens and Weppner (1973) found that 50 percent had continued to abuse heroin while on methadone maintenance and about 25 percent had used cocaine while in the program. Of these 101 "cheaters" 75 percent were male; 67 percent were black.

Chambers, Taylor and Moffett found a number of significant differences between cocaine "cheaters" and their noncheating counterparts. Cheaters were (1) significantly older than noncheaters, (2) more frequently black than white (96 percent of the blacks reported cocaine use at some time in contrast to 54 percent of the whites), (3) more often divorced or separated, (4) less frequently employed at time of admission, (5) had longer histories of drug abuse, and (6) more actively involved in continued criminal activities while on methadone maintenance. No significant differences were found between cheating and non-cheating patients with regard to sex, arrest histories, prior treatment histories, or adjustment characteristics. Similar findings have been reported among incarcerated drug abusers.

During this period cocaine was "rediscovered" and became popular among youth in the United States. A similar rapid increase in illegal use of cocaine had occurred in England during the early to middle 1960s (Connell, 1969; Wilson, 1968). Cocaine use in England, where the drug was used with heroin, became a matter of serious national concern. Bewley (1965) reported a 138 percent increase in the use of cocaine and heroin by youth from 1958-63, while use of heroin alone had only increased 15 percent during this period.

In the United States cocaine is currently controlled as a Schedule II drug under the Comprehensive Drug Abuse and Control Act of 1970 (Public Law 91-513). Schedule II drugs have acceptable medical use, but also have high potential for abuse which could result in psychological and physiological dependence. They include amphetamine, methamphetamine, and narcotics. Illegal possession, distribution, or manufacture of cocaine is punishable as a felony under federal law.

Woodley reported that as of 1971 only two companies, the Stephen Chemical Company and Merck and Company, were licensed by the Justice Department to import coca leaves to make cocaine. He noted that in 1969 268,679 kilos (kilograms) of leaves were imported to produce 1,184 kilos of cocaine, and 884 kilos of that were exported, primarily to Europe, where cocaine is more widely used as an anesthetic.

"In 1970 the United States accounted for 88 percent of the reported world imports of coca leaves. From imported coca leaves the U.S. produced 1,033 kilograms of cocaine and exported 725 kilograms. The [National] Commission [on Marihuana and Drug Abuse] suggested that some of the cocaine shipped out of the United States was diverted in the receiving countries and smuggled back into this country for illegal distribution" (Eiswirth et al., 1972, p. 155).

The increasing popularity of cocaine is documented by the incidence of its use at the Haight-Ashbury Free Medical Clinic in San Francisco beginning in 1970. Gay et al. (1973b) reported that interview data revealed that of 303 clients seen between March and September of 1971 10 percent reported moderate to heavy use of cocaine within the previous two months. With the 264 patients seen between September 1971 and January 1972 the number increased to 13.6 percent, and with the 147 patients seen between February 1972 and April 1972 it rose to 21 percent.

Phillips (1975) reports that in 1961 domestic seizures of illegal cocaine by drug enforcement personnel totaled six pounds. In the late 1960s seizures increased at alarming rates. In 1970 for the first time amounts of illegal cocaine seized exceeded those of heroin (Woodley, 1971). Phillips indicates that seizures by Federal authorities in fiscal years 1971, 1972, 1973, and 1974 were 787, 828, 1,125, and 1,651 pounds, respectively.

Olden (1973), Plate (1973), and Sabbag (1976) report that since the early 1970s cocaine has emerged unequivocally as one of the most popular illegal drugs in America—the drug of choice of such diverse groups as actors and actresses, dancers, symphonic musicians, editors and writers, models, television personalities and entertainers, socialites, professional athletes, successful salesmen, businessmen, bankers, corporation presidents, corporation lawyers, accountants, real estate brokers, stockbrokers, United Nations delegates and diplomats, press agents, college and high school students, middle class housewives, criminals, pimps and whores (and their customers), drug dealers, and so on. As both Plate and Sabbag have indicated, the only thing these groups may have in common is access to sufficient money to support their cocaine use.

Steele, Angrest, Monroe, Brinkley, Rogers, and Lesher (1977) report that an estimated 4.8 million Americans have tried cocaine. A more recent estimate places the figure at 10 million ("Conventional Wisdom" on Cocaine Dangers Challenged, 1979). They noted that the cocaine traffic has become at least a $1 billion-per-year business. By 1978 the smuggling of illicit cocaine into the United States had reached such proportions that Lester L. Wolff, Chairman of the House Select Committee on Narcotics Abuse and Control, was quoted as stating that existing law enforcement agencies cannot hope to seriously impede trafficking of the drug ("Enforcement can't impede S. American cocaine flow," 1978). Sabbag (1976) pointed out that the mathematics of the illegal cocaine trade is enough to keep the traffic alive forever. A trafficker will pay a South American farmer or *campesino* up to $350 for a kilo of cocaine paste. "A chemist, if he buys from a paste trafficker instead of directly from the farmer, may pay up to $1,000 a kilo for paste. Delivered in Latin America, a kilo of cocaine, 90 to 98 percent pure (as pure as it gets), costs anywhere from $4,000 in Lima to $8,500 in Buenos Aires. . . . When the cocaine leaves South America, the mathematics gets heavier. In New York, a kilo of coke sells for over $30,000. That is what a smuggler charges. But the kilo which the smuggler pays $6,000 for in South America is pure. He can put a full hit on it, turn it into *two* $30,000 kilos, and sell his product 50 percent pure, converting a $6,000 investment into a $60,000 product. And he can make more if he ounces it" (Sabbag, pp. 82-83). The street price of a gram of cocaine in 1979 has been estimated at $100 ("Conventional Wisdom" on Cocaine Dangers Challenged, 1979).

Cocaine's growing popularity in the United States may be a function of the fact that it reinforces qualities that have come to be admired as truly American: initiative, drive, optimism, the need for achievement, and the embrace of power (Sabbag, p. 87). Similar observations have been made about another powerful central nervous system stimulant, amphetamine (Edison, 1971). However, cocaine has unique attributes that may well make it more attractive for many people.

Pharmacological and Physiological Actions

The details of the physiological and pharmacological actions and effects of cocaine are currently matters of some debate. Only a sketchy survey of current knowledge is given below. More detailed discussion is presented in Chapter 13.

Clark (1973) states, "Chemically, cocaine (methylbenzoylepgonine) is an ester of benzoic acid and a nitrogenous base (epgonine) which differs from its nucleus, tropan, by two hydrogen atoms. There is a close chemical relationship between the nuclei of cocaine (tropan) and that of atropine (tropine), differing only in the radical at position two.

"Atropine and cocaine are tertiary aminoesters of aromatic acids. Many tertiary aminoesters of organic acids have both local anesthetic and antimuscarinic properties. However, atropine has only mild local anesthetic action and cocaine has little or no antimuscarinic action" (p. 75).

Cocaine has two distinctive pharmacologic actions: (1) as a topical or local anesthetic of high efficacy as well as high toxicity, and (2) as one of the most powerful central nervous system stimulants known (Eiswirth et al., 1972).

Most absorbed cocaine is hydrolized in the body to benzoylecgonine. Although it is thought that the liver is involved, the exact site of this hydrolysis is not known. Most cocaine is eliminated in the urine as benzoylecgonine within twenty-four to thirty-six hours after administration. Small amounts, usually less than 25 percent of a total dose, are eliminated unchanged in the urine of humans. The distribution of cocaine in the human body is unknown. In studies with dogs, Woods, McMahon, and Seevers (1951) found that cocaine has greater affinity for tissues than for plasma. After one to two hours in the body, most cocaine is concentrated in the spleen, liver, and kidneys.

Cocaine is said to produce remarkable euphoric reactions. While no *physical dependence* or tolerance evolves, intense desires for the drug and *psychic dependence* are associated with heavy use (Eddy, Halbach, Isbell, and Seevers, 1965; Isbell and White, 1953). Animal experiments show the drug to have pleasurable effects. Perry (1972) has reported that rats would press a bar 250 times to obtain caffeine, 4,000 consecutive times to obtain heroin, but 10,000 consecutive times to obtain cocaine.

Upon local application, cocaine is vasoconstrictive and blocks the generation and transmission of nerve impulses. However, once the drug is absorbed in the blood and distributed throughout the body the blocking action is reversed and the neurons return almost immediately to normal functioning (Eiswirth et al.). The duration of local anesthetic action ranges only from 20 to 40 minutes. Because they provide wider safety margins, Novocain, Xylocaine, or other synthetic derivatives are now more widely used in professional anesthesia (Wylie and Churchill-Davidson, 1966). The only current medical use of cocaine is in anesthetization of the mucous membrane in some oral-pharyngeal surgical procedures. Cocaine is rapidly absorbed following such application to mucous membranes (Adriani and Campbell, 1956); it may be detected in the blood within three minutes, reaches a peak plasma concentration in fifteen to sixty minutes, and may remain detectable for as long as six hours after application (Byck, Jatlow, Barash, and Van Dyke, 1977).

There seems to be general agreement that cocaine stimulates the central nervous system (CNS) from above, downward. Its effects begin in the cortical cells of the brain (Ritchie, Cohen, and Dripps, 1970) and are associated with euphoria, garrulousness, excitation, restlessness, and a feeling of heightened physical and mental power.

As dosage increases, stimulation of the lower brain centers may cause tremors and convulsions. "If overdose occurs, anxiety, depression, headache, confusion, dry throat, dizziness, and fainting are noted; hyper-reflexia appears and eventually clonic-tonic convulsions and respiratory arrest may follow. Such acute reactions, when accompanied by cardiovascular and respiratory collapse, constitute the prototype 'caine reaction,' and demand immediate supportive intervention" (Gay et al., 1973b, p. 421).

Clark (1973) has noted that different centers in the brain may be out of phase with each other in responding to cocaine. Thus, stimulation of the cortex is soon followed by depression. The higher brain centers are the first to be depressed "and this may occur when the lower portions of the cerebrospinal axis are still in the stage of excitation" (p. 75).

"The action of cocaine on the medulla results in an initial increase in respiratory rate; this soon changes to a rapid and shallow pattern. As depression increases, irregular or Cheyne-Stokes respiration may appear, and death may then ensue" (Gay et al., p. 421). Death from cocaine has been attributed to cardiac arrest, depression of the respiratory and vasomotor centers, hyperthermia, or convulsions (Van Dyke and Byck, 1977). However, Finkle and McClosky (1977) reported that in the cocaine-related deaths they studied, the terminal symptoms were entirely central-nervous-system mediated, usually being seizures followed by respiratory arrest, coma, and death; cardiac arrest was reported in three cases.

In 1975, Post presented a three-stage model of the development of "cocaine psychosis." This model hypothesizes that small doses of cocaine generate the first, *euphoric,* stage. With increasing doses, the euphoria shifts to *dysphoria.* As dosage or chronicity increases the dysphoric stage gives way to the full-fledged *schizophreniform psychosis,* characterized by ahedonia, disorientation, hallucinations, concern with minutiae, stereotyped behavior, paranoid delusions, parasitosis, insomnia, and a proneness to violence. Post noted that the specific effects would be influenced by genetic and environmental predisposing factors (such as type of psychiatric illness, if any, degree of recent stress or loss, occurrence of a vulnerable phase of a circadian or ultradian rhythm, the individual's expectations or mind-set, etc.). The testing of Post's model requires research with individuals who practice heavy, compulsive use of the drug. As shown in Chapter 13, the authors' studies presented herein provide data upon which elements of this theory can be tested.

Clark reports that cocaine increases body temperature. The drug does this in at least three ways: First, increased muscular activity increases heat production; second, vasoconstriction reduces heat radiation; and third, cocaine exerts a direct action on the CNS thermostat, setting it at a higher level.

Cocaine has powerful effects upon the respiratory and cardiovascular system. Post, Kotin, and Goodwin (1974) studied the effects of differing doses and methods of administration on sixteen depressed patients. Orally administered cocaine did not have marked or consistent effects on the patients' mood, body temperature, blood pressure, or respiration, nor did it produce changes in behavior. However, orally ingested cocaine did produce significant effects in sleep patterns, suppressing rapid-eye-movement (REM) sleep as well as the overall time patients slept. The investigators found an REM sleep rebound with termination of cocaine use.

In this study, intravenous administration of cocaine produced rapid changes in blood pressure, pulse, mood, and affective behavior. Patients varied in the dose required to effect changes (2 mg. to 16 mg.). Those doses which produced moderate physiological changes were generally accompanied by positive affective changes and a sense of well-being. However, doses which produced marked changes in blood pressure and pulse were generally associated with mixed states of agitation, dysphoria, and tearfulness inexplicable even to the patients.

Resnick, Kestenbaum, and Schwartz (1977) tested the effects of intranasal and intravenous administration of cocaine with nineteen volunteers having histories of frequent and regular cocaine use. Each subject received placebo, 10 mg., and 25 mg. cocaine. Twelve subjects received the drug intranasally and twelve received the dosages intravenously; five subjects participated in trials with both methods of administration. Intranasally cocaine produced physiologic and subjective effects only at the 25 mg. dosage, while both 10 mg. and 25 mg. intravenous dosages produced significant physiologic and subjective effects. The onset of intravenous effects occurred within two minutes after injection. The reports of the subjects indicated the 25 mg. intravenous dose produced a very mild and somewhat pleasant experience.

In a related study, Fischman, Schuster, Resnekov, Shick, Krasnegor, Fennell, and Freedman (1976) found that intravenous doses of 4 or 8 mg. of cocaine produced no effect on heart rate or blood pressure. However, after 16 mg. of cocaine the mean heart rate of the nine volunteers increased from a predrug rate of 74 beats per minute to 100 beats per minute. After 32 mg. of intravenously administered cocaine, mean heart rate increased from 74 beats per minutes to 112. Increases in heart rate began two to five minutes after injection and peaked at ten minutes regardless of the dose administered. Doses of only 16 and 32 mg. increased systolic blood pressure 10 to 15 percent above predrug levels. In the lower dosage ranges, these findings differ from those reported by Post et al., who found increases in both heart rate and systolic blood pressure with depressed patients following low intravenous doses ranging from 2 to 16 mg. of cocaine.

Cocaine affects the cardiovascular system by virtue of its capacity for central stimulation and peripheral potentiation of catecholamines. Small doses may depress heart rate, but large doses increase it. Peripheral potentiation of catecholamines results in vasoconstriction and hypertension (R. B. Smith, 1973).

Cocaine is absorbed at all sites of application. The drug produces vasoconstriction at the site of injection, which limits, at least temporarily, the rate of its absorption. Oral absorption is limited by gastric hydrolysis (Ritchie and Cohen, 1975) and results in greatly reduced blood concentrations and a shorter sojourn in the blood (Woods, McMahon, and Seevers, 1951). Neveretheless, the absorption of cocaine may easily exceed the rate of its detoxification and excretion. This is the cause of toxicity associated with the drug. Gay et al. (1973b) report that cocaine is detoxified primarily in the liver, by hydrolysis to benzoic acid and ecgonine. "Detoxification by the liver is estimated to be at a rate of 30 to 40 mg. per hour (considerably slower than most local anesthetics)" (Eiswirth et al., 1972, p. 156). This relatively slow process provides one explanation of why 1 to 20 percent of cocaine administered may be excreted unchanged in the urine (Fish and Wilson, 1969). It has been estimated that the liver can detoxify one lethal dose of cocaine per hour; in incremental, intravenous doses, the liver has a capability to detoxify as much as 10 g. of cocaine a day (Gay et al.).

The fatal dose of cocaine is difficult to specify, for cocaine is highly ideosyncratic. A review by Van Dyke and Byck (1977) reported that the fatal dose in humans has been found to vary considerably, ranging from 22 mg. (submucosal administration) to 2,500 mg. (subcutaneous injection). Most investigators agree that solutions of cocaine more concentrated than 20 percent should not be used in medical practice; 5 to 10 percent solutions seem more appropriate and minimize potential toxic reactions (Barash, 1977).

Barash (1977) reports that "When patients are receiving a number of drugs simultaneously, drug interaction with cocaine can be potentially lethal. Since cocaine interferes with the re-uptake of norepinephrine and potentiates the effects of exogenous catecholamines, it should be used with caution in patients receiving tricyclic antidepressants, reserpine, and the monoamine oxidase inhibitors guanethidine, methyldopa and dopamine" (p. 195). There is evidence that the practice of "speedballing" mixtures of opiates and cocaine is also hazardous (Finkle and McClosky, 1977), and cocaine may actually potentiate the lethality of heroin.

The fatal dose of cocaine (that dose which causes death 100 percent of the time) has been estimated to be 1.2 g. (1,200 mg.) after oral ingestion (Ritchie et al., 1970; Ritchie and Cohen, 1975). The lethal dose (which results in death

50 percent of the time) is approximately 500 mg. in a 150-lb. man (Eiswirth et al., 1972). However, after application to mucous membranes, doses as low as 20–30 mg. can cause death (Ritchie et al., 1970).

Scheppegrell (1898), Mayer (1924), and Wylie and Churchill-Davidson (1966) reported that deaths have occurred even with small dosages. However, by administering the drug at intervals, cocaine users can often inject amounts cumulatively larger than lethal dose requirements. Another factor that affects the probability that cocaine will result in death is the quality of the drug used. The quality of cocaine purchased on the "street" varies widely and is often low (Eiswirth, et al.). Wetli and Wright (1979) agree that the precise mechanism by which cocaine produces lethal effects is not known, but they note that cocaine-related deaths are on the increase, and they challenge the current popular belief that cocaine is a safe recreational drug.

Gay et al. have described the paradigm for treatment of acute cocaine toxicity: "Treatment in all cases is symptomatic, with special attention afforded the airways, breathing process, maintenance of blood pressure, and cardiac monitoring. Death from acute toxicity most often occurs within 2 to 3 minutes, but may be delayed as much as 30 minutes after symptoms develop. If a patient survives the first three hours after such an episode, he is likely to recover" (p. 424).

Social Usage Patterns and Effects

Cocaine, the "King," "Cadillac," or "Champagne" of drugs is distinctive in terms of the multitude of ways it has been introduced into the human body. The Andean Indians chew coca leaves in a bolus mixed with lime and a binding agent of cornstarch or guano. The upper classes there use it in a coca tea. In India cocaine is eaten in the betel leaf with small quantities of *catechu* (slaked lime), a little betel nut, or, sometimes, with spices such as cinnamon, cardamon, or ginger (Chopra and Chopra, 1958). Westerners have used cocaine in wine (even Champagne), liqueur, cigars and cigarettes, tablets, subcutaneous or intravenous injections, inhalant dispensers, ointments, salves, and syrups (Parke, Davis and Company, 1885/1974) as well as soft drinks and a variety of over-the-counter, nonprescription nostrums (Gay et al.). It has been thrust into the nose with a brush or employed as snuff, injected or rubbed into the gums, thrust into the urethra or rectum, soaked in wool-cotton and placed on carious teeth, and used as a throat spray (Lewin, 1924/1974; Scheppegrell, 1898). It has been rubbed on the head of the penis and on the clitoris to prolong intercourse and has been sprinkled on the genitalia to be licked off by the sex partner. Cocaine has been "cut" for sale with such substances as lactose (milk sugar), powdered milk, epsom salts, caffeine, talcum powder (which contains carcinogenic asbestos), sucrose, glucose, Mannite, quinine, strychnine, aspirin, vitamins, cornstarch, menita, inositol, mannitol, and even flour. Among the other compounds sometimes used as substitutes for cocaine are lidocaine, procaine, benzocaine, and tetracaine. The effects of these drugs on the central nervous system are different from cocaine, and allergic reactions to them are not uncommon (Hawks, 1977).

Although Eiswirth et al. (1972) indicated that high quality cocaine is rare, Siegel reports that the average purity of street cocaine in the Los Angeles area was 63 percent in 1977, while street samples in northern California averaged 53 percent purity. Waldorf et al. (1977), however, estimate street cocaine in the Bay Area to be of approximately 40 percent purity.

The price of illicit cocaine has increased steadily since the early 1970s. Gay et al. (1973b) reported that cocaine (of unspecified quality) could be purchased at street levels at about $50 per spoon (approximately a gram). In 1975 Ashley reported a price of $1,800 to $2,000 for a relatively pure ounce of cocaine. Somewhat later, Steele et al. (1977) stated the drug could cost from $1,200 to $2,500 an ounce at street prices, depending on its purity. In 1977 Waldorf et al. estimated the cost of cocaine in the Bay Area to range between $55 and $80 per gram, or $1,418 to $2,268 per ounce. These prices contrast sharply with current medical costs of cocaine. Pure pharmaceutical cocaine sells to medical institutions for approximately $20 an ounce!

Despite the proliferation of anecdotal reports, there is still little empirical information about who uses cocaine in America today. Perhaps Ashley (1975) described the "typical" user as well as anyone: He stated that cocaine users today represent a cross section of those who lead the "good life" in America's major cities. "Marijuana hadn't hurt them so they saw no good reason not to try cocaine. Moreover, the police and media had given it such an incredible reputation that it would hardly have been human not to give it a try" (p. 139).

Data obtained from clients entering federally funded drug abuse treatment programs indicate that cocaine users constitute a very small proportion of the patients entering such programs; their number has remained at approximately 1 percent for several years. However, 12 percent of all primary heroin users reported cocaine as a secondary drug problem (Greene, Nightingale, and DuPont, 1975). The majority of these cocaine users are young males, and slightly more than half of the males are white (Siguel, 1977). Data summarized by the National Commission on Marijuana and Drug Abuse indicates that 1.2 percent of junior high school students, 2.6 percent of senior high school students and 10.4 percent of college students have some experience with cocaine. Use seems to be higher among men, urban dwellers, western United States residents, and individuals with higher levels of income and education (Greene, Nightingale, and DuPont).

Ashley (1975) and Siegel (1977) describe a practice of smoking cocaine; apparently this practice is currently growing in popularity ("Conventional Wisdom" on Cocaine Dangers Challenged, 1979). Nevertheless at the present time, there are two other major ways of ingesting cocaine. By far the most popular method is "snorting," or "sniffing," the drug. Snorting consists of sharply inhaling cocaine powder through one nostril while holding the other closed. The material has usually been chopped up into fine powder on a hard surface (such as picture glass) with a razor blade or straight-edged razor. Typically, the user then arranges the coke in a series of fine "lines" or columns, three-quarters to one inch long. Waldorf et al. (1977) note that an effective line has approximately 1/40 g. (20 to 25 mg.) of cocaine. Typically, one or two lines are arranged for each person present. Once the lines are laid out the host starts the round by sniffing up the lines with a rolled bill or paper straw. . . . Each line is sniffed up with a single movement (often called a 'blow'). If there is a second line, it is usually snorted with the other nostril. Two lines, considered a 'good' dose, is approximately 40 to 50 mgs." (p. 30).

The second method is intravenous injection. This method reportedly produces an intense orgasmic "flash" or "rush" as well as ecstatic sensations of physical and mental power. Sensations of hunger and fatigue are abolished. According to Eiswirth et al. the user experiences exhilaration, euphoria, self-confidence, and accelerated mental activity. When the intense "high" wears off it is "replaced by nervousness and depression which can last for hours or days. Irritability, loss of temperature sensations and tightening of muscles often accompany cocaine's post-reactive depressive state. This depression is in such marked contrast to the previous pleasurable sensations that heavy users will continue to sniff or inject cocaine every ten minutes or so for several hours to avoid the onset of depressive symptoms" (p. 155).

There are two other variations of intravenous injection. The first involves the injection of a mixture of heroin and cocaine, the "speedball" which is popular among opiate users. Such a mixture apparently lengthens the euphoric effects of cocaine and buffers some of the adverse reactions. The second variant form involves the intravenous use of mixtures of cocaine and liquid amphetamine, the *"bombita"* said to be popular among Cubans and other Latin-Americans (Olden, 1973).

With high-dosage, compulsive use of cocaine, a full-blown toxic reaction can occur. The sympathomimetic signs include elevation of blood pressure, pulse, and respiration rates; sweating; exophthalmos; insomnia; and mydriasis. Signs of excessive central nervous system stimulation include increased deep tendon reflexes, twitching of muscles, spasms of entire muscle groups, and occasionally convulsions. Isbell and White (1953) state, "A characteristic toxic psychosis, characterized by paranoid delusions, usually develops. The addict feels that people are talking about him and that he is being watched by detectives. Sensations of insects crawling on the skin are very common. Shadows, windowpanes or mirrors may be misinterpreted as being the figure of a detective who is watching the addict.

"When psychosis develops, the cocainist is dangerous and may assault and seriously harm anyone, in the mistaken belief that he is a detective who is persecuting the addict" (pp. 563–564).

In the early 1900s and again more recently cocaine has been linked to violence and crime (Bejerot, 1970b; Chopra and Chopra, 1930/1931; Ludwig and Pyle, 1969). As noted earlier, Williams (1914) contended that an increase in violent crimes in the South was directly related to the increasing numbers of black cocaine "fiends." However, Kolb (1925a) asserted that efforts to identify cocaine as a cause of crime were absurd; the vast majority of criminal addicts were criminals before they became addicted. Kolb noted that because cocaine enhances mental and physical energy, the criminal who takes it might be more likely to convert abnormal impulses into action. "Beyond the point of maximum stimulation, the criminal and any other type of character becomes suspicious and fearful. They run away from imagined enemies, usually the police. They are in a paranoiac state, and in this state of fear might commit some act of violence if cornered. . . . Persons in this state are, of course, dangerous but any crime they might commit would be due to the frenzy of fear. Such a person would be incapable of planning and committing a deliberate murder or holding up and robbing a bank" (p. 76). The position of Dixon (1923) on the relationship between cocaine use and crime was similar to that of Kolb, though Dixon concluded that drug abusers were mental cases and should be treated as such.

Grinspoon and Bakalar (1976) assert that if one considers only its pharmacological effects cocaine has some potential for producing crime and violence. However, they conclude that when all the evidence is considered, cocaine is probably less dangerous in inducing violence and crime than alcohol, amphetamine, or barbiturates.

Although a number of studies (Edmundson, Davies, Acker and Myer, 1972; McLaughlin and Haines, 1952) show a high incidence of cocaine use among individuals incarcerated for criminal activity (or sentenced to treatment as an alternative to incarceration), there is no clear evidence that cocaine is criminogenic. The current position is that the paranoid delusions and hallucinations associated with toxic cocaine poisoning make the abuser dangerous and capable of antisocial acts and violence (Eddy et al., 1965; Isbell and White, 1953). Recent animal research indicates that cocaine by itself does not induce aggression; however, when aggression has been elicited by environmental events, cocaine may increase or decrease aggression (Hutchinson, Emley, and Krasnegor, 1977; Woods, 1977).

THE RESEARCH PROBLEM

The Need

There has been little up-to-date research on cocaine, its effects, hazards, and sequelae in humans. Byck (1974) described the state of our knowledge in the early 1970s:

"Strangely enough, there has been almost no recent research into the effects of cocaine on man. Even the literature of recent years on the effects of cocaine as a local anesthetic is sparse. If a search is made for articles about cocaine's psychopharmacological effects, no papers are to be found at all. The most recent edition of *The Pharmacological Basis of Therapeutics* (1970) does not give a single reference in the literature to document the central effects of cocaine in man" (p. xxxiv).

Although the general effects of this powerful CNS stimulant were known by the early 1970s, details of the physiological mechanisms mediating its effects are still incompletely understood. At that time, published work on the effects of cocaine in man was confined to clinical case reports describing individuals treated for acute or chronic cocaine poisoning in the early 1900s, incidental findings reported by investigators studying other drugs, a historical reference book focusing upon Freud's early work with cocaine, Chopra and Chopra's classic study of cocaine users in India, a few studies of cocaine use among addicts in methadone maintenance programs, a number of reviews, and several books for popular consumption.

Since 1974, however, work in this area has intensified. In 1975 Ashley published a thorough history of cocaine, which includes anecdotal data from a sample of cocaine users (primarily "snorters"). In 1976 Grinspoon and Bakalar published a book which included a comprehensive historical review, an extensive discussion of the legal and ethical issues associated with current policies toward cocaine, and phenomenological data obtained from seventeen users. Also in 1976, Sabbag published a book describing the experiences and activities of a cocaine smuggler and dealer. In 1977 Ellinwood and Kilbey published a collection of recent empirical studies on cocaine and other stimulant drugs. In this year Petersen and Stillman's *Cocaine: 1977* came out under the auspices of the National Institute on Drug Abuse (NIDA); it is a research monograph which provides a factual summarization of the history and some of the effects of the drug. Beyond this, well-designed studies and reports involving the use of cocaine in both animals and humans appeared in the research literature during this period (Fischman, Schuster, and Krasnegor, 1977; Fischman et al., 1976; Post et al., 1974; Post and Kopanda, 1975; Resnick et al., 1977; Siegel, 1977; Waldorf et al., 1977).

Despite the acceleration of research, however, most investigators agree that little is yet known about the effects of heavy or chronic use of cocaine in humans. This gap in knowledge has created considerable confusion and misunderstanding about the drug and its effects. It was with this gap in mind that the authors have conducted research on patterns and life styles of cocaine users/abusers, detailed reports of which are presented in chapters 3 through 11 below.

Essentially, the goals of our studies were to locate and select nine men who used and preferred cocaine over all other drugs, but who were different in many other ways. Once the men were selected, the *Representative Case Method* (see chapter 2) was employed to study them in depth, using a battery of dimensional, morphogenic, and sociopsychological measures. Each man was treated as an expert who could provide rich empirical and clinical detail with regard to both the personal characteristics of cocaine users and the situational context of their cocaine use. Data from the nine representative cases combine to provide a broad picture of men using cocaine in America today.

The Concept of Life Style

As used in these studies, the concept of *life style* refers to consistent patterns which find constant expression in diverse and even divergent areas of personal functioning, encompassing the intellectual, emotional, social, motivational, and even defensive life of the individual (Spotts and Mackler, 1967).

This definition of life style is similar, in many respects, to those suggested by Adler (Ansbacher and Ansbacher, 1956), Wertheimer (cited in Ansbacher and Ansbacher, 1956), Lewin (1953), and Allport (1937). All these theorists asserted that in the final analysis all behavior is guided and directed by one central need (Lewin), cardinal trait (Allport), superordinate guiding idea (Adler), or controlling goal (Wertheimer)—or a very small number of these in combination.

Life styles may be characterized as "standing patterns of behavior" (Barker, 1968). These are sets of activities that recur in the same form and retain their integrity even in the face of forces acting to change their features. Waves in the ocean, for example, form "standing patterns" that are independent of the specific molecules which compose them, and they tend to continue to move in predictable fashion despite obstacles such as ships and contrary forces such as underwater currents.

Theoretically, the concept of life style is more holistic than the concept of a *trait*, for it identifies the person as a system that is open to the environment. A life style is more external than a *personality* but more internal and individualized than a *social role*. A life style is the set of linkages relating the psychophysiological functions of a person to the external social and environmental conditions to which he or she adapts (Spotts and Shontz, 1974).

In the development of these studies we searched the literature for investigations bearing on the life styles of cocaine users, but with no real success. For example, early studies reported a high incidence of cocaine use among individuals with psychopathic or sociopathic tendencies. However, while the terms psychopath or sociopath have specialized meanings in psychiatric settings, they are diagnoses, not descriptions of life styles.

Chopra and Chopra (1958) pictured the cocaine "eaters" of India as persons whose "psychic condition is in an unstable state of equilibrium" (p. 17). They distinguished two types of cocaine abusers: (1) weak-minded, mentally dull and deficient individuals who use cocaine for its stimulating and euphoric effects and (2) irritable and nervous individuals of hypersensitive temperament who use the drug to help maintain some sense of balance or equilibrium in their lives. While these characterizations are interesting, they, like diagnoses, are not descriptions of life styles.

A number of investigators have attempted to describe some of the demographic and personal characteristics of individuals who use and abuse drugs in general, including cocaine. According to these investigators the typical drug abuser is probably male, in his or her early twenties, comes from a low socioeconomic status and is probably a member of a minority group, grew up under adverse conditions, probably came from a broken home and received inadequate parental control, grew up in substandard housing and came from a family with a high level of adult crime, is emotionally immature, introverted, and more frequently passive than aggressive, has difficulties handling anger and aggression, has low self-esteem, exhibits high levels of anxiety and a low frustration tolerance, did poorly in school or college and has limited vocational skills, is socially deviant and attracted to deviant peer groups, has some personality disorder and exhibits a history of antisocial behavior, such as truancy, even before taking drugs (Bender, 1963; Edmundson et al., 1972; Goode, 1971; Jaffee, 1970; Johnson, Abbey, Scheble, and Weitman, 1971/1972; J. R. Kramer, 1972; Rosenberg, 1968). This characterization differs from that reported by Minkowski, Weiss, and Heidbreder (1972), but does provide some picture of a typical (though hypothetical) drug abuser. Wilson (1968) described persons in England using cocaine with heroin as being seriously maladjusted individuals who display depression and dysphoria, distortions in reality testing, and disturbances in sexual identification and interpersonal relationships.

Studies of "typical" drug abusers describe some of the factors which contribute to drug abuse. However, such studies cannot define the life style of the user/abuser of the drug because: (1) they depict only a "typical" and hypothetical person and (2) many of the characteristics described are not life styles (which are general underlying patterns) but specific behavioral expressions of life styles.

A life style cannot be described by a number; it is a pattern, not a dimension. The complete study of a life style requires voluminous data on an individual. Ideally, these data should be "longitudinal" as well as cross-sectional, for a life style is time-dependent as well as a quasi-permanent entity. This research, therefore, consists of intensive and extensive studies of the lives and activities of nine persons who use or abuse cocaine. They are nine distinctive and separate, but interlocking, investigations. The functioning of these nine men as a group will then be examined on a variety of measures in chapters 12 and 13.

We make no pretense that these nine persons represent all possible life styles related to cocaine use. However, this research has attempted to systematically identify and study nine distinctive and strategically selected life adjustment patterns among male adult cocaine users.

Theoretical Assumptions

A variety of theories attempt to explain why people use and abuse drugs (Agrin, 1972; Jaffee, 1970; Kolb, 1925a, 1925b; Partridge, 1967; Rosenberg, 1968; Wieder and Kaplan, 1969). As valuable as these theories are in their appropriate contexts, none has seemed to suit the needs of the present project. We therefore have chosen to adopt no specific position. Instead, we have formulated four assumptions to guide our efforts.

Our first assumption is that people who use and abuse drugs do so in an effort to produce by pharmacological means personal states which they cannot achieve by their own efforts (Wieder and Kaplan, 1969).

Our second assumption is that there is no typical personality for drug users or even users preferring the same substance. Futhermore, we feel that no basis exists for assuming that drug usage alone is symptomatic of psychological pathology. As Wurmser (1968) has stated, "there is no pathology typical of all addicts (nor for all narcotic addicts alone)" (p. 75).

Our third assumption is that people who persist in heavy drug use gravitate to the regular use of the drug or combination of drugs that helps them most closely approximate desired personal states.

The fourth assumption is that even though drug users develop preferences, different individuals may use the same drug to fulfill quite different needs.

Method 2

THE REPRESENTATIVE CASE METHOD

The research described in this book uses the Representative Case Method, an approach that advocates the intensive study of individuals (Shontz, 1965; 1976). Philosophically, the Representative Case Method has its roots in the epistemological arguments of thinkers like Wilhelm Windelband, Wilhelm Dilthey, and Ernst Cassirer. In psychology, the method displays the seminal influences of such theorists as Wilhelm Stern, Gordon Allport, Robert W. White, and Henry A. Murray, to mention only the most prominent and well-known. Research on individuals has been advocated by many authorities (Allport, 1962; Bakan, 1968; Chassan, 1967; Davidson and Costello, 1969; Dukes, 1965; Mair, 1970a,b; Shapiro, 1961b; 1966; Shontz, 1965; 1976; Stephenson, 1953). Dukes (1965) found in the history of psychology a vast amount of influential research on single persons. However, not every study of one organism employs the Representative Case Method. Nor is the use of single subjects the only one of the method's characteristics. Succeeding sections examine the features of representative case research more closely.

Comparison with Conventional Methods

The classical approach in psychological science is to study large groups of organisms in an attempt to discover laws that govern average behavior. However, the goal of representative case research is to discover laws for each individ-

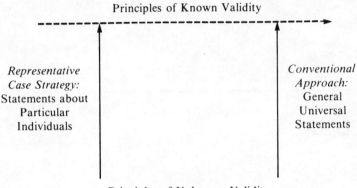

Principles of Known Validity

Representative Case Strategy: Statements about Particular Individuals

Conventional Approach: General Universal Statements

Principles of Unknown Validity

FIGURE 2.1. Relationship between Conventional and Representative Case Methods in Psychological Science.

ual. The Representative Case Method recognizes that a valid law of behavior may apply to everyone, to a few people, or only to a single individual. The degree to which the law may be generalized and the conditions under which it applies are limits to be discovered by empirical investigation. In Marceil's words (1977), the representative case approach is methodologically but not theoretically idiographic.

Figure 2.1 depicts the main difference between conventional research and the Representative Case Method. Both increase the store of valid principles (top of figure). However, the conventional approach (vertical arrow on right) seeks general laws from the outset, while the Representative Case Method (arrow on left) begins with the study of particular persons; this generates principles that are valid for each individual. The horizontal (dashed) arrow, pointing right at the top of the figure, shows the study of the particular leading to generalizations when supplementary studies of larger populations are conducted.

In conventional psychology, organisms are often called "subjects"; however, they are actually treated as objects (or respondents) and observed impersonally. The subject of such conventional research is not the person but a hypothesis. However, in the Representative Case Method the person participates in the research. He expresses himself in his own way; typically, he knows the purpose of the study and has every opportunity time and procedures allow to comment on the accuracy of the data and the investigator's conclusions.

Sample Size

The most common argument against such studies of individuals is that knowledge about one person cannot be generalized. This argument is valid for the type of research that samples populations. However, representative case research does not attempt to do this. An analogy is afforded by natural scientists studying the physical properties of a specific substance: A geologist (who does not perform representative case research) may concern himself with the substance's distribution in nature and the impurities with which it is usually associated; but an analytical chemist or physicist (who performs representative case research) would rather have one gram free of impurities than a ton of ore from the mine.

Obviously, to achieve a like purity in human materials is impossible. But as long ago as 1901, in *Varieties of Religious Experience,* William James pointed out that some personal characteristics may, when present in only moderate quantities, be difficult to recognize, but when present to an extreme degree are easily identified (James, 1901/1958). For example, a recognized saint is clearly a religious person, and what one can learn by studying a saint applies to the religiosity in us all. James's argument shows that a close approximation to "purity" can be obtained if cases are selected with sufficient forethought and care.

Specific Characteristics

Nearly all types of procedures, from laboratory experimentation to naturalistic case studies, may be applied to representative cases. The basic desiderata involve: the problem, the case, and the procedures.

The Problem

The Representative Case Method is better suited to some types of problems than to others. For example, knowledge of public opinion regarding religion can not be efficiently obtained by the intensive study of individuals; techniques for polling samples of large populations are preferable. Topics especially suited to representative case research are those which require the study of whole persons but which can be identified by readily recognized behavioral, affective, physical, or cognitive states. Such a topic is cocaine use.

The Case

A person must be selected as a representative case who has properties making him or her suitable for investigation. The person must present in clear, perhaps even exaggerated, form the exact condition under investigation. For example, to study anxiety it would be a good idea to select the most anxious person to be found. In the present research, the type of person needed is easily specified, though not easy to locate: someone who uses cocaine heavily enough to speak with authority about it.

Procedures

The person selected must be examined by techniques appropriate to the problem. Many case studies fall short because the investigator failed to ask clear questions before data were collected. A lack of objectivity or explicitness of procedure may in part result from such failure. Much of the current bias against single subject research (e.g., Holt, 1962) may stem, not from the small number of subjects involved but from the unsystematic way in which they are typically examined. The research reported here incorporates a broad range of measurement techniques, and treats the data they yield both quantitatively and qualitatively.

Overview of the Project

The merit of the studies reported here resides in their objective measurement of persons who display behavior of unusual interest but are beyond the reach of most investigators. The data also provide a base line against which users of other drugs and non-users may be compared. (Comparable data are already available on users of amphetamine, opiates, and barbiturates.) Most important, the data provide tests of hypotheses about the average effects of cocaine that have already been drawn from large-scale studies but cannot claim universality because they have not yet been validated by research on individuals (see chapter 13).

Uses of Data

1. *Intrapersonal study.* The data are first dealt with in nine separate studies, each an investigation of a cocaine user (chapters 3 through 11). These investigations penetrate into the individuals' lives. They are not clinical studies because they do not study patients, sickness, or maladjustment. And they are not intuitive or anecdotal because they draw inferences from objective data obtained in controlled situations.

2. *Interpersonal study.* Separate analyses examine the extent to which these individuals share behavior patterns (chapter 12). Despite our efforts to select persons with a wide variety of life styles, it may be that only one underlying life style can be inferred. At the other extreme is the possibility that each person is so unique that the hypothesis of a common life style must be abandoned. In between are the possibilities that a few life styles will emerge or that life style will be a function of type of measurement; that participants will group themselves differently on a morphogenic instrument, like the Q-Sort, than on a dimensional test like the MMPI (Minnesota Multiphasic Personality Inventory).

MEASURING INSTRUMENTS

The assessment methods used in these investigations are of two broad types: *dimensional* and *morphogenic*. The former measure along continua that are assumed to be the same for all participants. The latter describe patterns within individuals, and often use test materials constructed to reflect each person's unique characteristics.

The two types are not completely exclusive, for an instrument may measure along a single dimension (e.g., preference rankings), yet be used to study patterns within individuals. Similarly, a multidimensional instrument like the MMPI may be used in a somewhat morphogenic way if the interpreter focuses on patterns of scores rather than on the normative meaning of single score values.

Dimensional Measures

Intelligence

Two measures of intelligence are included: the Otis Quick-Scoring Mental Ability Test, and the Revised Beta Examination. The Otis scale is a brief paper-and-pencil test that emphasizes verbal and mathematical skills of the type taught in public schools. The Revised Beta Examination is a paper-and-pencil performance test that was originally designed to be more fair to persons whose exposure to training in conventional verbal skills is limited.

Personality

Two standard multidimensional measures are used. These are Form C of Cattell's Sixteen Personality Factor Questionnaire (Sixteen PF) and Form R of the MMPI. Each of these measures was administered at least once to every participant. Also administered was Form A of the *Eysenck Personality Inventory* (Educational and Industrial Testing Service) which yields extraversion, neuroticism and "lie" scores.

Three measures of sensation-seeking are included: the Novelty Experiencing Scale (NES; Pearson, 1970; Coursey and Gaines, 1974), the Change Seeker Index (CSI; Garlington and Shimota, 1964), and the Sensation-Seeking Scale (SSS; Zuckerman, 1970; 1971; Zuckerman and Bone, 1972; Zuckerman and Link, 1968).

The Novelty Experiencing Scale was administered in two forms. The "standard" form is an eighty-item paper-and-pencil test in which the person circles the word "Like" or the word "Dislike" to indicate preferences for different activities. The second, Q-Sort form of the instrument was designed for this research; it is morphogenic and is described in a subsequent section.

Drug Preference Rankings

Each participant ranked the following nine substances according to personal preference: amphetamine, beer, cocaine, hard liquor, heroin, LSD, marijuana, speedball, barbiturates. Rankings were obtained at all assessment sessions.

Morphogenic Measures: Structured

Q-Sorts

The Q-technique was developed by William Stephenson (1953). (Reviews of the technique have been provided by Kerlinger [1972], Nunnally [1970], and Wittenborn [1961]; a bibliography on Q-technique, covering the period 1935-67, was compiled by Steven R. Brown in 1968.)

The structure of the sixty Q-Sort items used in these studies is based on fifteen *content areas,* each of which contains two positive (desirable) and two negative (undesirable) items. White's (1951) value theory is the source of the content categories.

The fifteen areas are not independent. Some occupy complementary ends of bipolar categories (complements are indicated in the column on the right of table 2.1). For example, dependence and independence are logical opposites but are not mutually exclusive in a single person, and both have desirable as well as undesirable aspects.

In nine content areas, negative items describe a socially undesirable consequence of the trait (e.g., "stubborn" in the "independence" content area), while in the other six areas the negative form describes a socially undesirable consequence of a *lack* of the trait (e.g., "feeble, lax" in the "dominance" content area). One content area, "anxiety", is defined primarily by its negative pole. Its positive items do not represent "desirable anxiety" but rather a state which is the opposite of anxiety.

Two types of Q-Sorts are used here. One type is *standard*: It contains the same sixty items for all persons. The other is *individualized,* using separately constructed items for each participant. In both types, the number of items (N = 60) and the structure (fifteen areas, each containing two positive and two negative items) are the same.

To acquire items for the individualized Q-Sort, the participant was taken through from three to five administrations of the standard Q-Sort and then asked to generate his own items. The steps in this procedure were:

1. The person was given the title word for the content area and asked what the word meant to him.
2. If he could not generate items in this way, or if his definition seemed unclear or inappropriate, he was given a definition and asked to provide items on that basis.

3. If the person still could not generate items, he was shown the standard items and asked if those seemed appropriate.
4. The examiner insured that both positive and negative forms of the items had been generated.

Administration of Q-Sorts

Each person sorted the sixty items, which had been typed onto 3″ × 5″ white cards, into eleven piles. The piles ranged in meaning from "Most Uncharacteristic" to "Most Characteristic" and were assigned scores ranging from 0 to 10. The number of items to be put in each pile was: 1, 2, 4, 7, 10, 12, 10, 7, 4, 2, 1.

The standard items were sorted five times under different instructions to describe:

1. Your usual, typical self
2. Yourself during a cocaine high
3. Your ideal self
4. The typical cocaine user
5. Your usual, typical self

The order of the sortings was constant in all assessment periods and for all persons. The instruction to describe "your usual, typical self" was given twice, as both the first and the last sorting task, in order to permit evaluation of consistency of responses.

After the standard items were sorted, the individualized items were sorted nine times under different instructions to describe:

1. Your usual, typical self
2. Yourself when wanting cocaine
3. Yourself during a cocaine high
4. Yourself just after a cocaine high
5. Yourself during an amphetamine high
6. Your ideal self
7. Your bad or worst self
8. Most nonusers of drugs
9. Your usual, typical self

Again, the instruction to sort the items to describe "your usual, typical self" was given twice, as both the first and the last descriptive task.

Q-Sorts were obtained at all three assessment periods. The individualized items generated during the primary assessment were used without modification during the reassessments.

Role Construct Repertory Test

The Role Construct Repertory Test ("Rep Test") permits inferences of two types. First, it elicits the cognitive "constructs" that a person uses to describe

TABLE 2.1. Standard Q-Sort Items

Content Areas	Signs	Items	Complementary Content Areas
1. Achievement	Positive	1. Striving	Self-Satisfaction (Stasis)
		2. Accomplishing	
		3. Believe winning is more important than how the game is played	
	Negative	4. A work addict	
2. Affect	Positive	5. Happy	None
		6. Pleasant	
	Negative	7. Sad	
		8. Depressed, "got the blues"	
3. Anxiety	Positive	9. Mellow	None
		10. Peaceful, at peace with yourself	
	Negative	11. Anxious	
		12. Nervous	
4. Chastity	Positive	13. Chaste	Sexuality
		14. Faithful (sexually)	
	Negative	15. Sexually frigid or impotent	

			Opposite
5. Dependence	Positive	16. Afraid of members of the opposite sex	Independence
		17. Responsive to others, put others ahead of yourself	
		18. Accept help gracefully	
	Negative	19. Tied to someone's apron strings	
		20. Clinging	
6. Dominance	Positive	21. Strong, deep	None
		22. Influential, you impress others	
	Negative	23. "Wishy-washy"	
		24. Feeble, lax	
7. Excitement	Positive	25. Spicy (exotic)	Restraint
		26. Adventuresome	
	Negative	27. Violent, explosive	
		28. Impulsive	
8. Humility	Positive	29. Humble	Social Recognition
		30. Self-effacing	
	Negative	31. Often ignored or snubbed	
		32. Lonely	

TABLE 2.1. Standard Q-Sort Items *(continued)*

Content Areas	Signs	Items	Complementary Content Areas
9. Independence	Positive	33. Independent	Dependence
		34. Stand on your own two feet	
	Negative	35. Stubborn	
		36. Self-centered, determined to get your own way	
10. Knowledge	Positive	37. Wise	None
		38. Logical (you apply logic to personal and social problems)	
	Negative	39. Foolish	
		40. Unintelligent	
11. Restraint	Positive	41. Controlled, restrained	Excitement
		42. Certain, deliberate, intentional	
	Negative	43. Slow, dragging	
		44. Boring	
12. Self-satisfaction (Stasis)	Positive	45. Satisfied with yourself and the world	Achievement
		46. Easy-going	
	Negative	47. Lazy	
		48. Smug	

13. Sexuality	Positive	49. Romantic, physical, sensuous	Chastity
		50. Sexually stimulating or magnetic	
	Negative	51. Perform loveless sex	
		52. No favorite sex partner—"who" less important than "how often"	
14. Interpersonal Relations	Positive	53. Kind	None
		54. Friendly	
	Negative	55. Hostile	
		56. Cruel	
15. Social Recognition	Positive	57. Respected	Humility
		58. Well-known (famous)	
	Negative	59. Shamed	
		60. Laughed-at	

important people and roles in his life. Second, it reveals similarities among occupants of social roles, that is, it allows the investigator to infer which persons are seen as being similar to each other and different from others (Kelly, 1955).

The modified Rep Test in this investigation used twenty social roles:

Rep Test: Social Role Titles

1. Your usual self
2. Your ideal self
3. Your worst self
4. Your wife or present girlfriend
5. Your mother (or the person who has played the part of a mother in your life)
6. Your father (or the person who has played the part of a father in your life)
7. A person of the opposite sex with whom you have used cocaine (or with whom you would like to use cocaine)
8. A person of your own sex with whom you have used cocaine (or with whom you would like to use cocaine)
9. A person from whom you often get your cocaine (or from whom you have gotten cocaine most frequently)
10. An employer, supervisor, or officer under whom you worked or served and whom you liked (or someone under whom you worked in a situation you liked)
11. An employer, supervisor, or officer under whom you worked or served and whom you found hard to get along with (or someone under whom you worked in a situation you did not like)
12. The most successful person you know personally
13. A person who really drinks a lot of alcohol
14. The most interesting person whom you know personally
15. The person you dislike (or hate) the most
16. The person who needs you most (even if only just a little bit)
17. The person whom you would most like to be of help to (or whom you feel the most sorry for)
18. A person with whom you have been closely associated recently who appears to dislike you
19. A person who behaves or talks very strangely
20. Yourself when high on cocaine

It also used twenty-one cognitive constructs. Fifteen *individual* constructs were generated by each person during the first administration, while six *standard* constructs were supplied by the investigators. These were: kind (helpful), mean, selfish, strong, wise, sexy.

The twenty role titles were typed on separate 3″ X 5″ white cards. These were presented to the person one at a time. He read the "self" cards and was asked to recall what the appropriate self was like. The other cards required him to recall some person he had actually known and to put a name, set of initials, or other identifier on the card.

The procedures for administration were similar to those for the individual grid form described in Kelly (1955). The detailed procedures for the initial administration were:

1. *Label roles.* The person was given the role cards, one at a time, and asked to write an identifier on each appropriate card.

2. *Generate constructs.* The person was given thirty-two sets of three cards, one triad at a time, in the order shown in table 2.2, and asked:

· Which two are alike?
· In what way are they alike? (This provided the "construct.")
· How is the other different? (This provided the "contrast.")

Role card triads were presented until fifteen different constructs had been generated, or until all thirty-two triads had been presented.

3. *Sort constructs.* Each construct was written on a 3″ × 5″ card. For each construct the person sorted all twenty role cards into two piles: one for those roles to whom the construct did apply, and one for those to whom the construct did not apply.

The Rep Test was administered three times. However, individual constructs remained constant at the two reassessment sessions.

TABLE 2.2. Rep Test: Role Triads

Sort	Role Cards in Triad	Sort	Role Cards in Triad
1.	1, 2, 3	17.	6, 10, 11
2.	4, 5, 7	18.	9, 16, 18
3.	1, 2, 6	19.	9, 10, 13
4.	1, 3, 6	20.	4, 15, 19
5.	1, 3, 5	21.	1, 16, 20
6.	1, 2, 5	22.	7, 14, 17
7.	1, 6, 8	23.	7, 14, 18
8.	1, 8, 15	24.	11, 12, 16
9.	2, 8, 15	25.	1, 2, 20
10.	7, 8, 9	26.	1, 3, 20
11.	6, 9, 12	27.	2, 3, 20
12.	6, 9, 15	28.	5, 6, 20
13.	6, 9, 19	29.	7, 8, 20
14.	3, 8, 17	30.	13, 17, 20
15.	8, 19, 20	31.	4, 11, 14
16.	1, 13, 14	32.	4, 10, 20

Setting Survey

The Structured Interview of Environmental Interactions ("Setting Survey") was developed by William O'Connor (O'Connor, 1975; O'Connor and O'Connor, 1978) and described to us in a personal communication. It is used to describe the community (i.e., outside-the-home) subsystems which a person occupies during his regular activities.

At every assessment session each participant estimated how often in the preceding week he had entered eleven types of settings (work, social-recreational, commercial, etc.) and how many hours he spent in each. He also provided ratings of his degree of satisfaction in each and the level of independence of his actions.

Semantic Differential Ratings

The semantic differential was developed by Osgood, Suci, and Tannenbaum (1957). In the present research, ten stimulus terms were measured with twenty-six scales used by Halliday (1975) in a previous research. The stimuli were: drugs (in general), amphetamine, barbiturates, beer, cocaine, hard liquor, heroin, LSD, marijuana, and the speedball. The scales were self-anchored on a nine-point spread. Each participant's ratings were factor-analyzed to reveal his unique way of grouping drugs in his own mind.

NESQ

The Q-Sort form of the NES (see "Dimensional Measures," p. 00) is a morphogenic modification developed for this research. Each of the eighty items was typed on a 3″ × 5″ card; the cards were sorted by the subject into eleven piles, which were assigned scores ranging from 0 ("Very much dislike") to 10 ("Very much like"). The number of items to be put in each pile was: 1, 2, 5, 10, 14, 16, 14, 10, 5, 2, and 1.

Morphogenic Measures: Semi-Structured

The semi-structured instruments provided rich experiential detail on each participant. Although each instrument asked many specific questions, individual items served as probes as well as measures. That is, they served as a means of getting a participant to talk freely about himself.

Social and Drug History

This interview covered demographic information, family relationships, life crises, sex, education, employment, religion, politics, and drug use. A few projective items were also included.

Cocaine Experience Inventory

The Cocaine Experience Inventory made use of the expert knowledge of the participants concerning that drug. Effects of both snorting and injecting cocaine were noted, as well as cost and other factors.

Activity and Experience Audits

The Activity and Experience Audits were reports of the day-to-day behavior of the participants. In addition to noting every activity that each participant said he engaged in during his waking day, we elicited his spontaneous comments and feelings about the activities. Questions were asked to delineate the success of each activity (whether or not the person did what he set out to do) and feeling tone (if he felt good, bad, or indifferent during that activity).

PROCEDURES

The Assessment Situation

All assessments were taken individually. Generally, data were collected at the Greater Kansas City Mental Health Foundation, but other facilities were used when more convenient. Scheduling was flexible; some sessions occurred during evenings or weekends. The individual's social and drug history was taken first; otherwise, the order of presentation of instruments was flexible.

Legal Considerations

Cocaine use is now illegal. Therefore, if a participant reported that he preferred not to discuss the matter directly, assessments were obtained under special instructions, which had the participant respond as he would have when still interested in cocaine.

Reassessments

The first reassessment was at least one month after the start of the initial assessment and at least one week after the completion of the initial assessment. The second reassessment was at least three months after the start of the initial assessment and at least one month after the first reassessment.

TECHNICAL NOTES

General Features of Quantitative Analyses

The basic tool for performing analyses was Version 5 of the *Statistical Package for the Social Sciences* (*SPSS;* Nie, Bent, and Hull, 1970). Our computer work was performed by a Honeywell 635, located at the University of Kansas at Lawrence. The functions that were put to most use were the correlation and factor analysis programs. Factor analyses were conducted by the Principal Axis method, using communality values estimated from the data and employing an iterative procedure (up to twenty-five iterations) to produce convergence. Decision-making criteria were those built into the *SPSS* program as automatic default options. Extracted factors were routinely subjected to Varimax rotation.

Cluster analyses were performed by a special program (K-Means), available at the installation where these data were analyzed.

Data analyses other than those using programs described above were performed by hand.

Reliability of Q-Sort Data

A correlation between two sets of Q-Sort item sortings is an estimate of reliability only when the instructions require one person to describe corresponding patterns. For example, there is reason to expect high correlations between two sortings from the same person describing "yourself as you usually are"; however, the correlation between self-descriptions provided by different persons would not be an estimate of reliability. The same reasoning applies to the apparent "unreliability" of sortings provided by one person under different instructional conditions.

At every assessment session each participant provided two descriptions of his "usual self." Correlations between these sortings yield estimates of *intrasession* reliability. Correlations between descriptions provided at the three different assessment sessions yield estimates of *intersession* reliability.

Magnitude of Correlations

How closely must two sortings coincide if they are to be called reliable? There is no universal rule, but a glance at some hypothetical situations permits a reasonable judgment. If two sortings of sixty items were identical, the correlation between them would be 1.000. Sortings with average discrepancies of two categories per item would correlate .572. If an investigator wishes to merely describe coarse groupings of items (highest ten and lowest ten, for instance), reliabilities of this magnitude are adequate. (The value required for statistical significance at the .01 level is .325.)

In these studies the final version of a participant's "usual self" might be based on a composite of as many as six sortings. Composite scores are more reliable than single scores, and estimates of their reliability are available through techniques such as the generalized Spearman–Brown formula (Guilford, 1956, pp. 452–453). This formula indicates that (based on a single-sort reliability of .572) the combined reliability of two sortings is about .73; the reliability of six sortings is .89. These values far exceed what is necessary for purposes of the present research.

Person as Source of Reliability

Changes in the score on a stable characteristic may be ascribed to variations in the assessment situation or to temporary states of the examinee (fatigue, anxiety, distraction, etc.). However, reliability or the lack of it may also be characteristic of the person himself. In some cases reliability is generally low, regardless of instructions or assessment sessions. The hypothesis that participants may have misunderstood instructions is untenable: First, persons incapable of performing the tasks were not included; second, individualized items were provided by the participants themselves; and third, correlations among selected descriptions usually showed the relations expected in valid sortings. For example, "ideal self" usually correlated negatively with "worst self" while "usual self" correlated positively with "ideal" and negatively with "worst self." We therefore believe our data are valid, even when they reveal that a participant is unreliable. That is, the data always represent the best efforts of each of the nine participants to conform to instructions.

Factor Analyses of Rep Test Data

In the factor analyses of interpersonal constructs and interpersonal roles each construct was assigned a value of 1 for each of its applications to a role; otherwise its value was 0. When scores were summed across the three assessment sessions, the range of values in the cells of the construct-by-person matrix was 0 to 3. This is a narrow range for deriving correlation coefficients. Consequently, reliability values and factor loadings did not always yield easy interpretations. In general, factor loadings of .70 or greater were considered important, but quantitative outcomes were always regarded as suggestive rather than definitive, and raw data matrices were consulted to clarify outcomes.

Reporting of Interview Data

Much of the material in chapters 3 through 11 is presented in the participants' own words. However, the taking of complete verbatim records was out of the question, for several reasons. First, the need to preserve the confidentiality of the participants' identities precluded the use of tape recorders. Therefore, notes were taken by hand and later converted to a form containing as many of the participants' actual words as possible. Second, as anyone who has observed human speech knows, fully accurate transcripts of spontaneous speech leave much to be desired as a way of communicating clearly and efficiently. Consequently, in these reports actual speech was often modified to express meanings clearly but without any loss of characteristic vocabulary or style of expression. Finally, expository clarity required that information from all participants be presented in the same topical order. Paragraphs were therefore rearranged to fulfill this requirement.

As a result, the descriptive material in these chapters cannot be used as data for a study of language or speech patterns. The purpose of these chapters is to convey ideas clearly and with minimal loss of participant identity. The insight this provides into personalities compensates for the loss of technical detail.

PARTICIPANTS

Planning for Selection

This investigation was designed to identify up to nine life styles among men whose preferred drug was cocaine, and to study these intensively. The strategy for participant selection was developed from the following analogy.

Imagine that a spaceship capable of remaining in space for several months is orbiting another planet. Its mission is to conduct an intensive but time-limited investigation of the planet. Aerial mapping has indicated that the surface of this planet is variegated, with mountain chains, highlands, valleys, plains, marshy lowlands, and a number of large and active volcanoes. Stored in the ship's hold are nine scout-ships having accommodations for several scientists. Nine sites on the planet are therefore chosen for intensive examination. One team of scientists is assigned to study a site on the highest mountain chain, for example; others investigate other strategically selected sites. When analyzed and integrated, the information collected by the nine teams provides a comprehensive description of conditions on the planet.

This analogy of a planetary probe illuminates characteristics of the present research. A technology exists to study the problem at hand, the life style and correlates of cocaine use and abuse. The subject matter is an alien world with its own dynamics of sudden riches, euphoriant reactions, paranoia, and a labile and constant potential for violence. And the investigators chose not to examine randomly selected cocaine users but to study strategically selected ones intensively.

Identifying Target Patterns

We selected men with different behavioral adjustment patterns, as suggested by our initial perception of the world of adult male cocaine use. As described on p. 14 above, Olden (1973), Plate (1973), Sabbag (1976), and Woodley (1971) have presented an extremely variegated list of typical cocaine users from all walks of life. (These people do have in common a high enough income to support their heavy use.) Chambers et al. (1972) in the United States and Bewley (1965) and others in England described another group of users, namely, narcotic addicts in methadone maintenance treatment programs.

Seven life adjustment patterns were identified for examination. Two other patterns were formulated after the project was under way.

The first pattern was that of an individual representing cocaine use among upwardly mobile men in sales, managerial, and certain professional sectors that demand intense ambition and a willingness to pay a high price for success.

The second pattern was a ghetto pimp. Historically, the pimp has been an integral element in the mythology of cocaine. In fact, one slang expression for cocaine is "the pimp's drug."

The third adjustment pattern was that of a young adult, middle-class, blue-collar worker maintaining regular employment who accepts conventional societal values while taking drugs.

The fourth pattern was that of a successful black cocaine dealer. This pattern differs from that of the ghetto pimp. It provides a perspective that none of the others could match.

The fifth pattern was that of a man with a career in music, art, or the theatre. Given the reputed popularity of cocaine in rock bands, emphasis was placed on selection of a performing rock musician.

The sixth pattern was an adult male cocaine user engaged in a criminal career, but one not primarily associated with drug-related crimes.

A seventh pattern was that of a male cocaine user from a position of exceptional wealth and affluence. (The mythology associated with cocaine describes it as "the rich man's drug.")

The eighth and ninth patterns were discovered after the project was under way. The eighth was that of a marginal man exemplifying a group who, for diverse reasons, never achieve in life in any substantial way; this particular case also typified a person who speedballs mixtures of heroin and cocaine. The ninth pattern was that of an upper-middle-class white cocaine dealer who had no regular employment but had made large sums of money in this volatile occupation.

Emphasis was placed upon selecting persons who practice intravenous administration of cocaine. (We did, however, have one subject who is an intranasal user.) This decision was strategic, for it is among intravenous users that adverse reactions are most pronounced and the social correlates of usage show greatest variation. Also, there was thus a greater likelihood that the project could more readily confirm or refute some of the myths about cocaine by studying this group than by studying those practicing only intranasal use.

This project did not study cocaine use among women. That is not to imply that the problem is not important. On the contrary, cocaine use among women probably has its own dimensions and dynamics which merit separate investigation.

Selection of Participants

Screening and Choice

In July 1974 one of our staff members met with representatives of the criminal justice system and of several drug treatment programs in the Kansas City area. Discussions were also initiated with rehabilitated drug abusers and active drug users and abusers, as well as with local artists, musicians, and theatre people.

The selected life adjustment patterns were described and the individuals were asked if they could identify cocaine users fitting the patterns. Those who agreed were asked to screen their contacts and to keep identifying data to themselves.

Initially in this process a total of 537 adult male drug users were screened, yielding about 60 men with histories of cocaine use. Facts about socioeconomic background, occupation, age, patterns of drug and cocaine use, and the fit of each individual to the life adjustment patterns were reviewed, and the pool of candidates was thereby reduced to 28.

The individuals who had provided preliminary information then identified someone who had worked with the cocaine user or knew him well. Some of these persons functioned as intermediaries throughout the project. Others functioned in this role only for the initial contact, setting up the exploratory interview. Potential participants were told they would be paid $30 for the initial interview. Of the twenty-eight identified cocaine users, four could not be located, three had been incarcerated, and four declined to participate.

In each initial interview the investigators explained the project. The interviewer tried to answer all questions honestly and candidly. The matter of financial compensation and the steps which would be taken to protect confidentiality were explained. Candidates were told that if selected they would function as expert consultants on the subject of their experiences with cocaine and would be paid as such for their services. Each was told that he could maintain his alias or select a new one, the investigators did not desire to know his place of residence, all contact would be brokered by an intermediary of his choosing, he would provide aliases for parents, wives, siblings, associates, etc. The investigators pointed out, however, that if he agreed to participate he was expected to describe himself and his experiences as honestly as he could.

The investigators reviewed the initial interviews and four men were selected. Their intermediaries then made arrangements for the initial assessment session.

After the first four representative cases had been selected, the search was renewed. A finder's fee was offered to the person who located someone who fit the criteria and would participate. The search took on the characteristics of an enlarging spider web. One intermediary would exhaust his sources but would refer the investigator to another person with different contacts. The new intermediary would initiate his search, and so on. In some instances cocaine users who did not meet adjustment pattern definitions helped locate others who did. By the initial screening in early August eleven intermediaries had participated in the search. By the time the last case was selected in January 1975 the number of intermediaries had expanded to thirty-eight people.

All told, more than 800 adult male drug abusers were screened. There were no walk-in volunteers.

The Representative Cases Selected

Arky L. is the son of a white Arkansas sharecropper. He typifies the cocaine user from the deprived white strata of our society. Arky is an armed robber, although his criminal activity is not primarily drug-related.

Bill F. was reared in an upper-middle-class academic family. He is the only participant who practices exclusive intranasal cocaine usage. Bill does not use hard drugs other than cocaine, and he consumes the smallest amounts of cocaine of the nine men studied. Bill's vocation is important to our study: He is a musician in a well-known midwest rock band.

Tom P. had made a successful living as a white cocaine dealer. Many people who use illegal drugs also deal on the side; however, it is a different matter to do so exclusively, and live in an expensive apartment, drive new sportscars, travel extensively by air, wear expensive clothes, spend money lavishly, and court attractive women, while having no apparent means of support. Tom was such a man. He had practiced heavy intravenous cocaine use for eight to ten years.

George B. is a driving, ambitious, and successful salesman. He is one of the heaviest cocaine users in this project. One of George's other characteristics argued for his inclusion: He broke an intense dependency on cocaine and an addiction to opiates and methadone in a distinctive, but brutal, fashion.

Al. G., a black man, came from a background of poverty and was a long-term addict (fourteen years) who speedballed mixtures of cocaine and heroin. He made his living as a small-time gambler and street hustler. Al epitomizes a group of marginal men who never break out of their limited existences; men whom the world might consider as failures. Although Al never made it "big" in life, he was in many ways more successful than some who achieve much.

John B. is a blue-collar employee who works in a gas station. He is twenty-five, has used hard drugs for six years and cocaine for two years. He is a reasonably conventional person who wants children but loves drugs.

Willie M. is a forty-four-year-old black man who has been enmeshed in the drug scene for twenty-three years. He is one of the most successful dealers in the ghetto. If other investigators studied a ghetto dealer in Newark, Atlanta, Chicago, or Oakland, he would have much in common with Willie, for his survival would require many of the same characteristics.

Willie is eminently qualified to describe the physiological and psychological reactions to concentrated, daily drug use because he is one of the heaviest users of cocaine we discovered.

Fred S. came from an exceptionally wealthy family. He is twenty-one, the youngest man in the study. However, he has been a heavy user of hard drugs for four years and has been taking cocaine daily for three years. Fred maintains an extensive pharmacological library, is a walking compendium of drug information, and despite his youth is a person local drug abusers turn to when they want information about a new substance.

Rufus B. is a highly successful black pimp, bold and street-wise. Cocaine plays an important role in his life. He uses it regularly and (to use his terms) he has been "banging Girl" (cocaine) and mixtures of "boy" (heroin) and "girl" for ten years.

Demographic Characteristics of the Group as a Whole

In view of the fact that the representative cases were selected to vary in adjustment patterns, it is not surprising that they also varied in personal and demographic characteristics.

The nine cocaine users range from twenty-one to forty-four years of age and include both blacks and whites. (Although there is a small Latin-American population in Kansas City, we were unable to locate cocaine users from this group.) The participants have had from ten to thirteen years of schooling, and in socioeconomic background they range from sharecroppers' to millionaires' sons among whites and from poverty to the middle class among blacks. The occupational level of participants ranges from unemployed to holding positions of $35,000 per year. No income estimates were reported concerning persons whose primary occupations are illegal. Participants' police records range from one to over one hundred arrests. Some (for example, Arky L.) have often served time in prisons and penitentiaries; others (like Bill F. and George B.) have never seen the inside of a jail.

Confidentiality of Data

Several procedures were used to guarantee the anonymity of information reported by participants. First, no member of the project staff knew the true identity of any participant or his place of residence. All contacts between participants and project staff were brokered by an intermediary. Thus, if project staff wished to schedule an appointment with a participant, his intermediary was contacted; the intermediary in turn contacted the participant and a meeting was arranged.

Second, participant data were stored by a coded numbering system and kept under tight security. The numbering system was kept in staff members' heads.

Third, in the preparation of this book identifying data have been systematically masked.

Special Participant Problems

A special problem often associated with intensive, long-term research is participants' failure to keep appointments. As a group, these participants were notoriously lax; the no-show rate was approximately 60 to 70 percent. Most of these men live in a here-and-now world in which priorities and commitments constantly change. Sometimes participants had overslept; sometimes they were engaged in illegal activities; sometimes they were visiting or "getting high" with friends; and sometimes, even though they needed the money, they simply said, "To hell with it!"

One extreme example of failure to meet appointments was afforded by a man who dropped out from the research before data could be collected; he simply vanished. And there were in two cases other, grimmer reasons for not showing up: One man left town hurriedly with drug enforcement officers in close pursuit; the other was killed in a fight in a local bar.

Although the no-show rate for scheduled appointments was rather high, the men became involved in the study of their own lives and all but one participant completed the research.

_____ Part 2

Nine Cocaine Users

3

Arky L.

LIFE THEMES

Arky L. is a warm-hearted and congenial loner who has made his living as a thief, burglar, and armed robber since he was thirteen years of age. His life expresses six major themes:

- I am alone, an alien in a world I can't understand or find my place in.
- I don't like this world because it's so indifferent to me.
- I need love, affection, and care like a child; but
- I don't want to be dependent upon anyone ever again.
- I have a lot of explosive energy that must be released somehow; yet sometimes I want to give up and quit trying.

Cocaine Use in Relation to Life Themes

Arky is an intermittent, low-dosage, intravenous cocaine user. He prefers cocaine to a variety of substances that he uses, because it

- makes him feel powerful and independent instead of dependent and ineffectual,
- increases his sexual performance, reassuring him of his potency and masculinity,
- temporarily frees him from the anger he feels toward an indifferent world,

• provides a rare sense of well-being, euphoria, and freedom from discouragement, and
• helps him shake off loneliness and eases the attainment of closeness with others.

EVOLUTION OF LIFE STYLE

Introduction

Arky is a powerfully built thirty-year-old Caucasian. He wears a full beard and has shoulder-length hair usually topped with a crumpled blue painter's cap (with steel studs) set at a rakish angle. He looks older than his years, and when he sits slumped in the chair his countenance and tired, deep-set eyes remind one of the old warrior in Rembrandt's painting, *Man with the Golden Helmet.* Arky usually dressed in working-man's clothes: faded blue jeans, a T-shirt, a short and faded blue-jean jacket, and high-top work shoes. He is a relaxed person who displays little motor or skeletal tension, moving with the grace of an athlete. Arky identifies with ex-convicts and "street people," and his dress, carriage, and demeanor convey a rejection of social convention and middle-class values. Socially, Arky is poised, relaxed, and composed. He speaks freely and presents himself in a straightforward way. He answers questions directly and spices his comments with dry, homespun humor. He is a warm, gregarious individual who makes others feel at ease.

But Arky is a man of contrasting moods. Although he attempts to present himself as a warm and engaging person free from care and worries, this mood can shift rapidly to that of an exuberant boy telling about his adventures of the day. Yet, hidden beneath these impressions is a more persistent mood of somber concern, depression, and disillusionment.

Developmental Experiences

Arky was born and reared in rural Arkansas, the ninth (and youngest) child in an impoverished sharecropper family. His family was constantly faced with the problem of finding some way to pay the bills, feed and clothe the children, and keep a roof over their heads. When farming was bad, his father would work as a day laborer in construction, as a maintenance man, or on any other job he could find.

His father died when Arky was five years old. Arky remembers him as a hard worker, a kind and gentle man. Arky could not remember any time when his father disciplined him; this was understandable, because his father was always at work "trying to scratch out a living." His father's death was apparently a significant event; Arky remembers much more about the first five years of his life than about the period from six to eighteen years of age.

Arky describes his mother as small, warm, gentle, and honest. He says she was a good woman, "the greatest." She not only raised nine children but worked full-time outside the home. She had an eighth-grade education but limited occupational skills. After the father's death, she supported her family by working in a series of jobs as a waitress, a laborer, an aide in nursing homes, a fry cook, and in any other work she could find. Arky stated proudly that she sometimes held two full-time jobs and added, "Even though she is over seventy years old now, she is still working!"

Until he was about eight years old, his mother provided the only discipline he received. "She would whip me with an extension cord." She stopped attempting to discipline him after he was eight years of age because "by then I was bigger than she was." Afterwards, his mother would occasionally ask him to help around the house, but if he refused she would do it herself. He never saw her get angry about it.

Arky feels no attachment to his older brothers and sisters. As soon as they were old enough to work, they left the family. This made fewer mouths to feed, but did little else to relieve the mother's burden with the other children.

Arky said he was a lonely child. He managed to stay in school through the eighth grade, but he was laughed at and rejected by more affluent children for his hand-me-down overalls which had been patched and repatched. Some of the children stopped making such remarks openly "after I busted them. I always resented them rich kids; they had toys, nice clothes, and later even cars. I didn't have nothin'. We didn't have no car. I had to walk every place while them rich kids rode around in the new cars their dads gave them. Why did they make fun of a poor kid who didn't have nothin'? I hated them and still do!"

By the time he was ten, Arky had run away from home three or four times, usually hitchhiking two-hundred miles to his grandmother's house. He would stay with her until some member of his family came to take him back home. "I liked it there. She was good to me. I ate good, and sometimes my grandmother would buy me things; some little toys, candy, and sometimes even clothes."

At about twelve, Arky became involved in a variety of thefts and minor burglaries. Of this period he said, "Other kids had nice things. I wanted them too, so I took them! I wanted nice clothes and some money, so I stole it from them rich people!" From the age of thirteen until he was well into adulthood he was "raised" in reform schools and penitentiaries in Arkansas, Louisiana, Texas, and Oklahoma.

Arky does not remember much else about his life during the period from six to eighteen years of age, except that he did not want his mother to have to work so hard. Arky completed the eighth grade before quitting school, and later obtained his high school diploma while in the penitentiary. While in school,

Arky made mostly Ds and Fs. "I didn't even try. No, I tried to do good once, and, shit, the teacher made me stay in after school, so I just quit!"

Arky has held a variety of temporary jobs since he was eighteen years old. These included working in a service station, driving a winch truck in the oil fields for a pipeline company, working as an apprentice carpenter, as a laborer in a steel plant, and on an assembly line in a mattress factory. "I never stayed at none of them jobs more than a few months. I did like the job at the service station because I could visit and bullshit with people." Arky reported he was never fired; he would just grow tired of a job and not go back.

Arky lists his vocation as "robber." "I made my living stealin' and robbin'. The guys I worked with robbed in Arkansas, Texas, Oklahoma, Kansas, and Missouri." He admitted to twenty-five to thirty traffic arrests, two misdemeanor arrests (shoplifting), and twelve arrests for felonies. During the last eleven years, Arky received seven felony convictions and spent more than five years in state penitentiaries. He said he wasn't trying to get caught. However, when he counted up the months and years, he concluded, "I guess if you're looking for a loser, you found one."

Arky does not regard his time in prison as totally bad. "Hell, I had food and a place to sleep and everyone respected me because I wouldn't take any shit off anyone. I had more respect in the joint than I ever had on the outside!" Arky states he is tired of repeated incarcerations and would like to stay out this time if he could. "I would like to get me an education and be a counselor with juvenile delinquents, with poor kids. I know what it's like to be poor, and I think I could help them."

Arky married when he was eighteen years old. His first wife was a good woman and a good mother. "She was sort of a square gal. She didn't mess with drugs or alcohol or stuff like that." The marriage lasted two or three years but she divorced him because she grew tired of traveling and "couldn't take all the stealin' and robbin'." Arky has an eight-year-old son from this marriage. Arky says that he sends his wife and son money from time to time and has tried to take good care of them because "I didn't want them to have to go through what my mother and I had to go through." During the course of our research, Arky married a second woman.

Arky is a restless person. "I have always had to keep busy, keep movin', keep doin' something. Sometimes it makes me mad that I can't stop and take it easy, but I can't. I don't know why. It's like I have to. I've been that way since I was a kid!"

At the time of these studies, Arky was on parole and making a determined effort to learn to live in what was for him the alien "straight" world. He had a job and had even made an abortive effort to attend college. However he exhibited a fumbling "Buster Keaton" manner in his efforts to cope with his day-to-day problems of finding ways to get a check cashed, get his wife out of jail (where she was incarcerated for a traffic violation because she could not pay her fine), get his car fixed, see a doctor. If a problem is important and he has some knowledge about it, Arky will wrestle with it until it is resolved; however, if he is trying something new, is unsure of the eventual outcome or becomes frightened by an unforeseen contingency, he easily becomes discouraged and gives up.

Arky is apolitical and without religious affiliation. He wants nothing to do with politics. "Them politicians are more dishonest and crooked than us thieves. We only took what we needed. Them guys would steal everyone blind even when they don't need it. That's what that Watergate thing showed real clear!"

Interpretive Integration

Six major factors during his developmental years determined the evolution of Arky L.'s life style; these were

- poverty and economic deprivation,
- prolonged stress and discord,
- emotional and affectional deprivation,
- the absence of a masculine role model with which Arky could identify,
- ridicule and rejection by peers for conditions beyond his control, and
- anger and resentment toward people who had money and resources when he had nothing.

The loss of his father and the lack of direction and guidance contributed to the conditions adversely shaping an effective adjustment. It was consistent for Arky to develop a life style with the following characteristics:

- an underlying, persistent state of low-grade depression
- a superficial warmth, charm, and gregariousness, associated with difficulties in maintaining affectional bonds for long periods of time
- a rootless existence characterized by inability to remain long in one community, on one job, or with one group of friends
- a tendency to become discouraged when efforts are not immediately rewarded, and inability to sustain efforts toward long-range goals
- a disabling conflict between strong affectional needs and equally strong dependency strivings
- a hyperactive existence characterized by distractibility, impulsiveness and difficulties in delaying need-gratification
- deficiencies in ego development characterized by poor judgment and difficulty in conceptualizing life experiences and predicting consequences of actions
- lack of perception of long-term moral responsibilities or obligations
- a narrow time-life perspective, in which Arky is captured by events of the moment

· minimal guilt
· a relatively low level of anxiety

Arky has made his living as an armed robber. One could see such an existence as a reaction of vengeance and revenge against an insensitive world which would allow a helpless boy to be reared in poverty, be embarrassed by others, and grow up with limited love and affection. Arky states, "I just take what I need from them rich people" with such conviction that one gets the impression that Arky believes "them rich people" deserve it.

A major conflict which dominates Arky's existence is the clash over affectional and dependency needs. Arky wants to be loved and appreciated; at the same time, he wants to live a life in which he needs no one. He wants to be loved and cared for, but not to take any personal responsibility, make any personal commitment, or enter into any entangling alliances to obtain this. He said, "When I was little I decided never to depend on anyone ever again. You just get hurt if you do." Thus, while he has strong affectional strivings he equates love, closeness, and intimacy with a helplessness and dependency he cannot tolerate. His relationships with people mirror this see-saw struggle between contradictory needs. The closer and more intimate he becomes with people, the more frightened, insecure, and agitated he becomes. His typical solution is to break off the relationship and move on.

Arky is more comfortable with men than women. He is, nevertheless, sexually active and drawn to women for the affection and reassurance they can provide. Yet, because he fears "entrapment" in sexual relationships, his pattern is to engage in sexual liaisons with many women but never become emotionally involved with any of them.

Although Arky is basically a gentle and perceptive person, it is important to him that he not be seen as weak, ineffectual, or effeminate. Since acts of crime involve tests of courage and high risk, by committing criminal acts in which he takes his sustenance by force, Arky can assert his "masculinity" and "get back at them rich people." Arky admitted that he is not a remarkably successful thief. However, incarceration may provide one of the only ways he has to satisfy his dependency needs. In prison he can externalize his anger and resentment, yet be assured others must assume responsibility for his dependency needs. The penitentiary serves as a kind of mother surrogate or "home" to which he returns from time to time for support and nurture.

It is unquestionable that any person facing another with a gun is dangerous; however, Arky does not fit the stereotype of the armed robber. He is a man who needs and enjoys other people. One can easily imagine Arky with a fistful of money in one hand and a gun in the other, running the risk of capture while stopping to chat with the store owner about weather and fishing conditions. He states with pride that his vocation is that of a robber—one which may ultimately force him to injure or perhaps kill others or be killed himself—yet he became a vegetarian because, as he put it, "Why should something have to die so I can eat?"

Arky is growing exhausted by the constant activity of his existence. He knows he cannot win his vendetta against "them rich people" and sometimes wishes he could find more successful ways to get his needs met. When asked what kind of animal he would be if he had the choice, he stated, "I would be a kitty cat. They get a lot of attention and affection; I would be one of them." When asked what kind of flag he would fly from the antenna of his car to depict himself as a unique person, he said, "I'd have a flag of love. A scenery picture of a very peaceful and beautiful place where there is peace and quiet." When asked what kind of car he would be if he had his choice, he stated, "I'd be an old antique car, a big old Rolls-Royce that sets in the showroom and gets polished every day and doesn't have to put up with all the hassles in life."

FORMAL PSYCHOLOGICAL ASSESSMENT

Dimensional Test Findings

Intelligence Tests

Arky performs in the Bright Normal range on a standard intelligence test; however, other test data indicate that he is probably capable of performing at a Superior level. Arky has the intellectual capacity to complete college. He also has the intellectual ability to be a reasonably successful thief.

MMPI

Arky's scores on the Validity Scales of the MMPI confirm that he attempted to follow instructions and answer test items truthfully (Figure 3.1). The MMPI profile shows a personal adjustment characterized by low anxiety and guilt, freedom from hypochondriacal concerns, and absence of serious thought disorder. Test data also indicate that Arky's world view is cynical. He sees people as dishonest and hypocritical, motivated primarily by self-interest and personal gain. Arky expects people to take advantage of him and he feels justified in taking the measures he does to protect himself and his own interests.

The high *Pd, Ma* combination (Scales 4 and 9) indicate that Arky cannot successfully "bind" and delay the discharge of impulses. Rather, he will quickly move into action, whether appropriate or not. The MMPI Profile also substantiates the finding that Arky lives within a narrow time–life perspective, bounded by momentary needs and concerns. He frequently makes errors in judgment because he lacks skill in interpreting events within a larger social context.

MMPI results also depict Arky as an overactive and impulsive individual characterized by a high energy level and difficulty in tolerating routine activities. It is unlikely that Arky can remain at any job or physical location for long. He likes people but becomes easily frustrated with routine, and if not constrained

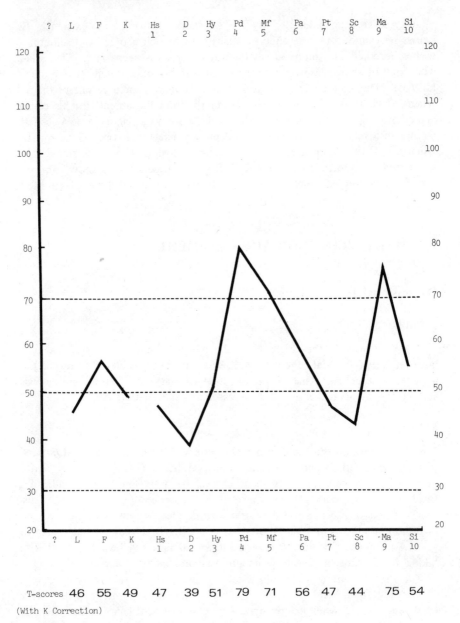

	?	L	F	K	Hs	D	Hy	Pd	Mf	Pa	Pt	Sc	Ma	Si
					1	2	3	4	5	6	7	8	9	10
T-scores	46	55	49	47		39	51	79	71		56	47	44		75	54

(With K Correction)

FIGURE 3.1. MMPI Profile: Arky L. *Reproduced from the Minnesota Multiphasic Personality Inventory Profile and Case Summary form, by permission. Copyright 1948 by the Psychological Corporation, New York, New York. All rights reserved.*

will either walk away or act out his frustration. A life style devoted to move-ment, constant activity, and action are hallmarks of Arky's existence. By keep-ing in action he attempts to block, avoid, or abort feelings of discouragement and personal inadequacy.

Unfortunately, Arky is a sensitive man who doubts his own competency and personal worth. He lacks confidence in his ability to cope with the world, feels discouraged, and would like to relax and find a more passive way of life. MMPI data do not indicate that he has been able to achieve this goal.

Sixteen PF

Table 3.1 presents a summary of the Sixteen PF (Cattell Sixteen Personality Factor Questionnaire) Test results. These demonstrate that Arky is not the carefree "stallion," "stud," or tough street man he would like to be. Though socially bold and unpredictable, he is not highly aggressive, self-sufficient, or competitive. On the contrary, the Sixteen PF portrays Arky as a gentle, sub-missive man who lacks the tenacity to pursue goals in the face of obstacles. Arky would like to be aggressive and potent, but he cannot stay in an arena and fight his way to success. He develops doubts about his competency, be-comes discouraged and disheartened, gives up, and withdraws.

The Sixteen PF Test substantiates the native warmth, charm, and gregarious-ness Arky displays in his interpersonal relationships. It also shows clearly the pervasive need to be cared for and nurtured which constitutes one pole of a major conflict in Arky's life. The test does not reflect so clearly the other pole of this conflict, the fear associated with accepting and acting upon such needs. The Sixteen PF also documents the fact that Arky's carefree, happy-go-lucky manner is the facade of a basically somber and pensive man wrestling with feelings of worry, self-doubt, and disillusionment. Arky frequently breaks the rules and social conventions, but not always out of anger or rebellion; social rules, conventions, and laws simply do not mean much to him.

The Sixteen PF profile indicates that Arky has difficulties in trying to under-stand and keep up with the world around him. Although warm, open and direct, he is insensitive to social nuances, misjudges other peoples' intentions, and lacks the savvy to accurately assess their reactions and motives. He becomes con-fused and frustrated by indirections and subterfuges, "games" and politicking, the status concerns and jockeying for position that are elements of so many social interactions. He is the perennial country boy living in a world that is just "too damn complicated."

Other Dimensional Measures

Arky obtained very low scores on all the Sensation-Seeking Scales. These results appear paradoxical. Zuckerman has hypothesized that people who score high on the General Sensation-Seeking Scale need varied, novel, and

TABLE 3.1. Cattell 16PF Profile: Arky L.

Standard Score	Low Score Description	Standard Ten Score (Sten) 1 2 3 4 5 6 7 8 9 10	High Score Description
9	Reserved, detached, critical, cool, aloof, stiff, precise, objective	A (8)	Outgoing, warm-hearted, easygoing, trustful, good-natured, participating
3	Less intelligent, concretistic thinking, less well-organized, poor judgment	B (3)	More intelligent, abstract thinking, bright, insightful, fast-learning, better judgment
8	Affected by feelings, emotionally less stable, worrying, easily upset, changeable	C (8)	Emotionally stable, mature, unruffled, faces reality, calm (higher ego strength)
4	Humble, mild, easily led, docile, accommodating, submissive, conforming	E (4)	Assertive, aggressive, stubborn, head-strong, competitive, dominant, rebellious
3	Sober, taciturn, serious, introspective, reflective, slow, cautious	F (3)	Happy-go-lucky, enthusiastic, talkative, cheerful, frank, quick, alert
4	Expedient, disregards rules, social conventions and obligations to people (weaker superego strength)	G (4)	Conscientious, persistent, moralistic, persevering, well-disciplined (stronger superego strength)
8	Shy, timid, withdrawn, threat-sensitive	H (8)	Venturesome, uninhibited, socially bold, active, impulsive
9	Tough-minded, self-reliant, cynical, realistic	I (9)	Tender-minded, sensitive, dependent, seeking help and sympathy
5	Trusting, accepting conditions, understanding, tolerant, permissive	L (5)	Suspicious, hard to fool, dogmatic
8	Practical, "down-to-earth" concerns, guided by objective reality	M (8)	Imaginative, bohemian, absentminded, unconventional, easily seduced from practical judgment

			Average			

#	Left pole	Right pole
1	Forthright, unpretentious, genuine, spontaneous, natural, artless, socially clumsy	Astute, polished, socially aware, shrewd, smart, "cuts corners"
4	Self-assured, placid, secure, self-confident, complacent, serene	Apprehensive, self-reproaching, insecure, worrying, troubled, guilt-prone
7	Conservative, respectful of established, traditional ideas	Experimenting, liberal, free-thinking, non-moralistic, experiments with problem-solutions
6	Group-dependent, depends on social approval, a "joiner" and sound follower	Self-sufficient, resourceful, prefers to make own decisions
6	Undisciplined self-conflict, lax, follows own urges, careless of social rules	Controlled, exacting willpower, socially precise, compulsive, persistent, foresighted
3	Relaxed, tranquil, torpid, unfrustrated, composed, low ergic tension	Tense, frustrated, driven, overwrought, high ergic tension

complex experiences. Thrill-and-Adventure-Seeking scores are reported to be higher for people who seek activities involving speed or danger. The Experience-Seeking subscale purportedly measures a need for a variety of inner experiences. The Disinhibition Scale is related to a hedonistic "acting out" life style. Boredom Susceptibility items center on a dislike of repetition, of the routine or predictable, of dull or boring people, and a restless reaction to monotony. Perhaps Arky scored low on these scales because he found all the items on them to be irrelevant, bearing no meaningful relationship to the world in which he lives.

Arky's score on the Novelty Experiencing Scale was similar to scores reported for airmen and male college students. One subscale score, External Sensation, was more than one standard deviation below the norm. This scale reportedly measures the need for physical excitement and danger, such as the risk floating down the Colorado River might provide. Arky L.'s low score on this scale does not mean he avoids external stimulation. All other measures indicate that he needs and requires it. The results do suggest, however, that Arky obtains such stimulation in ways not measured by this scale. It is doubtful that a career holdup man would find a guided Colorado River float trip exciting.

On the Change Seeker Index, Arky obtained an average score, as compared to those of college males and army men. Apparently, Arky's needs for stimulation, sensuous experiences, and change are comparable to those of other males.

When compared with adult industrial norms, Arky's Extraversion, Neuroticism, and Lie Scale scores on the Eysenck Personality Inventory fell into the forty-seventh, forty-eighth, and eightieth percentiles respectively. The inflated Lie Scale score suggests that Arky's scores may be invalid. However, the Extraversion Scale score is consistent with the Extraversion Index of 5.8 (Sten score) computed from Arky's Sixteen PF Scale. Together these data indicate that Arky is a stable individual who is not preoccupied with neurotic concerns and who presents himself as having an average level of extraversion.

Integration

The pattern of functioning which Arky evidenced on formal personality tests is congruent with information obtained from other procedures; the MMPI and Sixteen PF depict essentially the same themes. Nonetheless, there are some apparent inconsistencies in the dimensional test findings. For example, Arky was found to have considerably more intellectual ability than he demonstrates in his everyday behavior. These results can only mean that, given the events of Arky's developmental years and the pattern of functioning that evolved from these, he is unable to harness his native capacities in any consistent or effective way. Also, because of probable inappropriateness of items, results from the Sensation-Seeking, Novelty Experiencing and Extraversion–Introversion Scales are of limited value in supporting or rejecting hypotheses about Arky's life style.

Findings from Morphogenic Measures

Overview

Arky consistently presents himself as a person who wants to get along in life with a minimum of difficulties. However, he finds that he must always contend with contrary forces beyond his control. Some of these originate within himself; when they emerge, Arky covers them over as quickly as possible and tries to ignore them. Other such forces stem from other persons and are not so easy for him to manage or deny.

In the Q-Sorts, Arky described himself as carefree, happy-go-lucky, sexually active, and independent. However, this description turned out to be more a wish than a description of reality. Evidence also showed that another kind of person lies below the surface of Arky's personality. This person is tense, anxious, and ready to explode in hostile outbursts. Arky does not like this hidden self that keeps popping up, so he tries to deny it. When that fails, he takes cocaine to escape from it and restore the self he wants to be. Cocaine helps, but when it wears off Arky becomes uncomfortable, and the cycle begins again.

Q-Sort data also revealed that Arky does not have a high regard for his fellow human beings. He described other people (i.e., people outside the circle of his own friends) as snobbish, lying, cheating to get ahead, and lazy.

On the Rep Test, Arky almost acknowledged his weaknesses. He described the group to which he belonged in favorable and idealistic terms; they are warm, sweet, and trying to get ahead. However, he also described them as immature, dissatisfied, and as hiding from themselves.

The data suggested that Arky repeatedly lives through a succession of disillusionments. He starts a new project or friendship in high hopes that it will be ideal. He does not plan, but rushes in optimistically, expecting the best. Invariably, either his own impulsiveness interferes and destroys the relationship, or the actions of others cause Arky to realize that he was wrong for expecting them to be better than they are. When this happens, Arky turns to drugs to restore the self he would like to be.

Q-Sorts

Standard Items

Arky's sortings were highly consistent, yielding median correlation coefficients of about .70 both within and between testing sessions. Most of his sortings became more stable as the research progressed. However, one revealing exception occurred: In his first description of his "usual self," Arky admitted feeling anxious and nervous and having a tendency toward explosive violence. As if to conceal these admissions as quickly as possible, he changed his next self-description to one that is much less distressing. This relatively benign self-picture remained constant thereafter, but it obviously does not provide a complete description of Arky's personality.

Once he had covered over the admission of his tendencies to be anxious, nervous, and violent, Arky produced a remarkably strong correlation between his usual self and his ideal self (median r = .811). That is, he described himself as being highly self-satisfied. Although this result is often interpreted as a sign of good psychological adjustment, it cannot be taken for that in Arky's case, in light of the fact that his description of his usual self seems to be a facade.

Arky saw considerable similarity between the typical cocaine user and both his usual self (median r = .695) and his ideal self (median r = .687). Clearly, he made no effort to conceal his identity as one who uses cocaine, and indeed finds such use consistent with his own self-concept and ideal.

Factor analysis. Only one major factor appeared in Arky's standard-item Q-Sort data, and it was global in character. The results, therefore, indicated that Arky was providing essentially the same sorting of the items under all test conditions. A minor second factor contained only one heavily loaded component, namely, the self-description that Arky provided at the beginning of the first assessment session. Because so many sortings loaded heavily on Factor I, it was assumed to represent a general self-concept. Here, Arky endorsed statements which present him as a sexually potent male who is happy, peaceful, and easygoing. He rejected items communicating the ideal of sexual chastity and the thought that he might be hostile or cruel.

Factor II was identified with the one self-description in which Arky apparently admitted more than he wished. Here he endorsed statements that made him appear anxious, nervous, and explosive. The picture was far from that of a happy-go-lucky man at peace with himself.

Individualized Items
Most of Arky's descriptions using individualized items were stable over time, but some notable exceptions require comment. Most obvious was a reversal in his descriptions of nonusers of drugs. In the first reassessment period, Arky apparently shifted from telling how they would describe themselves to providing a description of what he thinks they are really like. As is shown in a subsequent discussion, his conception of them is none too flattering.

Arky described a cocaine high as similar to an amphetamine high (median r = .714). Futhermore, he described very little difference between what he is like when wanting cocaine and what he is like when taking it (median r = .813). These data suggest that his preference is for constant rather than episodic

TABLE 3.2. Individualized Q-Sort Items: Arky L.

Achievement
Positive
1. Reaching a goal
2. Become successful
Negative
3. Cheating to win
4. Lying to get ahead

Affect
Positive
*5. Happiness
6. Love
Negative
*7. Sadness
8. Hate yourself

Anxiety
Positive
9. Relaxed
10. Mellow
Negative
11. Scared
*12. Nervous

Chastity
Positive
13. Sexually innocent
*14. Faithful (sexually)
Negative
*15. Sexually frigid or impotent
16. Being a sissy

Dependence
Positive
17. Needs people
*18. Accept help gracefully
Negative
19. Unable to do things for himself
20. Inadequate

Dominance
Positive
21. Being a leader
22. Strong
Negative
*23. Dependent
24. Weak

Excitement
Positive
25. Being excited
26. Stimulated
Negative
27. Reckless
*28. Impulsive

Humility
Positive
29. Listening to others
*30. Modest
Negative
31. Shy
32. Withdrawn

Independence
Positive
33. On top of things
34. In charge of his own life
Negative
35. Snobbish
36. Looks down on others

Knowledge
Positive
37. Intelligent
38. Smart
Negative
39. Stupid
40. Dumb

Restraint
Positive
41. Patient
*42. Deliberate, restrained
Negative
43. Depressed, slow moving, lazy
44. Not caring about anything

Self-satisfaction (Stasis)
Positive
45. Feeling good
46. Carefree
Negative
47. Spaced out
48. Smug

Sexuality
Positive
*49. Romantic
50. Stallion, fox, handsome
Negative
51. Sex just for the sake of sex
52. Does sex with just any-body

Interpersonal Relations
Positive
*53. Kind
54. Charming
Negative
55. Being a jack-off
*56. Cruel

Social Recognition
Positive
*57. Well-known
58. Famous
Negative
59. Hated by most
60. Despised

Note: Items marked with an asterisk were not significantly changed from the original (standard) wording.

drug usage, and that he takes drugs not to produce a temporary state but to provide support for his basic personality.

Analyses presented later show that the state Arky is in after cocaine wears off is important in its own right. At first Arky did not admit that this state differs from the condition he is in *during* a cocaine high. By the time of the second reassessment, however, he was more straightforward about describing his less pleasant condition when without the drug.

Factor analysis. One major and two minor factors appeared in the rotated matrix of factor loadings. As was the case in Arky's sortings of the standard items, the first factor was a general self-concept. Again, sexual potency was dominant. Also important was feeling good and being in charge of his own life (positive independence). Arky rejected the idea that he might be sexually inadequate or cruel (negative interpersonal relations). This self-description is consistent with the one he provided when using the standard items.

Factor II is distinguished by its emphasis on listening to others and on being modest, and its more forceful rejection of such negative traits as being snobbish, looking down on others, cheating to win, lying to get ahead, and being depressed, lazy, or uncaring about things. This factor describes a "moral" self, a pseudo-ideal that Arky presented only at the first assessment session. The descriptions of "most people," which Arky provided in the two reassessment sessions, loaded negatively and strongly on Factor II. That means that Arky saw most people as immoral, just the opposite of this pseudo-ideal. In short, Factor II did not expose any desire on Arky's part to be moral himself; it reflected mainly his belief that most other people are immoral. The distinction is important, for it shows that, while Arky could articulate a set of moral standards, he applied them only to others and then in a condemnatory way.

Factor III contained two of Arky's descriptions of how he feels after the effects of cocaine have worn off. It is an uncomfortable state: Excitement and stimulation diminish, as do deliberateness and patience; anxiety increases, and so do dependence and weakness. Because these descriptions form a separate factor from the others, the data indicate that Arky regards this state as distinct from his usual self. His usual self is more similar to his description of what he is like *during* a cocaine high.

The data are consistent with the hypothesis that Arky takes cocaine because its effects support his self-concept and personal ideals. Without the drug, he enters a mood that is not compatible with his self-concept. He then seeks through cocaine to reduce anxiety and restore the excitement, freedom, and sense of independence which are crucial to the maintenance of his psychological integrity.

Rep Test

Role Groups

Arky's descriptions of people were generally consistent from one assessment session to the next. The overall median correlation among descriptions was .717, a value which is quite satisfactory considering the crudity of the data this test yields. He provided especially consistent descriptions of his ideal self, worst self, mother, father, successful person, interesting person, and person-who-dislikes-you. Least consistent were his descriptions of someone who drinks a lot of alcohol, a person you feel sorry for, and a same-sex cocaine friend.

The interpersonal constructs Arky invented are as follows:

Interpersonal Constructs

1. Being nice, saying the right things—being honest with people, open, honest
2. Sweet, gentle
3. Warm
4. Caring about others
5. Being a tough guy
6. Looking for the worst in others
7. Soft guy
8. Writes a lot of tickets
9. Hiding from themselves
10. Happy
11. Confused
12. Feeling satisfied inside, and knowing it can last
13. Immature
14. Trying to get on the top
15. Care only about the next shot

Factor analysis. The people in Arky's life fall into two distinct clusters. The first, bipolar, cluster contains ideal people and their opposites. People who are positive on this factor show many desirable characteristics: They are soft guys, nice, open, honest; they say the right things; they are sweet, gentle, warm; they care about others; they are kind, helpful, strong, wise, and happy; they feel satisfied inside and know it is going to last. Most representative of this cluster are Arky's ideal self, successful and interesting people, his parents, and a good boss he once had.

People whose traits are antagonistic to this cluster are tough guys who look for the worst in others, hide from themselves, and are mean and selfish; they "write a lot of tickets." The people at this end of the bipolar factor are all people Arky dislikes, including his own worst self. None of the people associated with drug use belong in this first factor, at either its positive or its negative end; this includes Arky's own "usual self."

For Arky, there are two kinds of society. In one, people can be easily divided into the very good and the very bad. The other kind of society is represented by Factor II, the drug people. They share many favorable traits of the people in Factor I; they are warm, sweet, gentle, care about others, and are honest. But people in this factor are also immature; Arky does not describe them as feeling satisfied inside and knowing it will last. Like the members of the negative group in Factor I they are hiding from themselves. Arky's description of his usual self has a much higher loading in this factor than in Factor I.

Construct Groups

Factor analysis. The interpersonal constructs devised by Arky were separated neatly into two groups by the factor analytic procedure. The first group of constructs was called *warmth* because that is the construct with the highest loading. Other constructs with positive weightings are "caring about others," "sweet, gentle," and "being nice, saying the right things—being honest with people, open, honest." Constructs with negative weightings (traits the opposite of the factor) include: "looking for the worst in others," "mean," and "writes a lot of tickets."

The second group of constructs described dissatisfaction and unhappiness. The highest loading is negative and is the opposite of "feeling satisfied inside and knowing it can last." Other high negative loadings are "wise, strong," and "hiding from themselves." Three constructs with positive loadings are worth mentioning: "immature," "confused," and "trying to get to the top."

The first of the two factors seems to represent a fictionalized ideal, the way Arky would like people to be. Factor II represents the bad things in people. To Arky, everyone is probably a mixture of these two factors. Perhaps he begins his friendships by hoping they will be like Factor I. When Factor II appears, he ends them.

Setting Survey

With regard to environmental settings, Arky's pattern of entry and occupation was stable from session to session, due largely to the fact that he consistently spent large blocks of time working and socializing.

Arky's Satisfaction ratings showed a slightly different pattern in the second reassessment session than in the other two sessions. The difference resulted from the fact that during the second reassessment he reported considerable dissatisfaction with a necessary but unpleasant visit with his parole officer.

As a general rule, two types of settings were most frequently entered by Arky: work and social-recreational. The latter were entered more frequently, involved more hours per week, and were more satisfying than the former. Arky does not keep his nose to the grindstone; his natural tendency is to feel pleasure in the company of others. However, he does not engage in religious or educational activities and does not belong to organizations.

Arky is not a leader; he has little authority or control in any setting. He would not like to be a leader; one could not appeal to him by way of his ambition. However, other data have shown that he responds to sympathetic social contact, even tenderness, and that is probably why he reacts with such great satisfaction to his mental health contacts. As brief as they are (less than one hour per week) they are the most satisfying times in Arky's life.

Integration

Arky tries to think of himself as a gentle, happy, easygoing fellow who is sexually active and lives an independent life. Underneath this wishful self-image dwell long-standing fears of sexual inadequacy and impulses toward explosive violence. These produce anxiety and nervousness, which Arky tries to cover up or escape from as quickly as possible. Arky wants others to be warm, sweet, and honest, and to care for each other, but he finds instead that they are selfish, ambitious, immature, snobbish, and undependable.

These patterns recapitulate most of the themes around which Arky's life is organized. They explain his feelings of loneliness and alienation as being a product of his disappointment in others. In response to his disappointment, he has come to regard the world as indifferent or hostile and himself as a stranger within it. He reacts by asserting that he is self-sufficient after all. This assertion is an angry reaction against a world that in his view does not allow him to live as he wants to live. Arky feels the resultant tension building and is frightened by its explosiveness. While he is not the kind of person to feel shame or guilt, he does not wish to be violent. He copes with this situation by channeling energy into pleasurable exictement and sexual activity and by taking drugs (especially cocaine) which make him feel free and provide enough pleasure to make life worth living again.

STYLE OF DRUG USE

General Pattern

Over the years Arky has tried most major legal and illegal drugs, with the exceptions of opium and LSD. (He has not tried opium because he never found it available; he has avoided psychedelics because "they make you crazy and I don't like trippin' like that!") Although cocaine is Arky's drug of choice, one could describe him as an intermittent polydrug user. He prefers certain drugs but will use, almost indiscriminately, what he finds available. When asked why he uses drugs, Arky stated, "It ain't very complicated, Doc. I just like to get high. Some people say they use drugs when they get depressed. Not me, I just have to wanna get high."

Table 3.3 presents the genealogy of Arky's drug use, his own estimates of its relative frequency, and his qualifying comments and remarks. He stated that the drugs he took were usually obtained from drugstore robberies, noting that utilizing these sources guaranteed access to "pure stuff, not the cheap shit you buy up here on the streets in Kansas City." Although he has snorted cocaine and taken amphetamine orally on occasion, he indicated he was primarily a shooter. "I was never afraid of the needle and you get better effects that way."

TABLE 3.3. Genealogy of Drug Use and Abuse: Arky L.

Drug Substances	Age (13–31)	Frequency of Drug Usage	Comments
1. Alcohol		Regular	I like beer and hard stuff too.
2. Barbiturates		Regular	Whenever I could get them in drug store robberies and holdups.
3. Amphetamine		Regular	I like amphetamine but drug store coke is better. You can relax on it, but not on amphetamines.
4. Cocaine		Regular	
5. Non-prescription, over-the-counter drugs Paragoric		Regular	I tried it as a kid.
6. Heroin		Intermittent	I never really got the habit.
7. Other opiates Dilaudid Morphine Codeine Demerol		Regular Regular Regular Regular	Whenever we could get it in drug store hold-ups.

72

		Frequency	Comment
8. Marijuana		Intermittent	I don't like it that much.
9. Psychotropics (Librium, Valium)		Fairly regular	I took them to relax.
10. Polydrug (amphetamines/ barbiturates, heroin/cocaine)		Regular	If you do much of one you have to do the other to balance it. Barbiturates make you violent.
11. Inhalants (glue, gasoline)		Intermittent	I tried them in the joint.
12. Illegal methadone		Intermittent	I tried it a while too.
13. Hallucinogens (psychedelics)		Never	It makes you crazy. I don't like "tripping" like that.
14. Other			

Legend

—— Denotes regular usage

- - - Denotes intermittent usage

73

Before he was seventeen, Arky had only experimented with alcohol, barbiturates, amphetamine, cocaine, heroin, and a variety of other opiates (Dilaudid, morphine, codeine, Demerol, and paregoric). Then, at the age of about seventeen, he settled into a pattern of heavy polydrug use with emphasis upon amphetamine, barbiturates, cocaine, some opiates, and polydrug mixtures of amphetamine and barbiturates, as well as of heroin and cocaine. His usage of these substances was based on their availability. Arky tried inhalants (sniffing glue and gasoline) while in prison and even tried illegal methadone for a while, before giving it up because he couldn't get much of a high from it. He has used marijuana off and on from the time he was seventeen, but has never "gotten into it" regularly as some of his friends did. Although he has taken heroin and opiates he never "used" them on a regular basis either. He reports that he has been drinking alcohol, particularly beer, since he was thirteen years of age; he likes hard liquor, too, but not as much as beer.

Arky has indicated that by and large the drugs he has used were obtained through robbery, at no cost. However, he admits that on occasion he has bought from other guys in "my line of work." The longest period of time he stopped using drugs by choice was three months.

Arky has never experienced an overdose on any substance.

Preference Rankings

Table 3.4 presents Arky's drug preference rankings. The data indicate that cocaine and amphetamine are his most highly preferred drugs. Opiates, barbiturates, and beer occupy the intermediate preference range, while marijuana, hard liquor, and LSD are the least desired. These data substantiate Arky's report that his drug usage is oriented towards the "lift" and "high" stimulants provide rather than the quiet "nod" produced by depressants.

TABLE 3.4. Drug Preference Rankings: Arky L.

Substance	First Assessment	First Reassessment	Second Reassessment	Mean	Composite Rank
Amphetamine	3	2	2	2.33	2
Barbiturates	6	5	5	5.33	5
Beer	7	6	6	6.33	6
Cocaine	1	1	1	1.00	1
Hard liquor	8	7	7	7.33	8
Heroin	4	4	4	4.00	4
LSD	9	9	9	9.00	9
Marijuana	5	8	8	7.00	7
Speedball	2	3	3	2.66	3

Ratings

On the semantic differential, Arky divided all substances into two categories, drugs and non-drugs; the only one he put in the latter category is LSD. Substances classified by Arky as drugs break down further into two classes, Amphetamine and Everything Else. Arky regards all drugs as "good, safe, beautiful, pleasant, right, valuable, and clean." Amphetamine is further distinguished by being "active, exciting, mighty, hazardous, bright, hard, fast, vigorous."

LSD achieved no distinguishing ratings, probably because Arky does not regard its effects as noteworthy.

Pattern of Use

Social Context

As a youth in the reformatory Arky dabbled with snorting cocaine, but all he remembers of that was that it gave him a lift. His first experience shooting it was while he was in prison. Another prisoner had smuggled in some coke and Arky tried some. Arky vividly and almost poetically describes the experience: "I still remember it and it was ten years ago. I felt like, Wow! I never had anything like this before! There was a *helluva* rush! I had this bitter, tingling taste in my mouth. My hair stood up on the back of my head, my arms, and even my hands! My chest was tight. My stomach was queasy. My ears rang, and my whole body just tingled. It was like havin' a big jolt of electricity runnin' through your body, but I was relaxed at the same time. It was the damndest thing I ever saw! After that first hit, I never did much more snortin'. It would be a waste!"

Arky loves cocaine because, in his opinion, cocaine is a mood drug. "Hell, man, it's the ultimate high. It gives you life. It's a flash of life! It's not like amphetamines. You can't relax on amphetamines but you can on coke. It will go with you wherever you want to go. Whatever mood you are in, it will carry it. If you want to listen to music, coke will go with you. If you want to do sex, it will go with you, unless you have had too much. It makes you feel great!"

Arky's typical pattern was to shoot up with a group of friends. The only time he used cocaine alone was when he was in prison (about 3 percent of his total usage). He estimates that half of his total cocaine usage was with one other male companion. The remaining 47 percent occurred in groups of two to six male companions. "Hell, when we would get cocaine in robberies, we would just fix and shoot for a couple days." On occasion he will still snort cocaine, with a woman when he wants to "do sex." He considers cocaine to be an aphrodisiac but feels it is more powerful for women than men.

Arky practices intravenous, but intermittent, low dose, cocaine usage. He estimates that over the ten-year period in which he has shot cocaine he only used it two to three times per month. "I would have done coke every day if I could, but you either gotta be rich as hell or do a helluva lot of robbin' and stealin' to get your hands on the stuff." Arky reports that his typical daily usage was a gram of pharmaceutical cocaine. (The largest amount he has ever tried was a quarter-ounce hit while he was on a run of several days usage; it almost "wrecked" him.) "I didn't do no more of them quarter ounce hits after that!"

"I liked to do runs for two or three days with my friends. We'd just hole up and fix and shoot and visit. We'd rest a while, then get up and fix and shoot again till it was all gone. It was great!" Arky has participated in from thirty to forty runs where all the participants were "fixing and shooting" for more than twenty-four hours without sleeping. "You don't get tired on coke. You feel like you could go on forever."

Arky states that his use of cocaine would always start in the evening. When asked why, he responded with some puzzlement, "Hell, I don't know. We just always started in the evening. When you're stealin' and robbin' you sure as hell ain't out workin' during the day like square Johns do. I don't know why we started at night."

When asked about the type of cocaine he used regularly, Arky states that from 80 to 85 percent was pharmaceutical cocaine obtained in drugstore hold-ups. "I have done some street coke but it has been stepped on so many times, it's just shit! Besides, I usually had access to stuff right out of the drugstore. That's hard to beat!"

Arky states the only way he can tell the difference between street and high grade cocaine is to fire it up (shoot it). "The rush is different and the taste is different. Good coke has a fume, a kind of bitter, tingling alcoholic taste to it. You have to shoot to know what you are getting." He states that while he has seen procaine he doesn't think he has ever taken any. "My friends told me the procaine rush is much harsher than the cocaine rush. They said you could tell the difference between cocaine and procaine by the difference in the rush."

Arky could think of no set of events—other than the availability of cocaine and the desire to "get high"—associated with triggering a cocaine run. "Some people want to fire up when they get down and depressed. I stay away from it when I am down till I get back up, then I do it." He could think of no life experiences or events that trigger his desire to do cocaine. "I just had to want to get high, that's all, and coke will sure as hell do it."

Arky asserts that on a run the dose of cocaine must be increased as the run progresses. "You're always trying to get back to the high of that first hit but you never do, even when you keep increasing the coke in the hits. He added that, after a two- to three-day run, "It takes approximately seventy-two hours, two good nights' sleep, and a lot of water to get the coke out of your system. After that, you can go back, start all over again, and get off good!"

Arky has experienced no withdrawal reaction after a two- to three-day cocaine run. "You are physically and mentally exhausted and tired as hell. Sometimes, I felt kinda depressed that I couldn't get any more coke, but if you can get some sleep—sometimes, you have to take tranquilizers or something to relax—you will be all right."

Reactions to Cocaine

Physiological Reactions

Table 3.5 indicates that for Arky, with his intravenous, intermittent, low dosage use, physiological reactions associated with stimulation of the central nervous system and sensitization of the autonomic nervous system always occurred when on cocaine. The sympathomimetic signs include elevation of blood pressure, pulse rate, respiratory rate, and heart rate; excessive urination and sweating; tightness in the chest; and increased sensitivity to light. In addition, dryness in the mouth and throat, loss of sensations of hunger and fatigue, ringing sensations in the ears, weight loss, and acceleration of mental activity were regularly associated with Arky's pattern of intravenous cocaine usage.

Other reactions, such as dizziness, goose flesh, nausea, flatulence and explosive bowel movements, itching sensations on the arms and hands, and headaches were frequently associated with intravenous cocaine use, but with less regularity than the first group of physiological reactions.

Arky reports that he did not experience signs of toxic central nervous system stimulation, such as deep tendon reflexes, tremors, twitching of muscles, spasms of entire muscle groups, or convulsions, nor did he experience numbness, fainting, hepatitis, inflammations, or abscesses at the site of injection which some users have reported.

Psychological Reactions

Table 3.6 indicates that Arky regularly experienced the following psychological reactions with intravenous cocaine use: increased restlessness and general excitement, intensified sense of well-being and euphoria, increased energy and perceived physical strength, the feeling that his mind functions more quickly than normal, a more active imagination, insomnia, sexual stimulation and prolonged sexual intercourse with more spectacular orgasms, intensified olfactory awareness and increased itching (possibly tactile hallucinations).

Increased anxiety, feelings of greater self-control, and increased loquacity or talkativeness were frequent, but were less regularly associated with cocaine usage than was the first cluster of sequelae.

Arky reports that his use of cocaine has *not* been associated with increases in optimism or personal courage, a feeling that everything is perfect ("Hell, I ain't no fool"), loss of ambition for work (he had no regular, legal employment during most of the period when he was taking cocaine regularly), a phy-

TABLE 3.5. Physiological Reactions to Cocaine Use and Abuse: Arky L.

Commonly Reported Reactions to Cocaine Use/Abuse	Reactions Observed Yes	Reactions Observed No	Percent/ Time Observed	Qualifying Comments and Observations
Dizziness — feeling of light-headedness	Yes		80	I get light-headed after I am "up" awhile. I get light-headed after a big shot. My whole body feels light.
Sweating — perspiration or increases in temperature	Yes		80	With good coke you sweat like hell, particularly in the summer.
Rhinorrhea — running nose		No		Not shooting, you get that snorting though.
Tremors — muscle spasms		No		I have gotten "chills" but I don't think it was the coke.
Lacrimation — tears to eyes		No		You get it snorting.
Mydriasis — dilation of pupils, light sensitivity	Yes		100	Bright light will hurt your eyes. After a while, your eyes get tired.
Gooseflesh	Yes		65	Yes, it's like an extra surge of electricity through your body.
Emesis — vomiting		No		You feel like you want to vomit, but you don't.
Reactive hyperemia — clogging of nasal air passages		No		It's a reaction to snorting coke.
Anorexia — loss of appetite, sensation of hunger	Yes		100	You are just not hungry.
Dryness of mouth and throat, lack of salivation	Yes		100	It's like having cotton in your mouth.
Increased heart rate	Yes		100	Your heart starts pounding like hell.
Tightness in chest or chest pains	Yes		100	A good shot will tighten you up across your chest and take your breath away.
Local anesthesia, numbness		No		You're not numb. Your body is like charged with electricity yet you are relaxed at the same time.
Nosebleed		No		No, snorters do sometimes.
Elevation of pulse rate	Yes		100	Yeah.
Increased respiration rate	Yes		100	You're breathing hard after a big shot.
Cellulitis — inflammation following administration		No		It happens with snorting if you don't rinse it out.
Infection of nasal mucous membrane		No		Same as above.

78

Symptom	Experienced	%	Comment
Yawning	Yes	50	It is like a yawn, but you are not sleepy.
Hyperphrenia — excessive mental activity	Yes	100	Your mind runs fast as hell.
Weight loss	Yes	100	You don't eat. If you did it regular, you would lose weight sure as hell.
Fainting	No		I heard of guys fainting, but it didn't happen to me.
Increased sensitivity to allergies	Yes	100	I guess that's what it is. It made my arms and hands itch. Sometimes I'd get a rash.
Diarrhea or explosive bowel movements	Yes	100	Sometimes when you shoot it stimulates your bowels. Gas builds up.
Hepatitis or liver infections	No		I had hepatitis in prison but not from coke.
Headaches	Yes	30	A big shot like a quarter ounce will cause a headache. The "rush" causes pressure.
Loss of fatigue	Yes	100	You don't get tired at all.
Ringing in the ears	Yes	100	With high grade coke every time.
Convulsions	No		I've seen people do crazy things but not go into convulsions.
Increased urination	Yes	100	If it is good coke it stimulates your kidneys.
Abscesses	No		I have never been "burned" on coke. I know guys who have, though.

TABLE 3.6. Psychological Reactions to Cocaine Use and Abuse: Arky L.

Commonly Reported Reactions to Cocaine Use/Abuse	Reactions Observed Yes	Reactions Observed No	Percent/ Time Observed	Qualifying Comments and Observations
Increased feelings of self-control	Yes		60	Coke "goes with you." If you are in control at the time, it increases it.
Increased optimism, courage		No		To me its a "mood" drug. Whatever mood you are in, it will carry it. You can relax if you want.
Increased activity, restlessness, excitement	Yes		100	You're restless and excited and feel like "going."
Feeling of increased physical strength or ability to do physical work	Yes		100	It makes you energetic. You get up in the middle of the night and clean house like hell. Whatever it is you are doing, you get carried away with it.
Intensified feelings of well-being, euphoria, "floating," etc.	Yes		100	If you have high grade coke, you have this fantastic sense of well-being.
Feeling that everything is perfect		No		I never felt everything was perfect. I am no fool, but you feel damned good on coke.
An exquisite "don't care about the world" attitude		No		You can get something like that with heroin, but not coke.
A physical orgasm in the "rush"		No		Never. It feels like electricity running through your body but no orgasm.
Increased thinking power and imagination	Yes		100	I don't know about your thinking, but you sure have a wild imagination!
Feeling that the mind is quicker than normal, the feeling that one is smarter than everyone else	Yes		100	I didn't feel smarter than other people but felt like my mind was quicker.
More talkative than usual, a stream of talk	Yes		50	If you get to talking, you "rattle" on forever. Sometimes you don't feel like talking though.
Indifference to pain	Yes		100	You don't notice it.
Decreased interest in work, failure of ambition, loss of ambition for useful work		No		You feel like you could work, but if you're on a "run," you're not interested in work, just the next "hit."
Insomnia	Yes		100	You need a tranquilizer or something to sleep.

Depression, anxiety	Yes	75	You get anxious. If you want to do something, you want to do it right now.
Prolonged sexual intercourse	Yes	100	You can go a long time if you can get up.
An aphrodisiac or sexual stimulant	Yes	100	If you don't do too much. If you do too much, you can't "get up."
Better orgasm on coke	Yes	100	It's more sensational, more intense. It's hard to reach a climax, but when you do, it's good.
Irrational fears	No		Not really.
Terror or panic	No		Not for me. I have heard of guys getting terrified though.
Tactile hallucinations — the feeling that insects are crawling on or under the skin (particularly fingertips, palms of hands, etc.)	Yes	100	I never felt any bugs or stuff like that, but my hands and arms would tingle and itch. I would scratch more than usual.
Changes in reality or the way a room or objects look — the wall waving or in motion, etc.	No		You might look at something, notice something in a picture you had never noticed before.
Paranoid ideas — the feeling that people are after you. You believe you are being watched, talked about or threatened, a wife or girlfriend is unfaithful, untrustworthy, etc.	No		I don't think it made me paranoid. You do wonder if the police are outside. Guys in my business who do coke are usually robbin' and stealin', and hell, you're always looking over your shoulder anyway. I don't know.
Causes one to carry a gun or run from imaginary enemies	No		Shit, we always carried guns anyway. That's how we made our living.
Visual hallucinations	No		I thought I saw a man behind a tree once when I was "doing" coke, but it was just lights and shadows.
Auditory hallucinations — hearing voices talking about you, threatening, etc.	No		I never did.
Olfactory hallucinations — new odors, smells, etc.	Yes	100	It intensifies all your body senses. Odors are more intense.
A trigger for violence	No		I have seen and lived with a lot of violent people, but I never saw anybody get violent on coke. I have never seen anyone "go off" on coke. It didn't affect me that way at all. It made me feel "mellow".

sical orgasm with the "rush," an increase in the incidence of irrational fears or panic, changes in perceived reality, visual hallucinations, paranoid ideation, triggering the release of feelings of anger, hatred, or violence.

It is difficult to interpret Arky's responses to the items involving paranoid ideas and visual hallucinations, for although he reported no such reactions, in the next breath he gave an example of each. Interpretation is complicated by the fact that people who pursue criminal careers necessarily live a paranoid existence. Even with extended inquiry, it was impossible to disentangle drug effects from the normal life style of the professional criminal on these two items.

Integration

Arky has drug preferences (cocaine and amphetamine), but he is not discriminating about the drug he employs to achieve a desired state. If one drug substance is unavailable, he will try another; if none are available, he might use beer or hard liquor. However, he avoids substances, such as the psychedelics, that would throw him into a "crazy" state or propel him onto a "mind-bending trip."

Although cocaine is Arky's drug of choice, his usage pattern is atypical. Many heavy cocaine users limit their social contacts during cocaine runs. As one individual put it, "The presence of another person only means you have another guy you have to be paranoid about!" However, a substantial proportion of Arky's cocaine runs involve from two to six other men. It appears that for Arky, lonely and rather isolated as he is, such experiences help him relax, be at ease, and achieve closeness. Cocaine facilitates periodic social cathartic experiences where he unloads his feelings so as to better tolerate what may otherwise be a bleak and lonely existence.

Cocaine meets other needs in Arky's life: It allows him, with his feelings of inadequacy and low self-esteem, to feel a sense of power, strength, and potency, and to experience what he calls "that fantastic feelin' of well-being you get with coke!" Along with bringing this sense of potency, cocaine also allows him to "escape" for two or three days at a time into a paradise where he "feels mellow," everything is fine, and he is free from the frustration he feels in the real world. Cocaine has a special significance for a person like Arky, who seeks excitement and arousal. As he states, "Coke's not harsh and raw like amphetamines, but it sure as hell fires you up!" Arky enjoys the physiological reactions that accompany cocaine use: the heart pounding, his breath sucked away in the rush, electricity running through his body, his mind moving quickly, and the flash of life that accompanies the rush. For a few brief moments he feels completely alive.

LIFE ACTIVITIES AND EXPERIENCES:
IN ARKY'S OWN WORDS

Overview

This section provides an account of two days in Arky's life. The first day was in October 1974; the second in April 1975. These days were selected because they typify Arky's pattern of day-to-day living.

The first day finds Arky trying to fix his girlfriend Nancy's car. (Actually, Arky spent more than a week trying to fix its cracked distributor cap.) His efforts took on the characteristics of an epic drama. On the first day, he involved Tom, a friend from his penitentiary days, and two giggly girlfriends. On subsequent days, two car loads of drug abusers, living in a halfway house treatment center, the house parent at the halfway house, and even his future father-in-law became involved as "consultant mechanics."

Arky was determined to fix the car. "I don't give a damn if it takes all winter. Somehow I am gonna make that damn car run!" In a sense, Nancy's car is symbolic of the world Arky lives in, because, as he said, "I simply couldn't figure out what the hell was the matter with it!" Arky's frustrated efforts to try to figure out how to get things done (fix a car, cash his checks, keep his appointments) is a recurring theme in his daily behavior. The quality of comic relief in Arky's artless efforts to solve these day-to-day problems covers an undercurrent of sadness in his life, revealing Arky as an impulsive, highly distractible, action-oriented man doing his dead-level best to make it in a world he really does not completely understand.

In the late fall of 1974, before the second day occurred, Arky married Nancy. We did not expect Arky to marry in traditional fashion, and he did not disappoint us.

"We got married last week! Why? It was my goddamn parole officer! The guy came by my place and found Nancy living with me. He said I couldn't do that because it would jeopardize my parole. I asked him how the hell that could be because we weren't botherin' anyone. He said that on my parole I had promised to obey all the laws and statutes of the state. He said there was an old law that says a man and a woman can't live in the same house unless they are married. I said, you've gotta be kidding! He said no, it was true. I said shit, do you want a piece of paper? He said, 'You mean you're going to marry her?' I told him that if such a dumb law did exist, I wasn't about to fuck up my parole! He said, 'you're crazy' and left."

"I took Nancy downtown that weekend and married her! Then I took the fucking license and all those papers over to his office and threw them on his desk and said, 'There are your fucking papers!' I was mad! He said, 'Hell, it's *your* marriage license. You keep it!' I said, 'No, it's your damn papers,' and stomped out of the goddamn place. So now I'm married!'"

In his description of the second day one can also see the emphasis upon restless action, movement and impulsiveness that characterizes Arky's existence. His pattern of living in a moment-by-moment action world with the foibles, mis-adventures, and frustrations associated with this style of life is displayed here in bold relief. No professional terminology or technical summarization could describe him more succinctly.

Activity and Experience Audits

First Day: A Thursday in October 1974

12:00 p.m.–6:00 a.m.
I was asleep at Nancy's house.

I had been out of the joint only a few months. I had gotten myself a job that was part of this drug abuse treatment program I am in—It's a good thing. This treatment program was paying me to work while I was trying to find something else. It helped me, because people don't like to hire guys coming out of the joint.

Well, I had this job (was doing okay on it, too), had been dating a bunch of gals around. This little gal, Nancy, took a shine to me; anyway, I was seeing a lot of her. Her car had broke down in the city. (She lived out in a suburb.) I brought her to her home and was going to take her to work the next day, take a day off my job and see if I could get her damn car running again.

6:00–6:30 a.m.
I woke up, got dressed, and washed up. I felt kinda blah like you feel in the morning.

6:30–8:00 a.m.
I drove Nancy to work. We were talking about what all I had to do to get her car fixed. On the way, we dropped Nancy's little girl (she's about two years old) at the babysitter's.

She said a girl (Linda) who she loaned the car to had told her the battery was down. Nancy gave me some money and the address where I could pick up an-other battery. I let her off at work and drove over to another halfway house (not the one I lived in) to pick up Tom, a friend of mine. I met him in the joint; we both got out on parole about the same time. The day before, he volunteered to help me work on Nancy's car.

8:00–9:15 a.m.
Tom and I drove down to this so-called "address," but the damn girl had

either given us the wrong address, because there wasn't no such place, or she didn't know what the hell she was talking about! I was slightly pissed about it all. Finally, Tom said hell, we could go out to his sister's place (she runs a gas station and store) and get a battery there.

9:15–9:45 a.m.
I was tired of driving around aimlessly, so Tom and I bought some beer and cheese for breakfast and took off to his sister's place. We talked about how screwed-up women can be sometimes. I enjoy being with Tom. He's kinda impulsive, but he's good people and I can be myself with him.

9:45 a.m.–12:30 p.m.
We got to his sister Marilyn's gas station. She has this kind of a station and store that's a kind of hangout for the kids in the area. Marilyn is a warm, friendly gal. She's easy to talk to. We have become very good friends. She loans me money from the "company" when I need it.

We asked her if she had a battery around the place. She said one of her customers had left a battery and we could use it if the guy didn't mind. Tom called the guy and he said it was okay. We put the charger on it and sat there visiting with Marilyn. The damn battery wouldn't charge! It had two dead cells. Shit, I was pissed!

We had been chatting with a guy at the station who had been in the joint with us. You may notice that guys from the joint kinda hang together on the outside —you do time with people, you know what they are like. The fact is, you can trust most of them more than you can trust a square John. Well, anyway, this guy said he had a battery up at his house.

We got up to the guy's house to get that battery, bring it down to the station, and throw a charge on it!

While we're waiting for the battery and bullshitting, well, two gals came in, Linda, a gal I was going with off and on, and her sister, Betty. They were laughing and cutting up. Linda was kind of bent; she thinks I'm spending too little time with her and too much with Nancy.

Well, *this* battery took the charge! Tom and I paid the dude and threw it in my car. The gals said they wanted to go down with us. We said okay, Why the hell not? We all piled in the car and took off.

12:30–4:30 p.m.
I drove down to where Nancy's car was sitting. Tom and the girls are smoking weed and chatting. I am drivin' and thinkin' maybe we'll get this damn car fixed yet.

Well, we put the new battery in Nancy's car and try to fire it up. The damn thing won't start! I am getting mad and frustrated with the damn thing!

The girls get to giggling at the problems Tom and I are having. They think it is all funny as hell! I didn't think it was very damn funny.

Tom and I decided there must be something wrong with the starter, because it just wouldn't turn over. So I walked up to a service station and bought a new starter. The guy let me borrow some tools and we came back. The girls are having a ball giggling and carrying on. I'm getting frustrated, but am thinking maybe this will do it.

Tom and I put the new starter in. It was a bitch! The tools didn't work worth a shit, and it had started raining. I am filthy, getting wet as hell, and the job is slow. I wanted to get it all over with!

Shit! The thing wouldn't start no matter what we did! Tom and I are both soaked. I am mad at the damn thing and pissed at the girls laughing at us out there in the rain.

Finally, I just said, "Fuck it!" I got some clean clothes out of my car and Tom and I walked back down to the service station. I gave the man his tools back and thanked him. Then I went back in the men's room and cleaned up. Tom sat out and visited with the guy who ran the station. He was not as filthy as I was; he'd been my assistant.

I felt better to be clean and have dry clothes on. I was cussin' the damn car. I simply couldn't figure out what the hell was the matter with it!

4:30–6:30 p.m.

We all got back in my car and picked Nancy up from work. I told her her damn car was a pile of junk! She laughed.

We drove on over to the babysitter's to pick up Nancy's daughter. (Everyone except me is smoking pot and having a hell of a time.)

We got the baby, then drove to my halfway house (I wasn't living there then, but I had to go see my counselor). They waited in the car while I met with him. The counselor is a young dude but an okay guy; I like him.

Then I drove Tom by the halfway house where he lives. The girls are still laughing and giggling and all. Tom had to "check in" so he wouldn't be in trouble there. This time I waited outside with the girls. I am feeling good now.

I drove us all back to Tom's sister's place. I am forgetting about Nancy's junk heap—even kinda laughing about the crummy day.

6:30–8:30 p.m.

We sat out at the station-store drinking beer, smoking pot, and having a good time. There are living quarters in the back—we're back there having a good time, relaxing, and enjoying ourselves. It was a pleasant change from the rest of the day. There were about twenty people in and out of there. They were nice. I felt good and enjoyed it.

8:30–10:30 p.m.

Nancy, the baby, and I left and started home. We were tired and relaxed.

We stopped for about thirty minutes at a drive-in and had some supper. We ate in the car. We drove on to Nancy's place from there.

I watched TV and chatted with Nancy's father. I talked with him about the damn car! He didn't know what was wrong with it either. We visited and watched TV till 10:30 when I went to bed. I had no trouble getting to sleep at all.

The Day: The part about working on the car was a bitch! The rest of the day was pretty pleasant.

Second Day: A Saturday in April 1975

7:00–7:30 a.m.

I woke up when the alarm went off, went to the bathroom, washed my face, dressed, and left.

7:30–8:00 a.m.

I walked down to the corner to a pay phone to call my boss. (Our phone's not in yet.) I called him, and he said there was no work for the day—I felt disappointed because he had promised me there would be work. I started trudging back to the house.

Lonnie came out of his place just as I got back (he rides to work with me now) and said he was ready to go. I told him there was no work today, but said I would drive him to work anyway.

Lonnie was talking something about a rock band he and Linda and my wife Nancy are going to see next week. I wasn't going. The ones you have here are so damn loud there is no way you can hear what they are singing. If they were good, I'd go see them but that's damn lousy acoustics they have at Cowtown!

I didn't mind driving Lonnie to work. Besides there was this little gal, Susie, I was going to drop by and bed anyway. I didn't want my wife to know about me going to see her.

8:00–8:30 a.m.

I dropped Lonnie off and headed out to this girl's house. I was looking forward to seeing Susie. My old lady is down on her—she thinks the girl is trying to take me away from her or something. Susie is about twenty-two years old, mixed up, and confused. There are a lot of mixed up, confused gals like that. Susie is a hustler and she gets strung out too much on drugs. (I was thinking on the way over about how Susie says she hates hustlin' yet she is not trying to do anything about it.)

I knocked on the door, then went around back and knocked on her bedroom window. Then I went back out front and beat on the door. Still no answer. I figured she must be really zonked out. Or maybe she got up early and had gone to get her methadone. Hell, maybe she stayed all night with some John, too! I didn't know. She is just a friend. I guess I have a knack for picking up a lot of "strays." This guy Loren moved in with me for a while; then another gal moved in (she was a runaway); then Susie moved in after she was dropped from the residential drug-abuse treatment program. She stayed with me a while.

I couldn't raise Susie, so hell, I drove home. It was no great loss. I'll go back sometime. She'll be there.

8:30–11:15 a.m.

I got home, went in the bedroom, took my clothes off, and went back to bed. It took me fifteen to twenty minutes to get back to sleep. I was thinking of nothing in particular.

Someone knocked on the door. It was the phone man coming to install the phone. I let him in, showed him where to put the phone, and sat down and bullshitted with him a while. He was talking about how Bell Telephone owns half the world and how they are trying to take over the other half; he said they're in security systems, burglar alarms, and all kinds of shit now. He left about 11:00 a.m. after he checked the phone out.

I was feeling okay after I got up the second time. I talked with my wife. She said she was going out to pick up a girlfriend and they were going to do some shopping or something. She asked if I wanted to go. I told her no, I was going to lay around the house and rest. (I was really waiting for Susie to come by. However, you can never tell about Susie. She might or might not show up.)

11:15 a.m.–12:30 p.m.

My wife left and I went in the bathroom and cleaned up.

Then I called Jack, a friend of mine, on the phone. He said he had wrecked his car and had to go to the insurance claims adjustor place at 1:30. The car still ran but was totaled. I offered him $50 for it because it was the same model as my wife's car and I could cannibalize it for parts. He accepted. I told him to come on by the house and I would go with him. He said fine.

I knew Jack in the joint. He's about the same age as I am. We did a lot of time together in the last eight to ten years. He's living with the first little girl I started out with when I got out of the joint, Betty. (Another friend of mine from the joint is going with this girl's sister. I guess guys from the joint stick together.)

My wife came back (luckily, Susie had not come by). I told her that Jack and Betty were coming by. I told her I was going to buy Jack's car that he had just wrecked for $50. She was pissed. I told her it was just like her car and I was going to take parts off it to put on her car. Hell, I told her a rebuilt transmission alone would cost more than $50 and we would get sort of a whole car for $50. She calmed down then.

12:30–1:00 p.m.

Jack and Betty came by. We sat there and drank a few beers and shot the shit. We talked about another friend of ours, Tom (the same guy I was with trying to fix Nancy's car), who is in jail and how stupid he was to get busted. Tom was in a bar, and then he drove off with another guy's car. The hell of it was that he drove the car back to the bar! The police had just come to answer the call and here he drives up in the car! Stupid!

1:00–2:15 p.m.

We all (me, Jack, Betty, my wife, and the baby) got in this "wrecked" car and drove off to the insurance place. We were still talking about Tom—we were talking about what a damn fool thing that was to do. If you are robbing, you may need an extra car if you don't have one. I could justify that, but shit, he had transportation! It was stupid!

We found the insurance place. Jack and I went in and talked to the adjuster; we were trying to get as much as we could out of it. He went out and looked the car over, wrote down the damages, and then called around town to see what it would cost to get it fixed. We kept laying it on the John (it was fun) and he ended up giving Jack more than he had paid for the car! He sat right down and wrote Jack a check. We all went away laughing and smiling at the deal.

2:15–3:00 p.m.

We drove back to our house.

My wife was going to go some place and check on some jobs, so Betty decided to go with her. Jack and I decided to go get some parts for his other car. My wife and I started looking around the house for some money. We found some, but didn't come up with enough. She took Jack's check from the insurance man and the check I had given Jack for the car. She said she would go by the bank and cash them both and give the money to Betty. (It seemed to make sense at the time.) While she and Betty cashed the checks, Jack and I would go get the parts for his other car and fix it.

I called some salvage places and we got some prices and figured out where we could get the parts cheapest.

My wife and Betty left and Jack and I got in his (no, *my* car now) and started to the salvage yard. We had not gone more than a mile before we realized we didn't have any money. Shit! I told Jack to drive us by my bank and I would try to get some money (my wife had both checks and our checkbook).

I went in the bank and talked to the lady there. I told her the situation, she checked our account, and then wrote out a blank check and put a tape of our bank account number on it. I finally got the money.

3:00–4:00 p.m.

Jack and I drove out to the salvage yard. We were chatting about what all we needed, and how stupid we had been to let the gals get away with all the money, and the checkbooks as well. We concluded we were a couple of idiots!

We got to the salvage place and told the man what we needed. He said he had some of the parts we wanted but the other parts we would have to take off the motors ourselves if we wanted them that day. In back of the building there is a damn mountain of engines piled up. We would have to climb up there and take the parts off ourselves. I was joking with Jack about how he used to lift weights in the joint—I told him he could just climb up there and throw those motors around!

We went out to get the tools out of Jack's trunk—and he didn't have any! We got to talking about how dumb we must be. (My tools were in my wife's car.) Jack had a couple wrenches, so we took them, climbed up on all those engines, and began pulling parts off. Its was hard work when you didn't have the proper tools.

About 4:00 it suddenly dawned on me that I was supposed to be in my counseling session at 3:30. We climbed down from the motors and went back up to the owner's shack. I called my counselor and told him where I was at and apologized. I told him we would be there at 4:40 or 5:00.

We hurried and got some of the parts we needed. We paid the man for them and told him we would be back for the rest of it later. We didn't have the tools to take them off anyway! After we paid the man he said, "Hell, why didn't you boys ask me. I have plenty of tools and would have let you use them." Shit!

4:00–6:30 p.m.

We drove to the center as fast as we could. (We were clear across town.) He was driving and I was navigator, giving him directions. There we were going like hell in a car that had just been totaled by an insurance company! Of course, it was smoking a little and the front end was out of line and wobbly as hell. We finally got there, though.

I talked to the director of the center for a minute. Then I had my counseling session. Jack sat outside and waited. My counselor is a nice guy, kind of tough on me at times, but that's okay. He gives me moral support when I need it. I haven't needed too much help from him. The important thing, however, is to know that he is there if I do need him.

Jack and I drove home. We talked about how we were going to get the rest of the parts for his car and when we were going to work on it.

6:30–9:00 p.m.

We got home. My wife, Betty, our baby, and Mary was there (the other girl was the one I always take to the doctor). We sat around bullshitting and drank a few beers. My old lady (don't know why I call her that, she's only twenty-one) took me aside and asked me if I was going to drive Mary home. I told her I didn't feel like it. She told me *she* wasn't going to drive her home! So I had to do it.

I drove Mary home. We made a stop at my in-laws' house to see if we had any mail. There was no one there, but I went on in and sure enough there was a stack of mail for us. I got it, locked up the house, and left.

I saw a doctor's office on the way and said, "I'm going to stop here and see about my ear. It has been sore as hell. I think I have a pimple in it."

I asked the receptionist how soon I would be able to see the doctor; she said 9 p.m., I said okay, and left. I jumped back in the car with Mary and drove her home. We chatted about her new boyfriend. She's a pleasant girl; you know, a pleasant fat girl.

We got to Mary's home and I sat down to watch TV. I drank a beer or two.

Mary and her hefty new boyfriend watched TV with me. We didn't say too much. He's on parole—I never found out what he's on parole for. Shit, we watched "Pretty Boy Floyd!" I didn't care much for it.

I played with another girl, Lana, who was living with Mary. She's an escapee from a girl's detention home; she is a poor little kid who ran away from home and got sucked into that concentration camp out there on Elm Street! She's real nice, just a teenager. She's not like most teenagers, she's got a good head on her shoulders. She is just a nice-looking sweet kid who ran away from a mess. I teased her about her hair—I was just bullshitting her. I was happier teasing her (she seemed to like it) than talking with the hefty dude on parole.

I left and drove back to the doctor's office. The whole side of my head was hurting. I had picked up my welfare card at my in-laws' place so I could get it free.

9:00–10:30 p.m.

I sat in the doctor's office a long time (it's a night doctor). I was thinking all these damn doctors are the same! They get you in their office and then let you sit there, those independent bastards!

I saw the doctor (it was a woman). She looked in my ear and said it was swollen. Shit, I knew that, but she said she couldn't see anything, any infection. She finally gave me some ear drops.

I told her to look again and pointed to where it hurt. She finally saw a pimple in there, but said it was not ready. I told her I wanted something besides aspirins. I suggested that maybe Demerol would help. She said she couldn't give it to me because it was a habit-forming narcotic. I told her I only wanted something strong to have around the house when I had earaches. (I used to get bad earaches in prison; every so often they would shake me down and find my Demerol and take it.) I told the doctor again I needed something strong so she gave me some new stuff she had (samples, I think). The amazing thing was that I took four of them and they helped quite a bit! It was some kind of non-narcotic stuff.

I left and drove home. I was feeling all right but kinda disappointed I didn't get what I wanted for my earache. She (the doctor) gave me a prescription but it was too late to fill it anywhere.

10:30–12:00 p.m.

I got home and laid down and watched TV for a while. The baby was in bed.

The medicine had helped my earache some so I was feeling better. I watched part of a movie. Then I went in and told my wife I was going to bed, laid down, and went to sleep.

12:00 p.m.
I guess you might say my wife woke me up and molested me.
Then I went back to sleep.

The Day: The day was a beautiful day, except I kept forgetting things; us letting the women get away with all the money and the checkbooks; us going to the salvage place with no tools—except for things like that, it was a good day!

4

Bill F.

LIFE THEMES

Bill F. is a guitarist in a well-known midwestern rock band. He is a pleasant and conscientious man who wants to build his career in the world of music. The major themes in his life are as follows:

- I desperately need to have everybody love me.
- I cannot oppose people, because they might withdraw their love.
- Through sensory (sensual) experience, I keep trying to create the childlike world I want to live in.
- I avoid penetrating deeply into experience because I might be forced to realize that my hoped-for paradise cannot exist.

COCAINE USE IN RELATION TO LIFE THEMES

Bill is an intermittent (two or three times per week), low-dosage, intranasal cocaine user. He uses cocaine because it

- increases his self-confidence in his interactions with others, socially and as a musician,
- enhances aesthetic experience and sexual relationships,
- perks him up and helps him play well when he is tired,

• helps him eradicate feelings of anger, so that he will not jeopardize relationships with people he cares about or needs, and
• helps him tolerate dull, routine life situations.

EVOLUTION OF LIFE STYLE

Introduction

Bill is a short, sturdily built twenty-three-year-old Caucasian. He wears glossy, well-groomed shoulder-length hair and a full, trimmed mustache. Bill usually wears a contemporary T-shirt emblazoned with a portrait of Beethoven, a Budweiser label, or some other such decorative motif; blue jeans; heavy, brown leather boots with brass buckles; and a wide leather belt.

Bill is a friendly and pleasant young man with a mobile and expressive face. He smiles frequently and conveys directly his desire to please and be cooperative. Motorically, Bill is rather restless and nervous; he squirms and moves about in his chair, leans over the desk to emphasize a point, strokes the hair on his arms and restlessly toys with the large signet ring on his finger. However, he speaks freely and answers questions in a direct and straightforward manner. Bill is sensitive to nuances in social relationships. He is alert to any changes in the expressions on his listener's face. If he thinks he sees a frown of doubt or misunderstanding he quickly asks if he was making himself clear, or else without inquiry restates what he was saying in different words.

His general mood is one of quiet, boyish optimism. One finds it difficult to avoid feeling parental concern as Bill talks about the problems he faces and his hopes and fears about the future.

Developmental Experiences

Bill's father teaches economics at a large midwestern university. "He was a pretty good father. He's fifty-three now. My father gets along with people easily. He had to work like hell to get his degree and support his family, too. He is still a hard worker because he likes his job, except when he has to travel a lot. He doesn't let work override his family, though. I remember when I was a kid he was going to Washington every week. He quit his job at that university and took another one that didn't pay as much so he could have time with his family.

"He is doing a lot of administration now; he seems to like it. He likes art a lot. He taught himself how to sculpture. He was pretty good at it, too. Then he learned how to paint and weave. He has a flower garden, too, and likes to work with his roses. The last time I was home, a year ago, he had bought himself a guitar and was teaching himself how to play it. He is a good singer, too."

Bill and his father are reasonably close. "We get along real well. He will talk a lot with me if he thinks I have problems. I can talk about anything with him. He is a pretty good father but sometimes I think he is overprotective; he worries about me. I decided I wanted to be a musician when I was eighteen, and I think he would have liked to have seen me go ahead and finish college. I went a year, but I wasn't ready. I want to get into the recording business, and he worries about that. It's a highly competitive business.

"My father is fairly affectionate. He hugs me when I come home. He talks a lot now with me about music. He is a pretty fair disciplinarian. My father was a little heavier at disciplining my sister and I than my mother was. Mostly it was spanking, but I only got a spanking if it was something serious; if the problem was not too serious, he would try to talk it out."

The most pleasant experience Bill remembers with his father is a trip they took together. "When I was about eight or nine years old, my father took me and several friends and drove us all three hundred miles to Chicago. We spent two or three days there going through all the museums. We all had a good time. I enjoyed being with him."

The most painful experience he remembers with him is an argument. "I was only about eight or nine years old. He was chewing me out about something; I think I had just learned what an abortion was. He was chewing me out, and I said, 'If you don't want me why didn't you have me aborted?' He got really upset, and I got a good whipping for saying that. I didn't say anything like that anymore. I remember that!"

When asked how he might change his father if he had his life to live over again, Bill stated, "I guess I wouldn't change much in him because he has been a good father."

Bill's mother is a teacher. "She's fifty and a neat person. My father is kind of a worrier, and she is more of a worrier than he is. She is fairly aggressive. For example, she wanted a college degree when I was in grade school; she got bored sitting around the house, so she went back to school, finished her degree and has been teaching ever since. She likes to work because she likes to keep busy.

"My mother is a very affectionate woman. She is much more demonstrative than my father. She is a hugger! She will do anything for her family. She has a good sense of humor and likes to joke a lot. However, she is very sentimental —she always cries when I leave."

"My mother didn't get angry often, but when she did she would really show it. Generally, though, she would try to talk things out with me. She would usually ground me or cut out TV time as punishment, but she would spank me if it was something serious. However, 'grounding' me or not letting me watch TV usually worked okay. Sometimes I would sneak out on her, though, and she would spank me if she caught me."

Much like his father, his mother has varied interests. "She likes to work, to teach, to do new things. She likes to travel and meet different kinds of people."

The most pleasant thing Bill remembers about his mother is her open expressions of affection—and the fact that she would make shirts for him. "I'd see one on a rock star and she would make one like it for me; I'd wear them to school and the other kids would ask where I got a shirt like that. The most unpleasant thing I remember with her was when I got lost on the way home from school—I was just fooling around. She came and found me and spanked me hard with a ruler. My feelings were hurt. I didn't know what I was being punished for."

Bill is closer to his mother than to his father. "In fact, I guess I am more like my mother than my father. She is kind of like me in that she is too easy on people sometimes."

When asked how he might change his mother if he had his life to live over, Bill stated, "The only thing I would change would be to make it so she wouldn't have to worry so much."

Bill has two older sisters, but only felt close to the younger one. "Betty, my older sister, and I weren't very close. She's twenty-eight now. I love her, but our interests were different. Susan and I were very close. Susan is twenty-five. As kids, we were interested in the same things. She is more affectionate than I am, but she looks up to me as a musician."

Bill describes his developmental years as being relatively peaceful and untrying. "We moved around a lot till I was about six. We moved twice after that. When I was four we moved to this college town where there were 40,000 students. We lived there ten years. I really liked that period. My father was always bringing all kinds of students home for dinner."

"I guess our income was about average for a college professor. We associated with a lot of faculty families. I didn't know any blacks till I was in the eighth grade. My father would bring all kinds of students home. I met a lot of interesting people who had traveled around. My first introduction to the hippie movement was there."

Bill ran away from home once. "We were watching TV, my sister and I. We wanted to watch different TV shows, and my parents let her watch what she wanted. I was seven years old. I decided to run away. I got my transistor radio and wrote them a note that I was going to the radio station to live. I left—it was raining—I got four blocks away before they caught me."

Bill's parents got along well. "They were pretty well matched and didn't have many conflicts, but my father and my sister, Susan, had real trouble. They are both stubborn. Neither liked to give in to the other one, and that would cause some tension, and fights, too. It really bothered me—I couldn't stand it! I didn't like to fight at all. Usually, even now, if I see a fight brewing between my friends, I will try to change the subject to avoid it. At times, people try to take advantage of me. For example, if I am selling something that I want a certain price for, I'll take their offer even if it is less than what I want.

I would like to learn how to be more aggressive at times, but I don't want hassles with people."

Bill states that his developmental years were stable. "The only problem was when my sister and father would get into a fight. We had a nice home and didn't have a lot of financial problems, and our family was pretty close and affectionate."

Bill enjoyed school and made good grades, "mostly Bs." He went to college for one year, then quit. "I know my father was disappointed, but I didn't feel like it was for me then because you had to put up with a lot of bull. So I didn't go back. I was nineteen."

Bill has been living on his own since he was nineteen. He has had several different jobs, including work as a fry cook, delivery boy, an apprentice carpenter in construction, and a janitor. For the last year, he has worked full time as a welder, playing guitar in his rock band evenings and weekends. "Basically I regard myself as a musician, but I have this conflict over whether I should work, because working forty hours at my job is mentally trying. I get home at nights and I really don't want to do anything. I should be practicing, but I am just wore out. Sometimes our band practices five nights a week. As we have become more popular, it takes more money to buy mikes and equipment, but I always have this conflict over whether I should quit playing and just work a while, or play and not work and use the days to practice, or keep on trying to do both. Our band makes enough money, I could live on it, but I am trying to save money to go to recording school, so I just don't know what to do sometimes."

"The only other problems I guess I have are with the band and this girl, Marian, I am in love with. She is the first girl I was ever serious about. She decided she wanted to travel—she wanted me to go with her but I couldn't—and is somewhere in South America now. I haven't heard from her in three or four months. I miss her a whole lot. She said she would come back, but she probably never will. It bombs me out that she doesn't communicate more often."

Bill does not see himself as a religious person. "I went to church regularly when I was a kid. In fact, I played guitar the first time in public at our church, but I don't go to church as regular as I used to. Politically I'm a liberal, I guess. I would vote for someone who was into freedom of speech and stuff like that, particularly if he were an anti-war candidate." When asked about his goals in life, Bill states, "I want to stay in music. I guess you could say my real career goals are to be a studio musician and eventually a producer."

Bill feels he is reasonably well prepared for such a career. "I've played in bands since I was thirteen years old and have made rather good money at it since I was seventeen. My mother started me on the piano when I was eight. Then when the Beatles came out I had fantasies about being a rock star; I took guitar lessions from the time I was twelve till I was eighteen. I regard myself as a musician, but it is a highly competitive field and sometimes I wonder if I will be able to make it. You have to take that chance, and maybe you will be at the right place at the right time and make it big.

"I must have played in sixteen to eighteen rock bands. I have been playing on the road for more than four years, on a regular basis. I like doing solos, but I am not sure I want to be the star of a band. I would like to play equal parts, or play for someone I really respect as a musician—one of my fantasies is to be a back-up musician for someone like Stevie Wonder. I would rather not be *the* member of a band. I don't think I would like to have a band of my own. I would rather be a member of a good band like I am in now than be *the* man."

"Being in a rock band, even a good one, is a hard life. You're on the road all the time, and in a band on the way up you don't go by jet, you go by van or bus. You ride six hours a day jammed in a bus to do a three-hour gig. You sleep in some crummy hotel, get up in the morning, get back in the bus with the other members of the band you were bored with yesterday, and drive all day to do your next gig—and it goes on and on. It's a hard life. A lot of people don't realize that."

"I can handle that part of the musician business. I am willing to do it for another four or five years if I have to, but I hope to move into studio recording. You can really do a lot with music in the studio; a lot of songs that ultimately became hits weren't worth a damn until studio musicians reworked them. In the studio you can get the exact sound you want, or you can add subtle little things that make the sound better. I don't know if I am a sensuous person, but I feel and think sensuous; I know good music that has balance or drive, and I think I know something about how to rework it and make it better.

"Music is somewhat like sex for me. I sometimes get goose bumps if I play well. Sometimes seeing a good band at work or listening to a good record will make me feel real high. Sometimes I like to 'limelight' a set or two, but sometimes I wish I were sitting in the back in a dark corner playing, because if you 'limelight' a lot you have to be a showman, not a musician, and you have to kiss the audience's or promoter's ass! I don't like that part, but someone has to do it. I'd rather not be the one!"

Bill is concerned about the future of his band. "We have been together for more than a year and have a real nice sound. We could make it big if it weren't for the hassles. They tear me up! It is hard keeping five musicians and a singer going the same direction. There are always a lot of little arguments between two members of our band—Bob, the leader, and Sonya, our singer. They fight all the time, and it tears me up! Bob is a hardheaded engineer and Sonya is a good singer, but she is self-centered. I try to keep them from fighting, but it doesn't work. Sonya just got an offer with one of the best bands in the midwest. I don't know what she is going to do, probably take the offer. I guess I can't really blame her if she does. It worries me a lot, but I don't know what to do."

Interpretive Integration

At least eight modal life events provide the framework for the evolution of Bill's life style. These are

- a secure and permissive childhood in an upper-middle-class professional family,
- emotionally stable parents pursuing professional careers and with diverse artistic and aesthetic inclinations,
- perhaps unfortunately, a family life characterized by the absence of parental conflict, disagreement, or confrontations,
- a relatively strong and enduring pattern of ethical and moral training,
- limited opportunities to learn how to compete with others,
- efforts by parents to stifle development of self-assertiveness, independence, or oppositional tendencies by threat of rejection or withdrawal of affection,
- an intellectually stimulating childhood with early musical training and contact with adults of differing life styles and experiences, and,
- in early adolescence, a proliferation of unconventional but highly successful rock bands which held out a model of a way of life Bill desired to emulate.

Reared in such an environment, Bill F. developed a pattern of adjustment characterized by

- strong aesthetic interests,
- rumination about acceptance, with strong needs to please others to gain love, acceptance, and approval,
- chronic fear of rejection and difficulty in opposing others, for fear of losing acceptance and approval,
- well-developed superego functions and acceptance of personal responsibilities and obligations to other people,
- lack of toughness, resiliency, and self-assertiveness due to preoccupation with gaining approval,
- suppression of feelings of anger, resentment, and hostility even when they are appropriate, and
- desiring to break away from parental control, go his own way, and somehow in the process find himself.

In summary, Bill is a gentle, sensuous young man who at age twenty-three is still going through adolescence. He is trying to determine what to do with his life and is wrestling with the problem of how to gain acceptance from others. In fact, his major life problem centers upon how to obtain the love and warmth he desperately needs. His major mode of adjustment is to *move toward others* by being lovable, modest, unpretentious, and self-effacing. When asked on the Metaphors Test what kind of animal he would be if he had the choice, he stated, "I'd like to be an eagle. They fly high and can see a lot, but I guess I am not an eagle yet. I guess I am a poodle—they're bright and they learn things fast to please their owners. I still would like to be an eagle, though, but I couldn't live alone—I would want other eagles around."

Bill becomes unnerved by open expressions of anger and hostility from others or by the emergence of these feelings in his own psyche. He would like to live in a fanciful paradise where people are loving and considerate and there are no disagreements, conflicts, or confrontations to shatter the warmth and tranquility of an idyllic existence. When others take advantage of him, he turns the anger he feels on himself and becomes depressed and self-deprecatory. If an argument develops between people he cares about, Bill attempts to abort or avoid it. He is capable of discerning disagreement between others perhaps even before the principals are aware of it, and his efforts at mediation may resolve some differences before they become acute. However, if these efforts fail all he can do is withdraw and suffer while the principals battle through to resolution.

Although Bill has chosen a career in the highly competitive field of music, he is not an aggressive individual who would exploit opportunities and claw his way to success. He is afraid to be the star—"the man"—because he feels he would have to become a manipulator and showman who could handle the audience, the promoter, and other band members. He fears this because he would have to be out front, take risks, be visible, and be vulnerable to being disliked. Bill is still too gentle and insecure for that. Rather, he will try to attach himself to a band he feels is on the way up and hope that his group will be discovered or lucky enough to "be at the right place at the right time."

Bill is aware of some of his limitations. This recognition may account, in part, for his decision to enter recording and become a studio musician or technician who is listened to by performing groups for his specialized knowledge, expertise, and exceptional ability to rework music and nuances of sound. This is probably an appropriate career choice for him.

FORMAL PSYCHOLOGICAL ASSESSMENT

Dimensional Test Findings

Intelligence Tests

Bill performs in the upper Bright Normal range of intellectual functioning. He has well-above-average intellect and can take an abstract, analytic approach to problems. He could easily have completed college had he chosen to do so. He certainly has the intellectual ability to handle the day-to-day problems of living effectively.

MMPI

Bill's MMPI Profile (figure 4.1) presents the picture of a socially sensitive, overactive man with strong aesthetic inclinations, but one whose life is characterized by an impulsive, hypomanic style of adjustment. There is no evidence of preoccupation with hypochondriacal concerns nor indications of a serious thinking disorder. The relatively low Validity Scale scores indicate that Bill attempted to follow the test instructions and answer questions honestly.

Bill is a gentle and idealistic man who lacks self-confidence and is prone to worry about himself and his relationships with others. He is sensitive, thoughtful, and imaginative, with strong and diverse interests in art, music, travel, and so on. Despite his lack of inner self-confidence, he is an energetic, sociable, and outgoing person who needs and enjoys contact with other people, makes friends easily, and would be described by others as warm, likeable, tolerant, and accepting.

The profile in Figure 4.1 also suggests that Bill is high-strung and impulsive, prone to leap into action when confronted with feelings of depression, discouragement, or dysphoria. He tries to avoid feelings of anger, resentment, and hostility by pretending everything is rosy and pleasant. Denial and impulsive flights into action appear to be his primary methods for handling stress, tension, and anxiety.

This is a sensuous man with a high energy level who may expend great effort to accomplish his desires but has difficulty in persisting at tasks imposed by others. While not self-assertive, Bill resents people in positions of authority—though he may not openly verbalize it. His world view is essentially cynical and he considers most people to be selfish, hypocritical, and preoccupied with the pursuit of their own affairs. He knows he must protect himself in such a world, but he is not certain how to do it.

Sixteen PF

The Sixteen PF (table 4.1) test depicts Bill as a warm, charming, and gregarious man who needs and enjoys interactions with other people. He is sensitive and perceptive, but easily upset by the frustrations, reversals, and adversities of daily life. Bill is a vulnerable person who can easily be intimidated and whose feelings are easily hurt.

The Sixteen PF shows clearly Bill's strong needs for affection and encouragement. It also depicts, but less clearly, his fear of anger, assertiveness, and aggression. Bill approaches new tasks with enthusiasm; however, if he does not receive encouragement and support he becomes discouraged, ruminates about his decision to attempt the task, and may give up or withdraw.

The problems Bill faces in attempting to get what he wants from life are not due to a lack of intellectual ability. He can see the "big picture" and grasp what must be done to achieve desired goals. The problem is that he becomes

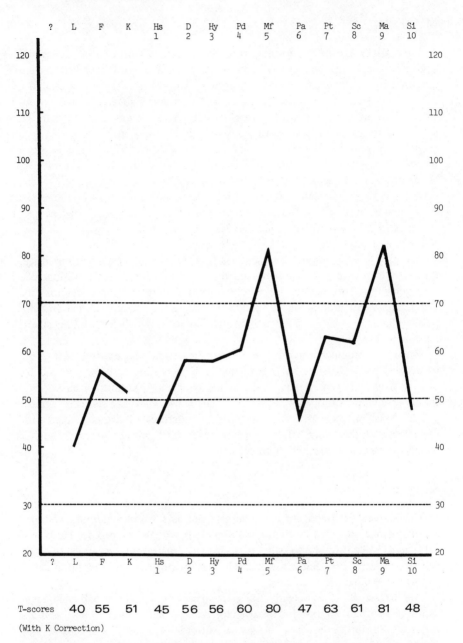

	?	L	F	K	Hs 1	D 2	Hy 3	Pd 4	Mf 5	Pa 6	Pt 7	Sc 8	Ma 9	Si 10
T-scores	40	55		51	45	56	56	60	80	47	63	61	81	48

(With K Correction)

FIGURE 4.1. MMPI Profile: Bill F. *Reproduced from the Minnesota Multiphasic Personality Inventory Profile and Case Summary form, by permission. Copyright 1948 by the Psychological Corporation, New York, N. Y. All rights reserved.*

neutralized in implementing the solution if confronted by adverse reactions from others.

The Sixteen PF depicts Bill as a person who follows his own impulses, ignores social conventions, and feels no particular moral or personal obligation to other people. This is somewhat paradoxical because Bill lacks the shrewdness and calculating, impersonal view of people which he would need to be able to manipulate or exploit others. In addition, he is too fearful of rejection to brazenly attempt such a thing.

Other Dimensional Measures

Bill's scores on the Sensation-Seeking Scales indicate that he has strong needs for novel and complex sensations and experiences. He obtained the highest General Sensation-Seeking score of any man we examined. These findings indicate that Bill is a restless and adventurous person who requires exceptional variety in his experiences and activities. He is a sensuous person who has wide aesthetic interests and would enjoy marijuana and hallucinogenic drugs, and association with unusual and unconventional people. Bill has difficulty tolerating routine people or situations, and becomes restless, anxious, and hyperactive when he finds things are not changing.

The results on the Novelty Experiencing Scales parallel the findings from the Sensation-Seeking Scales. The mean scores Bill obtained on the Novelty Experiencing Scales in every case were markedly higher than those obtained by comparison groups. His External and Internal Cognitive Scores were elevated but within one standard deviation of the means of the two normative groups. However, the Internal and External Sensation Scores were almost two standard deviations above mean scores for normative males. These results demonstrate dramatically that Bill seeks out and indeed requires active participation in stimulating and exciting activities, enjoys sensuous experiences, has an active inner fantasy life, and enjoys learning new things and tackling challenging intellectual tasks.

The score obtained by Bill on the Change Seeker Index is nearly two standard deviations above the mean of both comparison groups. These results indicate that he not only needs a high level of sensory input from both internal and external sources but also requires regular change and variety in his experiences.

Bill F. obtained raw scores of 12, 9, and 0 on the Extraversion, Neuroticism, and Lie Scales of the Eysenck Personality Inventory. These scores fall into the sixty-eighth, fifty-third, and ninth percentiles when compared with industrial norms. These results suggest he is somewhat more outgoing and extroverted than the typical industrial worker, and has no more disabling neurotic concerns and preoccupations than an average member of that group.

TABLE 4.1. Cattell 16PF Profile: Bill F.

Standard Score	Low Score Description	Standard Ten Score (Sten) 1–10	High Score Description
8	Reserved, detached, critical, cool, aloof, stiff, precise, objective	A	Outgoing, warm-hearted, easygoing, trustful, good-natured, participating
9	Less intelligent, concretistic thinking, less well-organized, poor judgment	B	More intelligent, abstract thinking, bright, insightful, fast-learning, better judgment
4	Affected by feelings, emotionally less stable, worrying, easily upset, change-able	C	Emotionally stable, mature, unruffled, faces reality, calm (higher ego strength)
4	Humble, mild, easily led, docile, accommodating, submissive, conforming	E	Assertive, aggressive, stubborn, headstrong, competitive, dominant, rebellious
8	Sober, taciturn, serious, introspective, reflective, slow, cautious	F	Happy-go-lucky, enthusiastic, talkative, cheerful, frank, quick, alert
1	Expedient, disregards rules, social conventions and obligations to people (weaker super-ego strength)	G	Conscientious, persistent, moralistic, persevering, well-disciplined (stronger superego strength)
4	Shy, timid, withdrawn, threat-sensitive	H	Venturesome, uninhibited, socially bold, active, impulsive
8	Tough-minded, self-reliant, cynical, realistic	I	Tender-minded, sensitive, dependent, seeking help and sympathy
5	Trusting, accepting conditions, understanding, tolerant, permissive	L	Suspicious, hard to fool, dogmatic

104

	Low pole		Score	High pole
	Practical, "down-to-earth concerns," guided by objective reality	M	6	Imaginative, bohemian, absent-minded, unconventional, easily seduced from practical judgment
	Forthright, unpretentious, genuine, spontaneous, natural, artless, socially clumsy	N	4	Astute, polished, socially aware, shrewd, smart, "cuts corners"
	Self-assured, placid, secure, self-confident, complacent, serene	O	6	Apprehensive, self-reproaching, insecure, worrying, troubled, guilt-prone
	Conservative, respectful of established, traditional ideas	Q	7	Experimenting, liberal, free-thinking, non-moralistic, experiments with problem-solutions
	Group-dependent, depends on social approval, a "joiner" and sound follower	Q	6	Self-sufficient, resourceful, prefers to make own decisions
	Undisciplined self-conflict, lax, follows own urges, careless of social rules	Q	2	Controlled, exacting willpower, socially precise, compulsive, persistent, foresighted
	Relaxed, tranquil, torpid, unfrustrated, composed, low ergic tension	Q	8	Tense, frustrated, driven, overwrought, high ergic tension

Average

Integration

Dimensional data reveal Bill to be a bright, intellectually able, gentle, and sensual man who is preoccupied with finding ways to obtain the affection and emotional support he needs from others. Apparently, he is willing to pay a high price for continued social acceptance. He is a "skimmer," fearful of the darker side of life with its anger, resentment, hostility, and strength; and, like the thirsty herd of cattle in the western movie, he is skittish and easily stampeded by shadow shapes and the unexpected. Bill's constant need for acceptance and reassurance and his fears of aggression leave him vulnerable to personal hurts as well as to manipulation and exploitation by more ruthless people.

Findings From Morphogenic Measures

Overview

This analysis of Bill's morphogenic data does not penetrate into the depths of his psyche. There are two reasons for this: The first is that Bill is untroubled by deep-seated conflicts rising ineluctably from his unconscious. The second, and related, reason is that Bill's personality does not in fact run very deep. He lives on the surface of life and runs away from his problems instead of facing them and working them out. For example, on the Q-Sorts he presented a favorable picture of himself stressing freedom, adventuresomeness, easygoing interpersonal relations, and rejection of personal hostility or aggression. There he said he is satisfied with himself as he is, but that when he takes cocaine he is even more so. He does not seem to need drugs, taking them to enhance experience, not to alter himself.

All in all, Bill's data fell neatly into place in exactly the patterns one would expect from a psychologically intact young man. He showed only one major, pronounced weakness, on the Rep Test: He seems extremely naive about himself and other people. Furthermore, he seems to want to remain that way. What he calls *freedom* is only the freedom to escape from personal entanglements or from situations where people are not nice to each other.

Bill is young, but his naivety seems strong even for a person of his age. One has the feeling that sooner or later he will be forced to face life in the real world. The data do not convince one that he will have the strength for it, and if he does not his reliance on drugs may grow. For the moment, however, as long as he can still run off or change his situation when things get rough he is surviving nicely.

Q-Sorts

Standard Items

Intercorrelations among Bill's repeated descriptions of the same Q-Sort concepts were uniformly high, higher in fact than is ordinarily expected. The median correlation between pairs of descriptions of himself as he usually is, provided at the same testing session, was .863. When sortings given under the same set of instructions were compared across testing periods, the grand median correlation was .794. Consistency values this high suggest that Bill was producing stereotypes rather than genuine descriptions of the concepts requested by instructions. As is shown in the next section, other comparisons confirm this suggestion.

Taken at their face value, the data indicate that Bill (1) is well satisfied with himself (median correlation between usual self and ideal self = .616), (2) regards himself as a typical cocaine user (median correlation between usual self and typical cocaine user = .643), (3) finds no conflict between his personal ideals and his use of cocaine (median correlations between ideal self and typical cocaine user = .565).

Factor analysis. Two factors emerged from the data, although loading patterns were somewhat diffuse, making factor identification difficult. Factor I seemed to be a self-description, but it also contained loadings in excess of .700 on all three descriptions of the typical cocaine user; loadings on all other sortings were also positive. Factor II combined Bill's descriptions of his ideal self and his self during a cocaine high. The implication is that Bill becomes most like his ideal when taking cocaine.

In Factor I Bill portrayed himself in a favorable light as one who wants to achieve, to live adventurously and independently, but who also wishes to be friendly, easygoing, and in control of himself. He rejects dependence and shame, does not like open, uncontrolled aggression, and rejects the thought of being foolish or unintelligent.

The qualitative differences between Factors I and II are subtle at best. Factor II appears to describe Bill's ideal, which is very much like his state when under the influence of cocaine. As compared to his usual self, his cocaine-related ideal is less subject to sadness and depression, more inclined to feel mellow and at peace, and less anxious, nervous, and lonely. None of these effects is powerful, and the data contain no evidence that Bill feels he desperately needs cocaine to achieve vital psychological or interpersonal goals. He takes it mainly because he likes the effects it produces. He could probably give it up easily and suffer very little for the loss.

Individualized Items

The overall picture is much the same as for the standard items: Bill's Q-Sort descriptions were all very reliable. As expected in normal cases, Bill's descriptions of his ideal self and of his bad self were virtual opposites, the median correlation between them being −.859. Because his descriptions of his usual self correlated positively with his descriptions of his ideal self (median r = .662), his description of his usual self also correlated negatively with that of his bad self. All in all, the findings indicate that Bill was making reasonable discriminations among item placements in responding to different sets of test instructions.

TABLE 4.2. Individualized Q-Sort Items: Bill F.

Achievement
Positive
*1. Gets things done
2. Getting your goal
Negative
*3. Believe winning is more important than how the game is played
4. Uses people to get ahead

Affect
Positive
*5. Happy
6. Feeling good
Negative
7. Bummed out
*8. Depressed

Anxiety Level
Positive
*9. Mellow
*10. At peace with yourself
Negative
11. Uptight
*12. Nervous

Chastity
Positive
13. Doesn't *use* others for sex
*14. Faithful (sexually).
Negative
*15. Impotent
16. Too shy to meet girls

Dependence
Positive
17. Works with others
18. Needs friends
Negative
*19. Tied to someone's apron strings

20. A leech

Dominance
Positive
21. Influential
22. Teaches others
Negative
*23. "Wishy-washy"
24. Unconfident

Excitement
Positive
25. Open to new things
*26. Adventuresome
Negative
*27. Violent
28. Doesn't think before leaping into things

Humility
Positive
*29. Humble
*30. Modest
Negative
31. Lacks close friends
*32. Lonely

Independence
Positive
33. Independent
34. Open, free
Negative
*35. Stubborn

36. Inconsiderate, because he must prove independence

Knowledge
Positive
*37. Wise
38. Creative
Negative
39. Dull, not smart
*40. Unintelligent

Restraint
Positive
41. Self-controlled
42. Thinks before actions
Negative
43. Dull, not interesting
44. Closed

Self-satisfaction (Stasis)
Positive
45. Feeling accomplished
46. Did what he set out to do.
Negative
*47. Lazy
48. Tired

Sexuality
Positive
49. Sensuous
50. Sexy
Negative
51. Does one-sided sex

52. Takes (sexually) and doesn't give

Interpersonal Relations
Positive
53. Easygoing with others
*54. Friendly
Negative
55. Inconsiderate
*56. Cruel

Social Recognition
Positive
*57. Respected
*58. Famous
Negative
59. A jerk
60. Foolish

Note: Items marked with an asterisk (*) are not significantly altered from their original (standard) wording.

108

Bill's descriptions of himself as he is before, during, and after a cocaine high did not differ greatly from each other or from his description of himself during an amphetamine high. These findings reflect the likelihood that he does not take either cocaine or amphetamine in quantities large enough to experience profound or differential effects. Finally, Bill described himself as being basically similar to people who do not use drugs (median r = .483). He regards himself as enough like others to ensure contact and communication, but dissimilar enough to retain his individuality.

Factor analysis. Three factors emerged from Bill's Q-Sorts of individualized items. The first factor was associated with his general self-concept (usual self) and his feelings about drugs. The second factor was bipolar, reflecting Bill's contrast between his ideal self (positive loadings) and his bad self (negative loadings). (This factor, of course, is independent of his usual self.) The third factor did not contain high loadings on any sorting, except perhaps Bill's first portrayal of nonusers (loading = .720). However, because all his descriptions of nonusers and of himself during an amphetamine high loaded at levels of about .60 on this factor, it merited closer examination, though it is not a major component in Bill's personality.

In Factor I (self), Bill says he is friendly and easygoing with others, adventuresome, independent, free, and open to new things yet having self-control, and the habit of thinking before he acts. He is not violent, impulsive, inconsiderate, or cruel, nor is he a leech tied to someone's apron strings. Four things stand out in Bill's self-concept: an insistence on freedom (along with its automatic rejection of dependency), a need for adventure and excitement (perhaps also a manifestation of the need for freedom), a need to retain self-control, and a need to be seen as easygoing and friendly rather than hostile or cruel.

Because Bill likes to stress the positive and because Factor II is bipolar, Factor II is analyzed here in its negative (bad self) form. (A simple one-for-one reversal produces Bill's picture of his ideal self.) At his worst, Bill is violent and thoughtless, and uses people to get ahead, focusing more on winning than on playing fair, and is dependent, inconsiderate, and cruel. He is not open to new things nor is he adventuresome. He is not friendly or happy, and he does not feel good. Bill always keeps this bad self under tight control, he does not appear to feel threatened by it at any time.

Bill feels that most people (Factor III) are achievement-oriented, happy, and have self-control. However, he also regards these people as being uptight and nervous (which is probably why his description of an amphetamine high also has a loading on this factor). To Bill, most people are also less interested than he is in adventure and new things, less independent, and a bit less likely to act foolishly or be "jerks."

Again, these data provide no basis for believing that Bill experiences serious psychological problems. He is like the young man in fairy tales who goes out into the world to seek his fortune—immature, perhaps, but he may grow out of it.

Rep Test

Role Groups

Bill's data here presented no serious reliability problems. Virtually all of his descriptions of important people were stable over time. The only person for whom consistency was somewhat low was "a person of the other sex with whom you take cocaine" (median r = .447). As it happened, this person turned up in a factor of her own in the factor analysis of Bill's Rep Test data.

As with Bill's other data, high reliability in and of itself is no evidence that careful discriminations were being made when different descriptions were required. It could be that Bill's descriptions were all the same description; perhaps he described not twenty people but the same person twenty times.

The constructs Bill created for use in describing people are as follows:

Interpersonal Constructs

1. Trying to be better as a person
2. I can talk to this person about anything
3. Tries to do many things, has many interests
4. Does not give up
5. Gets done what he (she) wants to do
6. Searching for something
7. Dedicated to music
8. Warm
9. Adventurous
10. Varied things in his (her) personality
11. An open person
12. Stubborn
13. Wants to travel, meet new people
14. Has a good sense of humor
15. Independent

Their content suggests that the idea—that he was describing the same person over and over—may not be too farfetched. Only one construct, "stubborn," was in any way derogatory, and that was not severely so. Many of the others seem either platitudinous ("has a good sense of humor") or vague ("searching for something") or both. Possibly Bill was trying to conceal his opinions; more likely, however, he is simply not insightful or precise in his thinking about others.

The lack of negative undesirable characteristics in Bill's list suggests that he tries to be non-condemnatory and to avoid unpleasantness. He does not face up to interpersonal problems but prefers to run away from them. This explains his desire for what he calls freedom and independence. What he really wants is to escape responsibility for managing interpersonal affairs on a long-term, intimate basis. He wants to meet new people all the time, because he tires of the old when relationships become too close. This lack of closeness to others is probably also associated with a lack of closeness to himself.

Factor analysis. Although factor analysis suggests that there are four main groups of persons in Bill's life, there is only one massive factor; the other three are distinguished either by the small number of their members or by the small number of constructs which apply to them. This outcome confirms the vagueness of Bill's perceptions of himself and others. It makes him seem so immature that one cannot but hope he will outgrow it before getting into serious trouble; Bill may be the young man seeking his fortune, but he also seems a babe in the woods.

The first factor contains twelve, out of a possible twenty, persons: his usual self, ideal self, worst self (negative loading), mother, father, person from whom you get cocaine, person of the same sex with whom you take cocaine, employer you like, successful person, interesting person, person you would most like to help, and self on cocaine. To these people Bill applied most of the fifteen constructs he had provided, all of them positive: trying to be better as a person, I can talk to this person about anything, tries to do many things and has many interests, does not give up, gets done what he (she) wants to do, searching for something, varied things in his (her) personality, an open person, has a good sense of humor, independent, and is not stubborn. Among the six standard constructs, Bill applied three to this group by indicating that they are all strong and wise but only his worst self (and *not* the others) is mean. Obviously, a factor this large does not leave room for variation among other people. In all the other factors, only a few distinguishing characteristics could be identified.

Factor II includes several people, two of whom Bill was required by the test instructions to dislike: employer you dislike, person you dislike, person who behaves strangely, and person who drinks a lot of alcohol. The worst he can say of these people is that they are stubborn, selfish, and get done what they want to do. Bill does not seem to want to admit any more intense feelings than this.

Factor III contains only a description of "person of the other sex with whom you take cocaine." This person is like the people in Factor I in most respects, but she is also dedicated to music, adventurous, stubborn, selfish, and sexy. In combination with Factor IV, discussed next, this factor suggests that Bill is having trouble in affairs of the heart and that sexual freedom and adventure are part of the independence which is of such personal importance in his life.

Factor IV contains a thought-provoking mixture: wife or girlfriend, father, and person who dislikes you. Even of these people Bill can say nothing bad. Though they are stubborn, they are searching for something, trying to be better, and are warm, kind, strong, and wise. This peculiar collection of people suggests again that Bill has dealt with domestic problems by running away from them. Apparently, he does this successfully, for he seems not to suffer greatly for it, nor does he admit to holding any grudges. One suspects, however, that someday he will either have to face these problems or find himself lonely. If the latter occurs, his relationship to drugs may become more intense.

Construct groups

Considering the way he grouped people, it would be surprising if Bill's inter-personal construct space were very complicated. Only two factors emerged: The first was a massive factor containing nearly all the constructs used to describe people in Role Group I. There is no point in repeating its contents here; suffice it to say that they are all positive, and nearly everybody he knows rates high on them.

The second factor has heavy loadings only on these two constructs: independent and does not give up. It has slightly lower loadings on these: searching for something and has a good sense of humor. One might suppose that if these constructs were presented to Bill, he could explain why they belong together. Aside from the possibility that they may present a picture of Bill himself, it is hard to make sense out of this factor.

In summary, Bill seems to be a naive young man incapable of handling the responsibilities of mature, intimate interpersonal relations. He maintains his image of freedom, independence, and of being easy to get along with by running away from difficult situations. Although this mechanism has worked well in his life so far, it leaves him deprived of the understanding of self and others essential to the successful conduct of life.

Setting Survey

Like everything else Bill produced, his Setting Survey data were highly reliable; not a single value was less than .900. Evidently, Bill has a schedule of constant activity and adheres to it closely. He reports a great deal of time spent at work, but he also enters social-recreational and organizational settings. He does not report entering settings devoted to either mental or physical health, as is consistent with our general impression that he is not in serious psychological difficulty. He also spends a lot of time "on the road" and playing in bars and night clubs.

Integration

Bill is not a person who delves deeply into the content or meaning of his own experiences. He understands his relationships with others only in the most superficial terms. In his Q-Sorts he produced stereotyped descriptions of himself which stressed friendliness, an easygoing manner, and a desire for freedom and adventure. He showed that he likes to think of himself as existing in an ideal state, without cruelty, sadness, hostility, or any other unpleasant emotion. The Rep Test showed that his views of others are similarly glowing and pleasant; none of the people presented to him as stimuli, even those he dislikes, were described as having any trait worse than that of being stubborn.

To live in such a benign world would surely be ideal, and Bill may be correct in his belief that he currently does so. Unfortunately, however, continued existence in such a happy situation is realistically impossible. Bill manages to stay within his idyllic state by ignoring unpleasantness when he can and when he cannot, by running away from it. Only as long as he can continue doing so will things go well for him. It is impossible to determine on the basis of morphogenic data alone what will happen if and when Bill's world falls apart. Because he relies so heavily on sensory experience (music, drugs), he might be expected to turn to these in greater desperation if stress ever becomes too severe. It is so important for Bill to stay out of touch with reality's unpleasant aspects that one suspects that his ability to deal with these when he must is too low. Eventual psychological maturity may not appear without considerable inner turmoil.

Despite these cautions and concerns, it would be wrong to assert that Bill is now in psychological difficulty. From a clinical point of view his record is clean; and so long as the balance he has achieved can be sustained he will remain in good mental health despite his use of drugs.

STYLE OF DRUG USE

General Pattern

Bill reports that the first drugs he ever used were marijuana and alcohol, at age fourteen (table 4.3). His first use of marijuana was experimental, but he began regular use at fifteen. "I like good grass. It helps me relax and be at ease with people." He began regular use of alcohol at seventeen. "I drink mostly beer but occasionally some hard stuff at parties or when our band is playing."

At fifteen Bill first tried LSD. He experimented with it for a couple of years. "Everyone else was doing it. I tripped maybe fifteen to twenty times; most of my trips were good. When I was seventeen, I did some MDA (3,4 methylenedioxyamphetamine). It was good, too, but I guess it was just part of growing up, because I quit when I was about seventeen."

At sixteen Bill tried amphetamine, but he stopped in less than a year. "This friend had some mini-whites he gave me, so I tried them—I ate them. They make you get right up and go, but I didn't like the speed feeling. They made me feel edgy, so I quit." During this same period, Bill tried smoking opium: "I only did it twice. It makes you feel pretty good but it's hard to come by. There isn't much of it so I never really got into opium."

Bill tried cocaine first at age seventeen. "The first time I tried, it wasn't so exciting, but maybe it was bad coke. Later I snorted some again. I started really using it when I was eighteen. Coke I like; I do it several times a week if it is available and I have the money."

Bill reports he tried eating some mushrooms—"they were no good"—and also drank cough syrup with codeine in it—"I didn't like the stuff at all; I only did it that one time."

TABLE 4.3. Genealogy and Pattern of Drug Use and Abuse: Bill F.

Drug Substances	Age											Frequency of Drug Usage	Comments
	13	14	15	16	17	18	19	20	21	22	23		
1. Marijuana		←—————————————————————————→										Daily	I like good grass. It relaxes me.
2. Alcohol		←——————————→								←————————→		Regular	I drink mostly beer but occasionally some hard stuff, too.
3. Hallucinogens (psychedelics: LSD/MDA)			←- - - - - - - - - - - - - - - -→									Fairly regular	I tried them awhile. Most trips were good. I liked it.
4. Other opiates (opium)				←- - - - →								Intermittent	I smoked some opium for awhile, but it is not often available.
5. Amphetamine				←- - - - →								Intermittent	I tried it but I didn't like it. It's too harsh.
6. Cocaine					←——————————————————→							Regular	I like it. It makes me confident. It makes it easier to work with people.
7. Non-prescription, over-the-counter												Intermittent	I tried some non-prescription

drugs (codeine)		cough syrup. I didn't like it too much.
8. Heroin	Never	I never did that and don't want to.
9. Barbiturates	Never	I don't like the idea of doing something that would make you feel down.
10. Illegal methadone	Never	I never tried it.
11. Psychotropics (Librium, Valium, etc.)	Never	I don't use them.
12. Inhalants	Never	I never tried, kids do though.
13. Polydrug	Never	I never tried it.
14. Other		

Legend

—— Denotes regular usage

- - - Denotes intermittent usage

Bill never tried heroin — "I don't want anything to do with heroin; I don't like the idea of punching myself with a needle" — illegal methadone, barbiturates — "I didn't like doing something they might get you for and I don't like to be depressed" — tranquilizers, inhalants, or polydrug mixtures.

Bill indicates that the cost of his drug use since the age of eighteen would probably not exceed two or three dollars per day. "I don't do that much stuff except coke and marijuana. Cocaine is expensive. It costs fifty to eighty dollars per gram, but I only do it two or three times a week. Generally, a gram will last me a month or so, unless we have a party or something. Besides, there are a lot of times coke is not available." Bill has never overdosed on any drug, nor has he ever been involved in any drug-abuse treatment program.

Preference Rankings

With the exception of the rankings of barbiturates and LSD, which showed modest variability, Bill's preferences are reliable (table 4.4). Cocaine, marijuana, and beer are most preferred. Hard liquor, amphetamines, barbiturates, and LSD occupy the mid-preference range, while speedballs and heroin are the least preferred overall. At this point in his life cocaine is the only "hard" drug for which Bill has a strong preference. He would rather do marijuana, beer, or hard liquor than amphetamine, barbiturates, heroin, or LSD.

TABLE 4.4. Drug Preference Rankings: Bill F.

Substance	First Assessment	First Reassessment	Second Reassessment	Mean	Composite Rank
Amphetamine	5	5	5	5.0	5
Barbiturates	6	7	6	6.3	6
Beer	3	3	3	3.0	3
Cocaine	1	1	1	1.0	1
Hard liquor	4	4	4	4.0	4
Heroin	9	9	9	9.0	9
LSD	7	6	7	6.7	7
Marijuana	2	2	2	2.0	2
Speedball	8	8	8	8.0	8

Ratings

Bill was cautious in his ratings of drugs, rarely using values near the extreme ends of the rating continua. He refused to rate "drugs in general" at all, assigning this stimulus neutral values on all twenty-six scales.

The nine specific substances fell into three distinct classes, each containing three drugs. The first class consisted of minor substances: beer, hard liquor, and marijuana. These he described as soft, clean, successful, and sheltered. The second class consisted of substances he regards as beneficial and desirable: amphetamine, cocaine, and LSD. He described them as strong, excited, refreshed, bright, and loud. The third class consisted of drugs he wants nothing to do with: barbiturates, heroin, and speedballs. Bill described this group as bad, dangerous, strong, hard, sick, and hazardous.

Pattern of Use

Social Context

Bill first tried cocaine at age seventeen. "I had heard and read a lot about coke. I was going to a rock concert with this girl that I liked, I wanted to be up, so I bought ten dollars' worth to snort. I tried it at home before I went to pick up this girl, I was expecting something like, Wow, but it didn't do that; nothin' dramatic happened. I was disappointed as hell! I wondered why something that gave you such a little return was so expensive. Well, I was in a good mood anyway. That's all I got out of it."

Bill says he now snorts cocaine because he likes the feeling. "It makes me feel more self-confident. It's easier for me to work with people, and I don't get so upset by things that would normally bother me. It sometimes makes me feel like I am floating. I am all pepped up, relaxed, and confident. If I am depressed or down it gets me into a better mood and peps me up."

Bill stated that about 30 percent of his cocaine usage occurs when he is alone. "I would do it alone if I was depressed, or sometimes before a date, or if we were doing an important gig." Forty percent of his coke usage is with one other person. "I do quite a bit with a friend of mine. We snort coke and just relax and listen to records. You feel good. You are able to pick out nuances in a record that you might not otherwise notice; the music is richer, fuller, and sounds better, too. I also did quite a bit with this girl I was dating; we would do coke with sex." The remaining 30 percent of his usage is with a few friends — "The guys in my band" — or at parties. "You're at a party and people are just drinking and having a good time. Toward the end of the evening the party begins to drag. The person having the party pulls out a bunch of coke and lays it out in 'lines' on the table and everyone starts snorting. The first thing you know everyone has perked up and is excited. Everyone is feeling good and the party is up and going again. Everyone is talking and having a good time."

As he said above, Bill likes to snort cocaine and do sex. "Both parties snort some. You're in bed, you have some good music on, you both feel good and have a warm glow inside. You can go on a long time and you don't get tired, you last longer and the orgasm is better for both of you."

Bill states that if good cocaine is available his pattern is to snort a quarter of a gram per day until he runs out. "The longest time I did coke every day was for a couple of weeks. I had gotten my income tax return and I just bought myself four grams. It cost me $280, but I just floated through life for two weeks." Bill's typical usage pattern is two or three times per week, mostly on weekends. The largest amount of cocaine he has ever snorted in a single day is one third of a gram — "I was feeling no pain that day." He has never done cocaine runs — "That's for shooters, I am a snorter; I don't want to mess with a needle." He indicates that if he had the money and cocaine was available, three circumstances would most likely trigger a desire to snort cocaine: having a party, being in a good mood and wanting to get high, and feeling depressed.

Bill reports no diurnal or nocturnal pattern in his use of cocaine. "I would do it day or night, but I always did more on weekends. That's when we would have parties or our band would be playing somewhere. I can play better if I am doing coke. Also, you can handle a crowd without getting your head messed up like you do on amphetamines. I do coke sometimes, too, when our band is on the road. You know, you did a gig the night before, you're in a bus riding 200 miles to the next gig, you're worn out and you have been cooped up for a couple of days with the other band members. They're crabby, bitchy, and bored, too. You are tired of looking at them, but you don't want a hassle because you have to play again tonight. I might snort the last hour or two on the road. Also, coke will help you play better if you are tired; however, if you are feeling good already it doesn't help you play better at all."

Bill reports that 90 percent of the cocaine he has used is "street coke." "It's what you buy from someone who is dealing. I would guess only 10 percent was pharmaceutical cocaine; that is a hell of a lot more powerful, but it is more expensive and harder to come by. Snorting a little bit of pharmaceutical coke is like snorting a lot of street coke. It kicks harder."

When asked how he discriminates between street and pharmaceutical cocaine, Bill stated, "It's partly the price. The dealer will demand more money if he has pharmaceutical coke. Also, pharmaceutical coke has more kick than street stuff. It's fluffy and glitters in the light. It has brilliance. It's nice to see those little crystals." When asked how he would discriminate between cocaine and procaine or benzocaine, Bill said he didn't think he could, adding that he may have used a synthetic drug sold as cocaine without knowing it.

Bill could not respond to the question of whether or not one develops a tolerance for cocaine. "I really don't think so, but I don't use enough to know." He stated that withdrawal from snorting cocaine was not remarkable. "I usually just feel tired and wish I hadn't come down so soon. That's about all there is to it."

Reactions to Cocaine

Physiological Reactions

Bill reports a limited number of physical reactions to cocaine. The most consistent (occurring 80-100 percent of the time) include numbness and dryness of the throat and mouth, clogging or distension of the nasal air passages, loss of appetite and of sensations of fatigue (table 4.5). A second cluster of reactions he reports, occurring about 40-60 percent of the time, include lacrimation, rhinorrhea, increased light sensitivity, yawning, and accelerated mental activity. A third clustering of reactions which are infrequently associated with cocaine use include increased heart, pulse, and respiration rates, mild tremors in muscle groups in his arms and legs, and occasional inflammation of the nasal passages. Given the intranasal method of drug administration and intermittent usage of street cocaine, it is not surprising that Bill reports such mild physiological reactions.

Psychological Reactions

Bill's most consistent psychological reactions to cocaine use, occurring 70-80 percent of the time, include greater self-confidence and feelings of optimism and well-being, prolonged sexual intercourse and a "better orgasm," increased sensitivity to odors, and sleeplessness or insomnia (table 4.6).

A second clustering of reactions, occurring 40-60 percent of the time, include restlessness and excitement, the feeling that his mind was quicker, increased imagination and thinking power, and talkativeness. In addition, cocaine sometimes makes Bill feel he is stronger and has greater ability to work. Bill has had no experiences of visual, auditory, or tactile hallucinations, anxiety or panic reactions, paranoid reactions, increased sense of self-control, changes in perceived reality, or indifference to pain. He does not consider cocaine a trigger for violence. On the contrary he feels it increases his alertness, self-confidence, and appreciation of sensuous experiences.

Integration

The reasons why cocaine is Bill's drug of choice are straightforward and uncomplicated: First, this somewhat shy and insecure man take it to increase his self-confidence, self-assurance, and effectiveness with other people, particularly on dates, at parties, or when his band is playing an important engagement. Second, he uses it to enhance his sexual performance. Third, he uses it to erase feelings of depression, which for Bill is a surrogate for anger. When Bill talks about feeling depressed he is really talking of his fears of his own anger flaring up and jeopardizing relationships with people he needs; he often fears that disagreements are in danger of bursting into angry confrontation. Finally, this stimulus-hungry young man uses cocaine to help him tolerate routine, dull, and boring life situations which cannot be avoided.

TABLE 4.5. Physiological Reactions to Cocaine Use and Abuse: Bill F.

Commonly Reported Reactions to Cocaine Use/Abuse	Reactions Observed Yes	No	Percent/ Time Observed	Qualifying Comments and Observations
Dizziness – feeling of light-headedness		No		I don't remember feeling like that at all.
Sweating – perspiration or increases in temperature		No		Not that I know of.
Rhinorrhea – running nose	Yes		50	It's pretty regular if you do much coke. You get the "sniffles."
Tremors – muscle spasms	Yes		10	If I do more than a quarter gram, my hands will tremble.
Lacrimation – tears to eyes	Yes		65	When I snort a big 'hit,' it makes my eyes water.
Mydriasis – dilation of pupils, light sensitivity	Yes		40	Lights bother me more when I am playing if I have snorted coke.
Gooseflesh		No		Not for me.
Emesis – vomiting		No		I never vomited snorting coke.
Reactive hyperemia – clogging of nasal airways	Yes		80	It makes my nose clog up for a couple of hours.
Anorexia – loss of appetite, sensation for hunger	Yes		80	I can eat snorting coke, but I am not really hungry.
Dryness of mouth and throat, lack of salivation	Yes		100	It is very dry and it also gets numb.
Increased heart rate	Yes		10	A big hit of pharmaceutical coke will make your heart pound some.
Tightness in chest or chest pains		No		I have never had that reaction.
Local anesthesia, numbness	Yes		100	My nose, mouth, and throat get numb, sometimes my gums, too.

Nosebleed	No		I never had it.
Elevation of pulse rate	Yes	10	You notice it with pharmaceutical coke.
Increased respiration rate	Yes	10	With pharmaceutical coke.
Cellulitis – inflammation following administration	Yes	20	You get nasal inflammation. I wash it out with water after snorting. It feels cool and refreshing.
Infection of nasal mucous membrane	No		I have never had a nasal infection.
Yawning	Yes	20	It makes me yawn sometimes.
Hyperphrenia – excessive mental activity	Yes	50	My mind does go faster.
Weight loss	No		I don't do that much.
Fainting	No		That's kind of silly.
Increased sensitivity to allergies	No		I am not allergic to anything.
Diarrhea or explosive bowel movements	No		Not for me, but it stimulates my kidneys. I have to go to the john more often.
Hepatitis or liver infections	No		I never had it.
Headaches	No		It doesn't cause headaches for me.
Loss of fatigue	Yes	100	You feel good. You are not tired at all.
Ringing in the ears	No		I have never had that.
Convulsions	No		Never.

TABLE 4.6. Psychological Reactions to Cocaine Use and Abuse: Bill F.

Commonly Reported Reactions to Cocaine Use/Abuse	Reactions Observed Yes	Reactions Observed No	Percent/ Time Observed	Qualifying Comments and Observations
Increased feelings of self-control		No		You just feel good.
Increased optimism, courage	Yes		75	I feel a helluva lot more self-confidence on coke. I feel more optimistic, too. I feel good all over. You glow inside.
Increased activity, restlessness, excitement	Yes		60	I get very restless and it makes me move about more.
Feeling of increased physical strength or ability to do physical work	Yes		25	It makes me feel like I can play better if I am tired.
Intensified feelings of well-being, euphoria, "floating," etc.	Yes		70	I feel good. I am relaxed, at ease with people, like everything is fine. Sometimes it makes me feel light.
Feeling that everything is perfect		No		That never happened.
An exquisite "don't care about the world" attitude		No		That didn't either.
A physical orgasm in the "rush"		No		It increases your endurance, but nothing like that.
Increased thinking power and imagination	Yes		50	If I am tired, it helps me think straighter, keeps me functioning together.
Feeling that the mind is quicker than normal, the feeling that one is smarter than everyone else	Yes		40	I can think faster and better on coke.
More talkative than usual, a stream of talk	Yes		60	I feel more confident and talk more with people, like at parties and things, yes.
Indifference to pain		No		I'm not insensitive to pain.
Depressed interest in work, failure of ambition, loss of ambition for useful work		No		Not for me.
Insomnia	Yes		75	It's hard to relax. It takes a while to unwind.
Depression, anxiety		No		It makes me feel good and relaxed, not depressed or anxious.
Prolonged sexual intercourse	Yes		80	You both have greater endurance on coke. You can go on a long time.

An aphrodisiac or sexual stimulant	Yes	80	It stimulates your sex drive, makes you "horny." You feel like it would be nice to have a girl around.
Better orgasm on coke	Yes	80	It's better. Coke enhances the whole general feeling.
Irrational fears	No		I've never had that.
Terror or panic	No		I feel good, not scared.
Tactile hallucinations — the feeling that insects are crawling on or under the skin (particularly fingertips, palms of hands, etc.)	No		I've never had any bugs. I have read about it, though, with shooters.
Changes in reality or the way a room or objects look — the wall waving or in motion, etc.	No		Colors are warmer and richer, sounds are richer and clearer, though.
Paranoid ideas — the feeling that people are after you. You believe you are being watched, talked about or threatened, a wife or girlfriend is unfaithful, untrustworthy, etc.	No		I wouldn't do it if I got that way. It wouldn't make me suspicious of people.
Causes one to carry a gun or run from imaginary enemies	No		No, Sir!
Visual hallucinations	No		It has never affected me that way at all.
Auditory hallucinations — hearing voices talking about you, threatening, etc.	No		Nothing like that.
Olfactory hallucinations — new odors, smells, etc.	Yes	70	It makes things smell sweeter for me.
A trigger for violence	No		It makes me more aggressive, but I am kind of not so sure of myself anyway. It never made me feel violent towards anyone.

LIFE ACTIVITIES AND EXPERIENCES:
IN BILL'S OWN WORDS

Overview

The following section presents an account of two days in Bill's life during a brief period from early February to March 1975.

On the first day, Bill tells what life on the road can be like. It is not much fun driving six hours in a snow storm in order to play three hours; the trip is cold and boring. He tells how he feels about the members of his band, particularly Bob, the band leader whom he has dubbed the "commandant." Bill resents him and appears to have little recognition that someone has to organize the group, take the lead, and make decisions.

On the second day in March, there is a snowstorm, but Bill goes to work at the plant anyway. He has to do a variety of jobs because many employees were unable to get to work. He visits with his friend Clyde, complains about the mismanagement of the plant, is then frightened by a VIP, but lasts the day. He goes home; he is tired, but he ends up going to a movie and later eating cake at Leonard's place and talking about the increasing price of coke.

The general impression gained from these days is of an untroubled but energetic adolescent. There is expressed, however, an undercurrent of fear of those in positions of authority. These feelings emerge not directly but by innuendo or as somewhat caustic asides: his comments about Bob, the band leader, concern over the ineptness and inefficiencies of the plant management, nervousness in the presence of the VIP, and so on. However, Bill also shows his boyish charm, need to be with people, and rather conventional life orientation.

Activity and Experience Audit

First Day: A Saturday in February 1975

10:00–11:00 a.m.

I woke up; I had a headache from the night before. I was woke up by two guys in the band, Bob and James, who wanted the truck to move our band equipment. (They wanted it to get ready to do a gig that evening.) They pounded on the door. I got up, gave them the keys, and they went off to get the U-Haul. I am more comfortable with James than Bob; Bob is the leader of our band but he is too technical. He always wants to be on time and gets upset if we dilly-dally around.

I got up, washed, and dressed. I felt OK except for the damn headache. My roommate Randy was still asleep so I walked down to the store to get some rolls and orange juice. I was thinking this gig is going to be a bitch because it looks like it's gonna snow.

I received a call from Bob, who said we had to leave earlier than planned because it was snowing. I was ready to go (I decided I would shave later). Sonya, our singer, called and said she wanted her boyfriend George to go along and wondered if anyone would mind. I said no and waited for the group to get to our place.

The others arrived at about 10:30. We loaded the van and left.

11:00 a.m.–2:00 p.m.

There we were, six people in the van — James, Bob, Randy, Sonya, George, and I — traveling to our gig. I played my guitar and sang a song we had written. The others just chatted or slept. I had seen another band the night before; we talked about them for awhile, they were good.

I dozed off to sleep for about half an hour.

It's not much fun bouncing over the highway into a snowstorm — that's what the radio said was ahead of us.

2:00–6:30 p.m.

We stopped for lunch. Jesus, it was freezing cold! We had some hamburgers, which were terrible! Mark Dairy Queen minus for that shit! However, it was something to fill our stomachs; I felt a bit better after eating.

We got back in the bus and started again. It was quiet and boring — I watched Randy play his magic tricks. I was thinking the damn road trips are a drag, a real drag. People don't think about this side of the business when they think about a rock band. Big-name bands go by jet but groups like ours have to go this way.

We stopped for gas and I went to the john and stretched my legs. That felt good. Then we got back in the bus again. Everyone had run out of things to say and the rest of the trip was boring. We just wanted to get where we were going and unload the bus and set up the equipment at our club. I was thinking, we had a good time playing there before; we had a good crowd and they liked us; we were fairly enthusiastic about it. Then we got our instruments out right there in the van and ran through a couple of tunes we would play that night.

6:30–9:00 p.m.

We hit town and checked into our hotel. It was freezing cold even in the hotel. We had two rooms; Bob and James were in one room, Randy, Sonya, George, and I were in the other. Finally I got to shave.

Everyone got dressed for the job. Musicians are kind of superstitious — they always wear something that they wore on specially good nights. I never go without my rings when we play. Everyone was relaxed, people were joking around — we were ready, this was what we had come to do. James came in and said, "let's eat." Bob, George, and Sonya didn't want to go out, so we decided to bring them something back. I didn't care whether we all went, I was hungry. I thought Sonya might get real hungry though.

Randy, James, and I drove to a restaurant and had a good dinner. However, it took a long time to get it! We talked about our food, about how the job was gonna go. We hoped it would be a good crowd and a good show. (The amount of money we make on this gig is contingent on the number of people that showed.) We were all feeling pretty good, no apprehension. We ate — I was glad to get some decent food in my stomach.

We drove back to the hotel. I took salads to the people. It was too late for Bob to eat. He wanted to keep his food warm so he sat it in a chair by the heater. I warned him it would be roasted. He gave me some damn physics explanation why it would not be burned. The ass!

James and I then jogged down the street to the club, one block away; the others followed. We set up and got in tune, got some beers, and chatted till around 9 p.m. when we had to play. Everyone was a bit nervous before we had to play. I had butterflies in my stomach — I always do before we play — It is a good sign. I understand old-timers don't get butterflies, they just get up and do their thing, but I am not an old-timer yet.

9:00–12:00 p.m.

We started. There were not many people in the place; still, I wasn't worried. I thought I played pretty good the first set. There was one blunder by the band in the last song — someone forgot one part of the song, I laughed it off. I would say we played average.

The break came and I got a beer and talked with the owner a minute. The crowd was a little bigger now, but not much. He said it was slow that night because a regional basketball tournament was in town. I nodded to a few people who were there.

We played the second set. It was pretty good till James made another mistake. I began to get a little edgy; it was the first time it had happened twice in the same evening. Towards the end of the set, the place was filling up. No one danced though — I was frustrated about that. I began to wonder what the hell was going on. I was thinking, what the hell does it take to fire up this crowd? Once in a while there was applause. However, it was just mainly people drinking beer. I played pretty good. The blunder upset me a bit, it was a real bad mistake.

At the next break the band got together and talked about our lack of enthusiasm and what the hell we could do about it. Then I talked with a couple at the next table; they wanted to sell us scented candles for a church group! None of us had any money for scented candles! We were joking about the place we had eaten: The food was good but it was really "low rent." The people in the next booth laughed at everything we said; I guess they figured they were supposed to. We all had two or three beers to loosen up. We then decided that

George should play with us on a couple songs — he's a damn good guitarist — to break the atmosphere. Bob and I switched guitars for that set.

We started the next set and it went! During this set people started dancing and that made me feel good. We all felt real good about it. Randy and I were making eyes at all the girls, but we didn't make any hits though. The set was good and the crowd liked us. We got better as the set progressed and went out in style!

12:00 p.m.—1:30 a.m.

We stuck around a while. The manager took the PA and said, "Thank you, band." He said to the audience, "Fill them up or we will pick them up! Five minutes to go." Randy went out and sat down with some people; he wanted to find some dope or a party to go to. I talked with two or three couples. They asked me where I was from and stuff like that. They said they liked our band, once we got started. I was pleased.

After awhile, we loaded our bus with the equipment. The work was cold as hell! We talked to the manager of the place for a few minutes. He gave us some beer to go and said the crowd liked us. He said we did good and that he hoped next time we would have a better crowd. He was real friendly.

I played a little better than average but not outstanding. It's a real funny thing; some nights you hit and everyone plays over their head. Other nights you have to work your ass off just to play an average evening.

1:30—2:00 a.m.

We went — literally ran — back to the hotel, Randy, James, and I. The others followed — walking — and froze! Bob opened the door and his dinner had burned up; the chair was about to catch on fire. The ass! I had told him! Randy, George, Sonya, and I went into our room and turned on the TV. We laughed over the program and made fun of the hotel.

Everyone got ready for bed. We went to bed but sat around telling jokes and laughing. Then I went right to sleep; I was damn tired, it had been a long day.

The Day: It was a typical gig. I was a little upset when we were making so many mistakes.

Second Day: A Monday in March 1975

6:00—7:00 a.m.

The radio comes on. I laid in bed awhile just listening. At 6:30 I listened to the weather report: We had a snow storm, the roads were terrible. I thought there would be no one at work but decided I better go to work 'cause I needed the money.

I dressed, washed my face, had a cup of coffee, and drove to work. I wasn't thinking of much of anything, just trying to stay on the road — it was slick.

7:00 a.m.–12:00 n.

I was three minutes late, but a bunch of people were coming in late because of the storm so the management was not bugging people about it. Only a third of the people were there. I went back to my department. We sat around till the supervisor decided what work needed to get out fastest. I knew no one would push us today.

The supervisor brought some work I had never done before. We talked about the weather awhile; then he explained what needed to be done. It was the final assemblies of the work. It was more difficult, more detailed work, but it was interesting because I had never done it before. It was nice! There would be nothing to distract me.

Break time came. I went into the coffee room and my friend Clyde was there. I didn't know he had made it in. I sat with him. The supervisor came in; he brought some donuts. We sat together and talked about how nice and quiet it was today! It was mainly small talk. One woman was bugging me and Clyde about a girl we wanted to put the moves on. She said our little "biscuit" wasn't there today — she was teasing us. We tried to make a snappy comeback, but she is always ahead of us!

I went back to work after about ten minutes. I was in a pretty good mood. The supervisor brought me a helper on the final assemblies; she was from another department. She is quiet, but we visited some.

My supervisor said Clyde needed help in the back. He and I went back. He explained what needed to be done and said I would be back there awhile. It was cold as hell! Clyde and I got the machine started and let it warm up; we talked while we waited about girls and music. We concluded you could understand music!

We started the work. The damn machine was screwing up a bit. We kicked it when it jammed. The maintenance man came by, saw us kicking the machine, and said he would be by to fix it. He asked us to run it while he watched; he concluded it wasn't running right! We laughed like hell! We decided it was not our problem if maintenance didn't fix it, they are the ones losing money. It worked pretty well after that!

12:00 n.–1:00 p.m.

An announcement came over the speaker: Everyone was to come up front. The department head — who had been wandering around all day — said my line had been awarded the plant's "Neatness Award." Whee! I thought it was funny! There was also the "Grotty Award," given to the maintenance man's office. We clapped and cheered! The department head said a VIP was gonna be there later on that day. He told us he had come before and found some workers lax and fired the whole line and the supervisor. The department head said look good if you have nothing to do. Clyde and I went back and shut down the machine for lunch.

We went to the lunchroom. My supervisor's wife had made some soup; he brought that for seven of us. We ate with him and others from all over the department. We all talked about how good the soup was. The supervisor told us horror stories about the VIP who was coming. Aside from that, it was small talk.

1:00–3:30 p.m.

I went back to the machine. Clyde had gone home for lunch; he said the roads were real bad. We turned the machine on and warmed it up again. We finished the work we had started that morning. Then we had to clean up, but the cleaning liquid didn't work. More inefficiency! It took longer and didn't do as good a job.

At the break, I got something to drink with Clyde. We talked about the weather; small talk. I am feeling pretty glad the VIP hasn't arrived.

Hell, he comes in right at the end of the break! We split for work; we were looking very busy! Clyde and I started cleaning the assemblies and filling out paperwork.

My former supervisor came down. He wanted us to get some new cleaner, but there wasn't any. He said the VIP had been in his area and was acting real nasty. He told us to be prepared for anything that might happen. The VIP walks in right then and commented on how cold it was. He saw a chart hanging on the wall and asked us what it was; neither of us knew. He wrote something down in his notebook. He said the area was dirty, and told us we should keep the mass welder cleaner. He apparently knew I didn't work there regularly because he asked me my classification. I told him; he made a note of it and told me I was supposed to go back to my job out front.

I went back to the job. I felt nervous. I thought he might get real upset; I was working above my classification. I think he gave the department supervisor hell! I think this is the reason the guy asked me if I wanted to be trained for that job classification.

I did my regular work, that I had been doing that morning, till 3:30. Then I punched out!

3:30–6:30 p.m.

I drove home. It was snowing, about to storm. I thought I would spend the night at home; a bad storm was coming, I was real tired. I laid down, started to read, and fell asleep.

6:30–10:30 p.m.

The phone rang; from another friend of mine, Leonard. He is a little older than me; he is a bandsman, though. He wanted to go to a movie. I asked how the roads were; he said bad, but he is a good driver. I said OK.

I ate some supper and had a cup of tea. I sat around till Leonard came in. He had a joint in his mouth and wanted to get high before we went to see the movie. So we smoked some joints. It was good reefer!

We left for the movie — he drove. The roads were bad and slick! I wasn't worried, he was a good, good driver. He was saying that his girlfriend had made a cake — we could eat after the movie — I had to try it. She is good at baking things.

We got our tickets and went in. There were not a lot of people there. It was a murder mystery, a pretty interesting story with a trick ending, but it moved slow. Another fellow we know sat with us. He had just been busted the day before and was out on bond; he was telling us he decided he was gonna give up dealing. That's not surprising, he's in trouble with the law. We watched the movie.

After the movie we said goodbye to the guy and left. It was really cold! We drove to Leonard's house and had some of that cake he was talking about — real good! Leonard said there would be some good weed coming into town. He asked about some coke, less than seventy dollars a gram. He heard of some for about sixty dollars that might be pretty good; he said he would check on it. We complained that prices are getting too high. Then we listened to a couple of records. He gave me some music and told me to learn some of the songs and I could jam with his group.

I said I better get home.

10:30–11:00 p.m.
Leonard drove me home. I told him I would see him in the next few days. I went up and went to bed; it only took 20 minutes getting to sleep.

The Day: Pretty good day in general.

5

Tom P.

LIFE THEMES

Tom P. — an angry, volatile, lonely, troubled, unhappy man attempting to sort out the pieces of his life and find something worth living for — was a successful cocaine dealer for five or six years.

Five central themes were dominant in Tom's life:

- I want to love my father and I want him to love me, but no matter what I do I end up hating him.
- Because I am so much like my father, I hate myself; but I'll never give in, I'll never allow myself to feel guilt or shame.
- I am going to be the meanest, most daring person in the world; I'll get the attention I deserve if I have to kill myself for it.
- I am always ready to explode.
- Normal life is not possible for me; if that's the way it is I'll live abnormally.

Cocaine Use in Relation to Life Themes

Tom was an intravenous, daily, heavy-dosage cocaine user. Cocaine was his preferred drug for several reasons:

- It helped ward off the pervasive depression and dysphoria permeating every aspect of his life.

· It provided him temporary relief from a harsh and unforgiving conscience.
· It eliminated feelings of inadequacy and self-doubts and made Tom feel invincible, a Titan who can accomplish any task.
· The strength and self-assurance he obtained from cocaine contributed to his success in a dangerous occupation.
· Use of cocaine helped him manage the rebuffs he felt from other people.
· The drug helped keep him from going crazy.

EVOLUTION OF LIFE STYLE

Introduction

Tom, a twenty-eight-year-old Caucasian of average height with a sturdy build, wore his hair in a mod, curly, natural style, had a full, close-clipped beard and mustache, sharp, penetrating eyes, and a full, sensuous mouth. He dressed casually, in quiet good taste; he typically wore tailored, double-knit slacks, a long-sleeve sport shirt, a fashionable sportcoat or jacket, and expensive loafers. His manner was intense and watchful; his demeanor generated an aura of tension, even of malevolence. Viewed across the table, Tom's countenance could stimulate fantasies of the Borgias.

At the outset of the initial interview, Tom stated, "I wouldn't have come down here, but my friend [his intermediary] said you were square but honest. He said you want to work with guys who are experts on cocaine, and I don't know anyone who knows a hell of a lot more about cocaine than I do." In a subsequent session, Tom casually reported that he had checked us out in Washington and felt reasonably certain we were not law enforcement personnel.

It took Tom some time to relax. However, once he was able to do this he was cooperative. Tom revealed himself to be impatient and angry with himself and the world. "Sometimes I get so pissed at people and at myself that I feel like I will explode." It was difficult for him to sit through the assessment sessions. Consequently he was repeatedly filling his coffee cup, going to the restroom, pacing the floor, and taking "stretch breaks." Yet Tom needed to talk with someone; he was unhappy and frightened by his own anger and impulsiveness. His inability to establish a meaningful relationship with his father was a topic that surfaced repeatedly. He could not understand it, but neither could he let it go; he seemed compelled to reexamine it.

Developmental Experiences

Tom was born in North Carolina, the youngest son of an Army officer. At the time of this research he had an older brother, age thirty-eight, and a sister, age thirty-five. Tom described his father as an unusual man. "I love him, I guess, but I hate him too. We're not really close; I wish we were. My father is a big man. Shit, he'd make two of me. He's about six-foot-three, has short, steel-gray hair (he still rinses it), weighs about 220 pounds, and doesn't have an ounce of fat on him. Even though he is sixty now, and retired, he still does calisthenics every day. He looks like what you imagine an officer should look like—big, powerful, trim, and ramrod-straight. He is a sober and serious man—even cold. He is all business except when he drinks; then all hell breaks loose.

"When he walked out of the house every morning, everything about him was perfect: His shirt and trousers were creased just right, his boots were shined to a tee, and he looked like a million. I liked and admired that. I guess I learned that from him, because I take pride in the way I look and the way I dress.

"He's super intelligent. He can figure algebra and mathematical problems in his head and is always right. He is twice as smart as I am. He got mad as hell at me when I almost flunked algebra in high school — the big son of a bitch told me I was stupid! I guess he just automatically figured that because he could do it so easy, I should be able to do it, too. I couldn't, even though I tried like hell.

"I couldn't describe my father as an affectionate man at all. Shit man, he was *cold*! He was a hell of a disciplinarian, particularly if he had been drinking, which was often in those days. He's a bourbon man, and he would take his fists to me if I had done something wrong — he'd beat the shit out of me with his fists. I was afraid of him! I was relieved as hell when he would be out in the field or go overseas. That's a hell of a thing to say about your father, but that's how it was. Hell, when he was home it was like being in the army your-self. My room had to be kept clean and my clothes hung up — hell, he'd check on it! I had to dress just right, look just right when I went out, keep my shoes shined. Shit, when I was in high school, kids started wearing long hair. Not me, I kept mine cut short and still do; I knew that if I had asked him if I could wear my hair long he would have beaten the hell out of me!

"My father is strange. When I was a kid, he would bring me nice gifts when he came back from overseas or wherever he was, but he wouldn't do anything with me. He did take me fishing once in Colorado, when I was about thirteen, but he was cold and remote and would be on my ass if I didn't tie the flies right.

"Of course, my father had to work long hours. He was a field soldier, not a garrison man. He liked to be out commanding troops, out in the field training his men and on maneuvers a lot. He drove them like hell, but they all respected him because he wouldn't ask any soldier to do something he wouldn't do.

"Even though he was out in the field he would still get on my ass! He would call my mother to find out how things were going. If she told him I had screwed up on something, he would get me on the phone and tell me he was gonna knock the shit out of me when he got back, and he would do it — even if it was six or eight months later! My father would do what he said he would do, sure as hell!"

When asked how he might change his father if he had his life to live over again, Tom stated, "I admire my father and look up to him. He's a helluva man, a man's man. I would want him to be warmer and more affectionate with me and do things with me, like other guys' dads did. I would want him to be more patient with me; he is not very patient and neither am I. He is cold.

"My father's career was everything for him. He wanted to be a general, but he didn't make it. The last time he was in Nam, they had this Cong stronghold surrounded. He and his best friend, Major Smith, were waiting for reinforcements to arrive. A sniper shot Major Smith. My father just took his men in and wiped out the fucking village. There was an investigation; he was cleared by the review, but they raised some questions about his judgment. He just went into action faster than his superiors planned.

"I haven't seen my father for five years. When he retired, they moved to Santa Fe. I lived with them there for a while after I came out of the service. I had gotten into drugs and I was doing cocaine pretty heavy then. My father found out about it and told me to get out. He said he didn't want to see me again. I cried, but I left. I have been back to see my mother, but not when he's around. Sometimes, I lay in bed and think of things, plot and scheme about what I will do to get even with the son of a bitch! I think revenge could be sweet."

Tom described his mother as a "good gal." "She is a warm, affectionate woman who would do anything for me. Like a lot of mothers, she thinks I can do no wrong. She is fifty-eight now but still good-looking. She was a good mother, I guess. She talks a lot and can't take too much pressure. However, she pretty well raised us kids alone because my father was gone a lot. They had trouble when I was about twelve; my father was stepping out on my mother. He never stayed with any of the broads, I guess he just wanted the lay. He always came home to my mother. They fought about it but she put up with it. She is a very religious person, goes to church every Sunday. Sometimes my father went too if he was home.

"My mother is sharp. She went to college but stopped when my brother was born. My mother really couldn't manage me when I was a kid; she is soft and it was easy to manipulate her. I wish she had been less easy to con, but shit, she had her own problems. We must have moved eleven or twelve times when I was growing up. It is hard on a woman to pull up her roots, move some place else, and start all over again knowing that in a year or so you'll be moving again.

"She was protective of her children, though. I'd get thrown out of school for fighting, and she'd go down there and get me back in school. I don't know how she did it. We are pretty close, but she would play games with me: She would tell me how she would not let my father hit me again, but as soon as he came home she would back off, because he could intimidate her. My father would never hit my mother, he would just intimidate her. The worst thing she did was to keep that damn club over my head — if I didn't do what she wanted, she would threaten to tell my father. I knew that if she did I'd be beat up again, so a lot of times I had to play along with her. She tried to discipline me by grounding me, but it didn't work, I would just sneak out on her. I learned how to manipulate her, to con her so there wouldn't be too much risk she would turn my father loose on me."

Regarding his brother and sister, Tom stated, "Bart is sharp like my father. He's a salesman for a big computer firm in New Orleans. He has everything I would like to have: a good wife, a nice home, a good job, and two beautiful kids. He and my father had it out when I was eleven or twelve years old. Bart left and has never been back. He sends my mother tickets to fly down and visit for a week or so every year, but he has never invited my father. My mother says my father would like to make up with Bart, but he is too proud.

"My sister, Mary Ann, is not at all like me. She is quiet and reserved, a gentle woman, more like my mother than any of the rest of us. Mary Ann and my father were pretty close; he listened to her where he wouldn't listen to me. Maybe she was the favorite, I don't know. I do know she talked my father out of beating me several times and I appreciated that. We were pretty close as kids. She made almost straight As in school, got a degree in education. She never did teach though because she married an architect, right after she got out of college.

"She looks down on me now; she thinks I am always high and makes sarcastic remarks about me being a drug addict. Shit, it seems like everyone has done okay except me! Here I am twenty-eight years old, and I don't have a fucking thing to show for it except the money I have stashed away. My father was a captain by the time he was twenty-eight. What the hell do I have to show?"

Tom described himself as a hell-raiser when he was growing up. "I went to good schools, but, hell, I never had a lot of close friends because we were always moving. I must have gone to eleven or twelve different schools growing up. My father wasn't home a lot, so I was sort of raised by women. I didn't like that worth a shit! I would get out of the house as much as I could. I really confided more with my friends than my parents.

"I was an angry kid. Shit, I am still a very angry person! A lot of the crazy things I did as a kid — like fighting and drinking — were done partly in anger, but they were also a way of letting people know I was around."

Tom described his family as above average in income. "We always had enough money, we didn't suffer financially." He felt that his family was stable, but not close. "My mother was very affectionate and I am pretty close to her, except I can't talk to her about things that bother me because she gets too upset. My relationship with my father is nowhere."

Tom stated he was never interested in school. "I mostly made Cs, with a few Ds like that damn algebra course, but you couldn't say I was a scholar because I never did any homework. I graduated from high school and went to the university for a year. I got by the first semester but the second semester I didn't go to class much. I was too busy screwing, drinking, and just raising hell in general. I flunked out the second semester. My father was mad as hell because he was picking up the tab. Maybe I was trying to screw him, make him hurt some like he hurt me. I know that I need attention, and if I don't get enough I will do something to get it, even if it means being kicked out of school. When we would have parties in high school, I would get drunk out of my mind just to be noticed. When drugs came out, I had to get into it heavy to be noticed. I am not a person who can be easily ignored! I hate to think I make a fool of myself in front of other people; sometimes that gnaws at me, but I will screw myself up if no one else does."

After leaving college Tom worked for a while as a warehouseman, then enlisted in the army. "I thought that maybe if I did okay in the army my father and I might have more in common. Besides, I would have been drafted anyway. I applied for the airborne, but couldn't pass the physical. I got shipped to Nam. We were in a lot of combat and, crazy as it sounds, I enjoyed it. I was scared shitless, but there was a lot of action. I killed me some Cong! I was close enough to see them sometimes. I just shot the shit out of them! I liked going out on patrols. Some of the other guys thought I was crazy as hell, but I liked it. I got a Bronze Star for one firefight we got into.

"Maybe I should have stayed in the army. It was okay in the field, but when your unit was pulled out of combat there was always some asshole, a sergeant or a smartass lieutenant, on your back all the time. I didn't like that, so when my enlistment was up I got out. The army was good for me. It was the only thing I have started on my own and finished." Tom stated proudly that while he had done a lot of drugs in Viet Nam, he was never discovered, and his discharge was an honorable one.

After returning from the service, Tom searched for employment. "In a period of a year I had three or four jobs. I worked on an auto assembly line for a while — that was a bitch! They work you like an animal, so I quit. I worked for a while in a department store, but got bored. I drove a delivery truck a while, but that is back-breaking work. I really wanted to be a salesman, and I finally got a job in sales for this company. I was heavy into coke then. I sold the merchandise like crazy, but I would take my receipts, buy coke with it, and then run like hell the rest of the week to get my money back out before I had to turn the receipts in on Friday. I did well at it for a while. I was an ounce dealer then, but I sure as hell wasn't getting any sleep keeping that game going. I made good money and only missed turning my receipts in by Friday once; I gave the supervisor a cock-and-bull story and turned the money in Monday, but they began to watch me closer. I showed up late for a couple of sales meetings; I was bombed out of my mind, and they let me go."

After this experience, Tom drifted into dealing. "I had developed some good contacts. The money was good, and it was exciting. Fuck, you never got bored in that business! You have to enjoy the cops-and-robbers game though. Cocaine is my speciality, I have dealt all over the midwest. I only do kilos now. I have good contacts on the coast and the border towns. I think a guy could stay in this business forever if he was careful. Besides, you can always buy information; you can buy someone in the narc's organizations to keep you informed. Shit, they will even call and tell you when they're gonna make raids, so you can warn your friends, as long as you keep movin' the money to them."

Tom stated he had been very successful as a cocaine dealer. "I have made a lot of money in coke, but you have problems. You can't go to a bank and deposit $10,000 to $15,000 every month without getting your ass in trouble, so most of my money is in Swiss banks. It's awkward, but it's safe. The other thing is there is always the risk of some son of a bitch trying to break in and take your coke, your cash, and your life. So you move around a lot, keep your eyes open, and protect yourself: You never use the same motel or hotel more than once, and you never let yourself fall into a pattern – that's deadly! I may work out of four or five different motels. You never use the house phones. Shit, maybe you read in the paper where that big car dealer's son was picked up for selling heroin out of a motel. I know that dumb son of a bitch! He was setting up sales from his motel room using the house phone! That bitch working that switchboard has nothing better to do than just listen in on calls; she called the police on the S.O.B. He deserved it for being so stupid!"

"As I was saying, there is always some S.O.B. who wants to take your money or your coke or your life. I shot three of them, not in Kansas City, but down on the coast. I didn't kill them, but I shot the bastards. I wouldn't tell you if I did kill them anyway, would I? After a while the word gets around that you're not a person to be fucked with. That makes some of the bastards keep their distance."

When asked what he wanted to do with his future, Tom stated, "I would like to retire from the drug business; I'd like to live a respectable life. I have made a lot of money. I would like to find a good woman that I could love and who would love me – I was engaged to a gal like that when I was in Nam. When I came back she was dating another guy. I damn near beat the S.O.B. to death. She said I was an animal, and that was the end of that. I have balled a lot of broads, but I have never found a woman like her. I date and ball a lot with good-looking chicks and broads; they like my car, my money, and my pad. I even liked some of them, but you never let one of those bitches get close to you, because they can fuck you up fast, man. Broads could have narcs on your ass in a minute, so I never date any broad very long, but shit, there are always more of them to be had."

"I would like to have a job with variety, like sales, because I get bored easily, and when I get bored, I get mean. I have problems with anger, too. I get angry at myself very easily. I know my capabilities, but I haven't been able to break out of drugs – that makes me mad as hell! People who don't understand me make me mad, too. I like it when things go smoothly, but if things don't go just right I say fuck it, I am going to get high! I don't like people crowding me. My friends say I am too critical of other people, but I am just as critical of myself. I know my problems, but I won't do anything about them. I am probably one of the best escapists from reality around. I would like to really want to change, but I have always looked for the shortcuts. For the past six or seven years, there have been three things in my life — drugs, money, and broads. How do you change all of that?"

Interpretive Integration

At least seven modal factors in Tom's early life provided the framework for the evolution of his life style:

- Being reared primarily by women in a financially secure family
- Regular moves by the family from one military base to another, which limited, if they did not preclude, enduring relationships with peers and contemporaries
- Absence of a positive relationship with his father who was a harsh disciplinarian, who demanded much but gave little of love, attention, support, encouragement, or time to his son
- A loving but weak and manipulative mother whom Tom could feel affection for, but did not respect
- A consistent psychological climate of friction, emotional stress, and frustration.

Reared in such an environment, Tom as an adult displayed a pattern of adjustment characterized by the following:

- Nagging self-doubts and deeply hidden, but nonetheless powerful, feelings of inadequacy
- An enduring undercurrent of unhappiness, depression, and malaise
- A high level of tension, with easily mobilized rage toward himself, his parents, and the world
- A negativistic world view in which people are seen as being hypocritical, uncaring, and motivated by selfish interests (Tom expected people stronger than him to take what they wanted from him by force and those weaker than him to exploit him by manipulative ploys, deceit, and subterfuge.)
- Strong dependency needs but an inability to tolerate intimacy
- Basic suspiciousness and distrust of others
- A repetitive life pattern characterized by (1) events which reinstate basic feelings of inadequacy and (2) subsequent feelings of depression and dyshoria which in turn trigger (3) impulsive outbursts of rage
- A decision that if he was unable to obtain attention (or other substitutes for love and affection) by legitimate means he would take it by deceit or force and by being the misfit, the criminal, the bad son.

Tom's existence was torn by powerful contradictory strivings. His psyche was a battleground where the divisive elements of his own personality raged back and forth in constant warfare: Sometimes he would have liked to have had a wife, family, and a good job, yet he knew he could not. He would have liked to have found peace and happiness, but he was chronically unhappy, discouraged, and depressed. He wanted a meaningful relationship with his father, yet knew it could never be. He would have liked to have maintained legitimate employment yet knew he was abrasive, impatient, and could not tolerate routine or authority. He would have liked to be a "success," but considered himself a failure. Tom had strong dependency and affectional needs, yet could not tolerate intimacy or closeness. He would have liked to have found someone he could trust, yet knew he must trust no one. He sometimes felt weak and inadequate but knew that in his occupation these feelings might cost him his life. He would have liked not to be upset by other people, yet his anger and contempt were almost uncontrollable. He would have liked to relax, but he was a driven man who had to be constantly moving. Critical of others and deprecatory and contemptuous of himself, he knew he had problems but felt helpless to solve them. He would have liked to be able to give up drugs but knew he could not. He would have liked to "succeed" but knew with certainly that if no one else prevented him from doing so he would do it himself.

Tom stubbornly attempted to make his life style one of defiant, lonely, self-sufficiency work. When asked what kind of animal he would like to be, Tom stated without hesitation, "I'd be a tiger! They are powerful, strong, and self-sufficient to the maximum. They are good-looking, graceful animals. People respect them — no one is going to fuck with a tiger! I'd be a tiger." When asked what kind of car he would be, Tom stated, "I would be a red Ferrari. They're fast, sleek, handle well, and not very many people have one."

Finally, when asked what kind of flag he would fly from the antenna of his car to communicate his uniqueness and individuality to the world, Tom provided a picture which summed up his position: "It would have to be something people would notice. I would want that damn flag to be bright red! I would have a white hand with a middle finger sticking straight up! That would tell people where I was at! If and when I ever do change, I don't intend to be humble about it!"

FORMAL PSYCHOLOGICAL ASSESSMENT

Dimensional Test Findings

Intelligence Tests

Tom's test scores show that he operated within the Average range of intellectual functioning. Given these findings and Tom's chosen occupation, the fact that he was never arrested for other than traffic violations and avoided apprehension by drug and law enforcement personnel seems remarkable.

MMPI

The outstanding features of Tom's profile are his strong but unstable sociopathic orientation, his paranoid suspiciousness and distrust, his hyperactivity, and his tendencies toward ruminative worries (figure 5.1). The Validity Scales indicate that Tom answered test questions with reasonable honesty, although the *F* Scale value is somewhat elevated.

Tom lived with intense feelings of tension, frustration, and inner turmoil which he discharged through restless and reckless physical activity, brooding worry, and rumination. He could form relationships with other people; however, these tended to be superficial and manipulative. Few people knew Tom well, because he kept them at arm's length. He was suspicious, distrustful, even contemptuous of most people, viewing the world as a predatory place and tending to divide people into two types: those who take what they want and the "chumps" who are their victims. Tom did not want to be a "chump."

Tom was sensitive to slights and rebuffs, but he was not empathic; on the contrary, he had little regard for others' feelings and would probably be described by them as cold, exploitive, unpredictable, and dangerous. Behind his social facade, he was a lonely, alienated man, frightened by his own volatile anger and impulsivity. Self-critical and self-deprecatory, he saw himself as a screw-up, a failure, a loser. He wished his world were different, but since it was not he suffered bouts of depression in which he felt helpless and hopeless.

Usually Tom attempted to approach people and situations in a planned way. However, with his low frustration tolerance, if things did not move as he thought they should he reacted to the immediate and transitory pressures. Tom felt like a walking volcano. His suspiciousness frequently led him to misinterpret events. In such instances he took no chances but struck out quickly with verbal abuse or even physical attack.

Sixteen PF

The profile in table 5.1 depicts a man at war with himself. These data show Tom as a tense and angry person living with a high level of inner turmoil, driven, and finding little peace in life. This is a moody man with an active fantasy life, brooding and worrying about the slights, hurts, and disappointments he has experienced and his hopes and fears for the future.

Tom lived a delicately balanced paranoid adjustment; He was chronically suspicious and vigilant. He needed others yet feared them. He wanted to be understood and appreciated yet felt he was not; this only increased his anger,

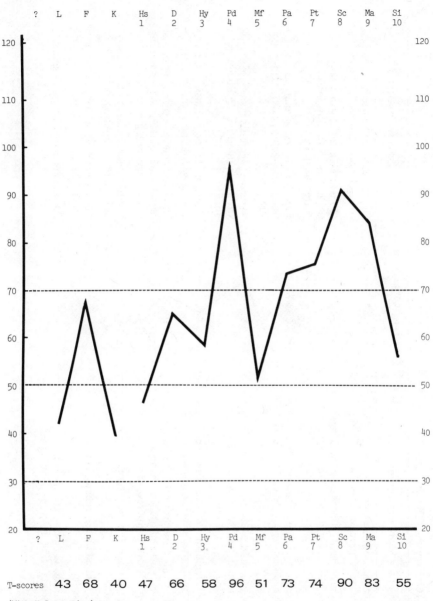

	?	L	F	K	Hs 1	D 2	Hy 3	Pd 4	Mf 5	Pa 6	Pt 7	Sc 8	Ma 9	Si 10
T-scores	43	68	40	47	66	58	96	51	73	74	90	83	55

(With K Correction)

FIGURE 5.1. MMPI Profile: Tom P. *Reproduced from the Minnesota Multiphasic Personality Inventory Profile and Case Summary form, by permission. Copyright 1948 by the Psychological Corporation, New York, N.Y. All rights reserved.*

TABLE 5.1. Cattell 16PF Profile: Tom P.

Standard Score	Low Score Description	Sten (factor)	High Score Description
6	Reserved, detached, critical, cool, aloof, stiff, precise, objective	A = 6	Outgoing, warm-hearted, easygoing, trustful, good-natured, participating
3	Less intelligent, concretistic thinking, less well-organized, poor judgment	B = 3	More intelligent, abstract thinking, bright, insightful, fast-learning, better judgment
1	Affected by feelings, emotionally less stable, worrying, easily upset, changeable	C = 1	Emotionally stable, mature, unruffled, faces reality, calm (higher ego strength)
8	Humble, mild, easily led, docile, accommodating, submissive, conforming	E = 8	Assertive, aggressive, stubborn, headstrong, competitive, dominant, rebellious
6	Sober, taciturn, serious, introspective, reflective, slow, cautious	F = 6	Happy-go-lucky, enthusiastic, talkative, cheerful, frank, quick, alert
7	Expedient, disregards rules, social conventions and obligations to people (weaker superego strength)	G = 7	Conscientious, persistent, moralistic, persevering, well-disciplined (stronger superego strength)
6	Shy, timid, withdrawn, threat-sensitive	H = 6	Venturesome, uninhibited, socially bold, active, impulsive
5	Tough-minded, self-reliant, cynical, realistic	I = 5	Tender-minded, sensitive, dependent, seeking help and sympathy
10	Trusting, accepting conditions, understanding, tolerant permissive	L = 10	Suspicious, hard to fool, dogmatic

Standard Ten Score (Sten): 1 2 3 4 5 6 7 8 9 10

142

Left pole	Score	Right pole
Practical, "down-to-earth concerns" guided by objective reality	8	Imaginative, bohemian, absent-minded, unconventional, easily seduced from practical judgment
Forthright, unpretentious, genuine, spontaneous, natural, artless, socially clumsy	4	Astute, polished, socially aware, shrewd, smart, "cuts corners"
Self-assured, placid, secure, self-confident, complacent, serene	5	Apprehensive, self-reproaching, insecure, worrying, troubled, guilt-prone
Conservative, respectful of established, traditional ideas	4	Experimenting, liberal, free-thinking, non-moralistic, experiments with problem-solutions
Group-dependent, depends on social approval, a "joiner" and sound follower	5	Self-sufficient, resourceful, prefers to make own decisions
Undisciplined self-conflict, lax, follows own urges, careless of social rules	3	Controlled, exacting willpower, socially precise, compulsive, persistent, foresighted
Relaxed, tranquil, torpid, unfrustrated, composed, low ergic tension	10	Tense, frustrated, driven, overwrought, high ergic tension

Average

143

hostility, and resentment. He found it difficult to confide in others. When he did, he expected to be betrayed. The friendly stranger attempting to initiate a relationship with Tom did so at considerable risk of insult, verbal abuse, or physical attack.

Tom felt alone in an alien world. Therefore, he attempted to take what he wanted rather than negotiate for it. He was aggressive and headstrong and forced his will because he trusted no one to deal with him fairly. His approach to life was undisciplined and unconventional, with little care for the opinions and values of others. Tom tended to be concrete and dogmatic; this left him few options for dealing with the world and meeting his needs. Poorly organized and frequently exhibiting poor judgment, he got by because of his willingness to play for stakes higher than those most others could accept.

Other Dimensional Measures

On the Sensation-Seeking Scales Tom obtained below-average scores on the General, Thrill and Adventure, and Boredom Susceptibility Scales, but above-average scores on Experience-Seeking and Disinhibition. The relatively high Experience-Seeking score indicates that Tom needed intense stimulation and change, whether through association with unconventional people, the use of drugs, or rapidly changing activities. He enjoyed heavy drinking, variety in sexual partners, and an unconventional way of life. Although impulsive and distractible, and describing himself as having a low boredom tolerance, he scored well below the norms on the Boredom Susceptibility Scale.

Tom's performance on the Pearson Novelty Experiencing Scales was not remarkable, except for his External Cognitive Score, which was more than two standard deviations below the means of the two comparison groups. This suggests a concrete person, not one taking pleasure in intellectual pursuits or attempting to understand the meaning of events and activities in the world. This low score is consistent with Tom's self-observation, "I can't sit still long enough to read a book. I can relax and watch TV sometimes, but I probably have only read one or two books in the last year. I am a kind of driven person; I just have to keep moving. I always think of Satchel Paige's comment that you have to keep movin' and not look back, because if you do you might find it is gaining on you. I don't know what 'it' is, but I am a person who has to keep moving."

Tom's remark verifies the remarkably high score he obtained on the Change Seeker Index. This score is almost three standard deviations above the mean for army males and more than two standard deviations above the mean for college males. These data leave little doubt that Tom was a restless and hyperactive man who required not only heavy and constant stimulation but also constantly changing stimulation for him to maintain his desired level of arousal.

Integration

The dimensional measures substantiate the picture that Tom presented in interview situations, but reveal a paranoia, a penchant for violence, and an intense inner turmoil and personal suffering sometimes masked in one-on-one discussion. Tom was lonely, but he trusted only an isolated self-sufficiency. He felt inadequate, but lived in a world where a man with a weakness is a victim. This volatile and angry man found little rest, peace, or happiness in life. His paranoia and suspiciousness, willingness to act quickly and harshly, his cunning and street savvy had thus far saved him. Tom believed that he could stay in his business forever, perhaps live to a ripe old age, and retire to the Riviera. However, given the self-destructive overlays in his personal makeup and sheer probability such an outcome never seemed very likely.

Findings From Morphogenic Measures

Overview

Tom's behavior on the morphogenic tests was chaotic. Although some of his data were consistent and reliable, other material was not merely internally inconsistent: It contradicted itself at every turn. On the Q-Sorts, Tom sometimes seemed self-satisfied in the sense that he described himself as being similar to his own ideal. This seems reasonable enough until one discovers that at other times Tom described his usual self as the opposite of his ideal. Furthermore, Tom consistently identified closely with his bad self. Sometimes, it is true, he said he wanted to be good, and sometimes he said he wanted to be bad. But whatever he wanted, he described his actual self as being consistently bad by any standard of morality. In the final analysis, his data seem to make sense only if Tom is regarded as compulsively evil. Never did he describe himself as being like other people; in fact, one surmises that his sense of selfhood depended upon being unlike them in every possible way.

On the Rep Test Tom blunted the edge he displayed in the Q-Sorts; here he showed his capability of recognizing warmth and affection in others. But he seemed to feel these qualities would not change his behavior; he wanted to be loved in spite of his actions. Also, his descriptions of people hinted that he recognized and was bothered by his inability to understand and communicate with them.

The data lead inexorably to the conclusion that Tom was engaged in an effort to be as unlike the ideals and moral standards he was taught as possible. Thus, Tom emerged as a paradox — a man with a conscience so demanding that he could become an individual only by defying it at every turn. He was a man who needed others, but who had been hurt by them so deeply that his independence could arise only from rebellion.

Q-Sorts

Standard Items

Due to the fact that Tom did not participate in the second reassessment, reliability data were somewhat abbreviated. Within the two sessions in which he did participate, Tom's descriptions of his usual self were consistent (median $r = .696$). Across sessions they were less so, being on the borderline of what is psychometrically acceptable ($r = .511$). Other reliability values were not only low, one of them ("self during a cocaine high") was negative ($r = -.508$). In short, most correlations among the same instructional conditions are so low as to cast doubt on their meaning.

However, Tom's self-descriptions on all morphogenic measures displayed a different type of consistency, one that does not appear in standard analytical procedures but which overrode other formal considerations. At both assessment sessions, Tom described his usual and ideal selves as being similar (median $r = .693$). Ordinarily this is a favorable sign, because it suggests that a person is satisfied with himself. However, two factors speak against this interpretation in Tom's case: First, as is shown in a subsequent discussion, Tom was not always this self-satisfied; in fact, at times he was quite the opposite. Second, also shown in a subsequent discussion, the self with which Tom expressed satisfaction is no paragon of virtue; indeed, it is the type of personality most people reject out of hand.

Tom's data did not suggest that he was intellectually unable to be consistent nor did they suggest he was incapable of appreciating the requirements of the task. Rather, they presented a picture of a person who recognized and admitted his own uncontrollability and whose values shifted from admiring himself for being "Big Bad Tom" to hating himself for what he does.

Factor analysis. Tom's descriptive sortings yielded two factors, but the structures of loadings were not sufficiently patterned to permit analysis. Except for his description of himself while on a cocaine high, all of Tom's sortings during the first assessment session formed a single factor. However, the loading of sortings at the next session (first reassessment session) were so scattered that factor identification was unfeasible.

Because no patterns could be found in the factor analytic outcome, all of Tom's sortings were combined into a single overall composite. This composite showed that Tom presented himself in totally negative terms: He described himself as stubborn and self-centered, hostile and cruel, sad and depressed. He said that he is not wise, logical, independent, able to stand on his own two feet, happy, friendly, or respected. This is scarcely the picture of a person who is satisfied with himself; it is more that of a person trying to put up a strong front who sees himself as mean, violent, and uncontrollable, and is not sure he wants — or is able — to change.

Individualized Items

Tom's use of individualized Q-Sort items (table 5.2) was markedly more reliable than his use of the standard items. Again, his descriptions of his usual self were consistent within sessions (median *r* = .602) and between sessions (median *r* = .624). Several of his other descriptive sortings also reached acceptable levels of consistency.

However, Tom's description of himself as he is during a cocaine high was as unreliable as when he used the standard items (*r* = −.508). Even more important was the radical shift in Tom's description of his ideal self at the first retest (*r* = −.637). Obviously, when Tom changed something he did not go halfway. Also typical of Tom was the rapid swing from the strong negative correlation between usual self and ideal self at the first assessment session (median *r* = −.712) to a moderately positive correlation between the same two sortings at the first reassessment (median *r* = .590). This change took place because of the unreliability in Tom's description of his ideal self. While he consistently identified his usual self with his bad self (median *r* = .643), the correlation between his descriptions of his ideal self and his bad self swung from −.660 (about what one would expect in a normal case) to +.637. Tom had changed his description of his ideal from a rather conventional one to one more consistent with his actual self.

No one can say that Tom distorted psychological facts. He seemed to know what he was like, and was perfectly aware of conventional standards. Furthermore, he seemed to accept as a fact that he could not live according to those standards. His reaction was not to change himself, but simply to change his ideals and make himself feel good about being bad. Naturally, this arrangement is not conducive to the development of any feeling of unity with others. Indeed, Tom not only felt different from most people, he felt himself to be their psychological mirror image; whatever they are, he was the opposite. The median correlation between his descriptions of his usual self and that of most nonusers of drugs was −.590.

Factor analysis. Two factors were extracted from the data (As with the standard items, however, the identity of the factors was not clarified by examining the factor loadings.) The two factors could only be called Self-Presentation I and Self-Presentation II.

Self-Presentation I looked like a virtual repetition of the self-description Tom provided with the Standard Q-Sort items. He said he is vicious and hostile, uptight and anxious, "wired" and violent, yet sad and depressed. He said he is *not* happy, joyful, wise, intelligent, mellow, or calm.

Tom's second Self-Presentation (Factor II) still stressed selfishness and stubbornness, sadness and depression, as well as viciousness and hostility. However, *anxiety* was out of the picture, and Tom put heavier stress on getting ahead by stepping on others and making money, even on a job he hates. He was more rejecting of positive restraint (being patient and self-controlled), desirable methods of achieving success, and positive sexuality (which for Tom meant being sexy, a stud). This self-picture is even nastier than its Factor I counterpart.

TABLE 5.2. Individualized Q-Sort Items: Tom P.

Achievement
Positive
1. Trying to get ahead
2. Putting forth efforts at your tasks and succeeding
Negative
3. Getting ahead by stepping on others
4. Making money but hates the job

Affect
Positive
*5. Happy
6. Joy
Negative
*7. Sad
*8. Depressed

Anxiety
Positive
*9. Mellow
10. Calm
Negative
11. Uptight
*12. Anxious

Chastity
Positive
13. Not doing sex when confined
*14. Faithful (sexually)
Negative
15. "Pussy shy."
16. No sex because he is repulsive

Dependence
Positive
17. Shares the load to get the task done right
18. Needs help, like a child
Negative
19. Leech
20. Grown up but still immature

Dominance
Positive
21. A leader
22. Leader of the pack
Negative
23. Meek
24. Weak

Excitement
Positive
25. Electric
26. Vibrant
Negative
27. Wired
*28. Violent

Humility
Positive
*29. Humble
*30. Modest
Negative
*31. Ignored
*32. Lonely

Independence
Positive
*33. Independent
34. Makes his own decisions
Negative
35. Selfish
*36. Stubborn

Knowledge
Positive
*37. Wise
38. Intelligent
Negative
39. Ignorant
40. Not bright

Restraint
Positive
41. Self-controlled
42. Patient
Negative
43. A drag
*44. Boring

Self-satisfaction (Stasis)
Positive
45. Self-satisfied
46. Content
Negative
47. Dormant
48. Rigid, stationary

Sexuality
Positive
49. Sexy
50. Stud
Negative
*51. Loveless sex
52. Does sex just for the sake of getting off

Interpersonal Relations
Positive
53. Considerate
54. Forgiving
Negative
55. Vicious
*56. Hostile

Social Recognition
Positive
*57. Respected
58. A star
Negative
59. Sucker
60. Patsy

Note: Items marked with an asterisk (*) are not significantly altered from their original (standard) wording.

Here, Tom seems to have added purpose to his violence, to be more deliberate. His rejection of sexuality may be a way of saying that in this self-presentation there is no time or energy for pleasure. If Tom's self-presentations on the Q-Sort are accurate, he must have been, on some occasions at least, a formidable person indeed.

The Q-Sort data did not permit clear inferences about how drug usage fit into Tom's life. It is easy to understand his preference for drugs that kept him at a high pitch of excitement and staved off the depression lurking underneath the surface of his life. Downers could not have appealed to him; their effects would have been the opposite of what he needed. Drugs were as much a part of Tom's life as food and clothing; he would get them one way or another, under any conditions and with no guilt over doing whatever must be done to get them. This self-image as a big bad man might have been inflated by Tom in order to preserve his own self-esteem; there is every reason to believe, however, that, even if overdrawn, the image is accurate in essence.

Rep Test

Role Groups

Like everything else Tom produced, his descriptions of people were either highly reliable or nearly totally chaotic. None of the reliability values fell in the low-to-moderate range of .400 to .500; there was a large group of fifteen reliable descriptions (correlation values from .615 to 1.000), and a smaller group of five unreliable descriptions (correlation values from .067 to .369). But no obvious basis could be found for these five descriptions being as unreliable as they were. Perhaps if Tom had been able to participate in one more reassessment session, additional data would have helped clear up the confusion.

The constructs Tom created to describe people were these:

Interpersonal Constructs

1. Hustler
2. Warm
3. Respected
4. Honest
5. Close friend
6. Like him (or her)
7. Successful
8. Happy
9. Legitimate
10. Knows how to handle himself (herself)
11. Hard to understand this person
12. Selfish
13. Hard to talk to this person
14. Dislikes what I do, but loves me
15. Basically nice

Factor analysis. Fifteen of the twenty people Tom described were separated by factor-analytic procedures into five groups, varying in size (according to loadings on each factor) from one to six. Though the first group (Factor I) was small, it was bipolar, and Tom regarded seventeen of the total of twenty-one interpersonal constructs as applying to these role members. The strongest loading was negative and consisted of Tom's description of himself on cocaine; in other words, when Tom was on cocaine he was the *opposite* of the two people who make up this factor. Positive loadings appeared on Tom's descriptions of his mother and of "the person who needs him most." Tom described people at the positive end of this factor as having a host of desirable characteristics: warm, respected, honest, close friends; he likes them, and they are successful, happy, legitimate, know how to handle themselves, basically nice, kind, helpful, wise, and strong. They are *not* (as Tom must therefore be when on cocaine): hustlers, sexy, selfish, or hard to understand.

Factor II contained only two persons: person of the other sex with whom Tom takes cocaine, and person who behaves strangely. The main feature of this factor was that Tom used relatively few constructs to describe these people: basically nice but hard to understand. Since neither of these statements is very profound, Factor II must be written off as a source of useful information.

Factor III contained six persons and it dealt with success and failure. At its positive end Tom placed: an employer he liked, his ideal self, a successful person, an interesting person, and a person of his own sex with whom he was in the habit of taking cocaine. At the opposite end of this bipolar factor he put his description of his worst self. People at the positive end of this factor were: respected, successful, happy, honest, and legitimate; hard to talk to or understand but not mean or selfish.

The ideal self Tom described on the Rep Test differed from descriptions of the same concept he provided with Q-Sort items. Since his Rep Test ideal is conventional and middle class, this shows Tom was aware of conventional values and sometimes applied them to himself. A peculiar aspect of the data is that Tom's description of his usual self loaded *negatively* on Factor III as well as on Factor I (which consisted of people he liked). It did not load positively on any factor. That implies that Tom defined himself not by what he *is,* but by what he is trying *not to be,* i.e., not like his mother (lovable) or father (successful). These data hint that the sadness and depression Tom complained of on the Q-Sorts is the despair of a life empty because built on opposition, not on creative enterprise.

Apparently, Tom was having domestic problems at the time of this investigation, for one end of Factor IV contained both a girlfriend and "a person who dislikes Tom." At the other (negative) end he placed "the person from whom he gets cocaine." The most distinctive characteristics about the people at the positive end of this factor were: hard to understand and hard to talk to. That, of course, is not surprising. Tom's forte was direct action; he did not analyze feelings or meanings. Though he admitted to not understanding his girlfriend, he did not say he regarded her as selfish or as a hustler; he reserved these traits for the person at the other end of this factor, "the person from whom he gets cocaine."

One descriptive construct did not turn up in any role groups or person factors: the construct "dislikes what I do but loves me." Tom used this construct to describe both a girlfriend and his mother, but not his father. Tom's father was given a factor to himself. In most ways, he showed up as the standard image: respected, honest, legitimate, strong, and wise, is basically nice and knows how to take care of himself. But Tom also described him as hard to talk to, and for Tom this seems to imply a fundamental disagreement between the two men. The nature of the disagreement was not revealed, but we know that his father had little use for his behavior and that Tom was unable to communicate with his father because he had relatively little to say that his father could understand.

Construct Groups

Although our factor-analytic procedures extracted four factors from Tom's data, only two were major components of his interpersonal space. The first cluster consisted of items describing friendly, affectionate relations or traits: close friend, like him (her), warm, basically nice, kind, helpful, not mean or selfish. The second cluster consisted of items all of which described conventional success or achievement: respected, successful, strong, wise, honest, legitimate, knows how to handle himself, *not* a hustler.

Setting Survey

Tom's quantitative indices on the Setting Survey were remarkably reliable. However, these findings are almost totally meaningless, since Tom's data appeared to be reliable only because he reported so little activity. There are two possibilities here: Either Tom did virtually nothing or he did not want others to know what he was doing. The Setting Survey data may reflect Tom's general psychological defensiveness. However, they may also result from unwillingness on Tom's part to describe activities that might be incriminating. One may be sure that Tom did many things that would not stand the light of public exposure — even for the benefit of science.

Integration

It seems strange that Tom's Q-Sorts should place such heavy stress on violence, hostility, and badness, while his responses to the Rep Test stressed affection, conventional success, and difficulty in understanding and communicating with people he loves. The following theoretical construction helps resolve this discrepancy.

Tom was brought up in a family in which parents placed stringent but perhaps contradictory demands upon him and offered inconsistent examples for him to follow. Further, he received comparatively little reward for conformity to conventional social rules; he gained more attention for deviation from conventional behaviors. Indeed, he may have sensed that he was surreptitiously admired for it. Although his parents may have truly loved him, after their fashion, they did not use this powerful lever to teach him the difference between right and wrong. They used it in the wrong way, or, perhaps, in too many different ways simultaneously. It seems that Tom found he could get his most consistent reaction from them by being bad.

It may be that as a child he felt that his parents hated him. As an adult he may have come to feel that they really loved him; but by then it was too late for Tom to change. Tom could have developed the capacity to take love from others, but giving it would always have been difficult. He could have learned to admire others' successes, but he would hate himself because he lost all chance for it on his own. And in the final analysis it is himself he hated most of all.

To complete the picture requires recognizing that Tom needed to present himself as a man without a conscience precisely because he had a conscience, strong and strict, that in his experience had given him nothing but misery. He would not yield to it, so he fought it. A person who is truly without a conscience would be indifferent to morality or the feelings of others. Tom was not indifferent, he was antagonistic; he identified what is normally expected of him and automatically rebelled against it. Jean Genet maintains, in *The Miracle of the Rose,* that it is possible to discover truth by experiencing what is wholly and purely evil; but Tom had not reached a level of philosophical sophistication where he could see beyond his rebelliousness to some more fulfilling future possibility. Perhaps if he had had time he would have made it.

STYLE OF DRUG USE

General Pattern

Tom began drug use with alcohol at age fifteen (table 5.3). "I started drinking beer in grade school and got heavy into hard stuff — bourbon and Scotch — during my sophomore year in high school. I'd go to class bombed out of my mind! My mother thought I would be an alcoholic, but what the hell, my friends were doing it too! I didn't stay with it too long. I still like beer; in fact, I have started drinking more beer since I've been trying to quit drugs. It's as if my body has to have something in it. Otherwise, I feel empty."

Until he was eighteen, alcohol was the only drug Tom had tried. Then he tried LSD, mescaline, and psilocybin — "I did acid two or three times but I didn't like it; all the trips I had were bad ones" — marijuana — "I don't use it like I used to, but it relaxes me" — and inhalants — "I tried gasoline sniffing but all I got out of it was drunk and a helluva headache; I only tried that twice, that was enough for me!"

At age nineteen, Tom tried Robitussin — "I drank it a couple of times. It almost made me sick" — and experimented with barbiturates — "I shot them but I gave them up because they make you drunk and you act like a slob, a blubbering idiot!"

At age twenty-one, Tom began heavy use of hard drugs. "Hell, I tried them all: I did heroin when I was twenty-one; I was hooked on it when I was twenty-two. It was hard, but I drove the shit out of my system with cocaine and got off. I did Dilaudid, morphine, and even some opium while I was in Nam. (I still do heroin or Dilaudid once in a while, coming off a cocaine run.) About that same time, I shot methamphetamine, but the crash you get when you're coming off amphetamine is a real bitch! I don't even like speed, it's raw. Then I got into *my* stuff, cocaine. I have been banging cocaine and speedballing coke and heroin ever since. The other drugs — unless it is the kind of heroin you could buy in Nam — don't even compare with good cocaine. Cocaine has been my thing for six or seven years — I love it!"

Tom stated it was difficult to calculate a daily cost figure for his drug use: "I don't know. When you are dealing, you always skim coke off the top for your personal use. Then you cut it, sell it, get your money back and make a profit, too. I am just pulling a figure out of the air, but it cost me maybe twenty-five to thirty dollars a day. It sure as hell didn't cost me any more than that."

Tom stated that he had only overdosed once. "I thought I was having a heart attack! I almost blacked out. A friend shot some heroin into me and I began to feel a little better after a while. My chest kept hurting, though, the next few days, and I had a high fever for three or four days; Finally, I had to go to the doctor. I had a staph infection, and shooting all that coke every day had spread it all over my system. He gave me penicillin for almost a month. I had a helluva time clearing it up. As it is, the staph damaged my heart valve. They want to replace the valve, but I won't let them. I have to take it easy, though, and I'm afraid to shoot as much coke as I used to."

The longest period of time Tom stopped using cocaine during the last few years was no more than four or five days. He stated that although he had twice become addicted to heroin and other opiates, he had driven the opiates out of his system with cocaine; he was never involved in any drug-abuse treatment program. "In my business, you can't afford shit like that. It is dangerous as hell, anyway. The feds keep informants in all of those programs; they pay addicts to watch the guys who come and go in those programs. As it is, I have never been picked up by the police except for three or four traffic violations. On one of those I had half a kilo of coke in the car, but I was very polite and talked my way out of it. That cop had a chance to get himself a promotion, but he fucked it up, like they usually do."

TABLE 5.3. Genealogy and Pattern of Drug Use and Abuse: Tom P.

Drug Substances	Age																Frequency of Drug Usage	Comments
	13	14	15	16	17	18	19	20	21	22	23	24	25	26	27	28		
1. Alcohol																	Regular	I like beer. I have been drinking more beer since I quit the other stuff.
2. Marijuana																	Intermittent	I don't like weed like I used to.
3. Hallucinogens (psychedelics—LSD, mescaline, psilocybin)																	3–4 Times	I didn't like the stuff. It scared me.
4. Psychotropics (Librium, Valium, etc.)																	Intermittent	I used Valium once in a while to relax.
5. Inhalants																	1–2 Times	I tried it but didn't like it.
6. Non-prescription, over-the-counter drugs, cough syrup																	1–2 Times	I tried cough syrup, too.
7. Barbiturates																	Daily	I shot them a bit, but they make you act like a slob.

154

		Usage	Comment
8.	Cocaine	Daily	I love cocaine. It's my thing. You feel ten feet high.
9.	Amphetamine	Intermittent	No thanks, the crash on "speed" is something else.
10.	Heroin	Regular	I used it to "come down" off coke. It's the best.
11.	Polydrug (cocaine/heroin)	Intermittent	I did some speed-balling.
12.	Other opiates Dilaudid morphine opium	Intermittent	I used them to buffer coke when heroin was not available.
13.	Illegal methadone		
14.	Other		

Legend

——— Denotes regular usage

– – – Denotes intermittent usage

Preference Rankings

The data in table 5.4 substantiate Tom's report about his preferences. Cocaine, a speedball of cocaine and heroin, and heroin alone are most preferred. Tom's rankings also indicate he preferred beer, hard liquor, and marijuana to amphetamine and barbiturates.

TABLE 5.4. Drug Preference Rankings: Tom P.

Substance	First Assessment	First Reassessment	Mean	Composite Rank
Amphetamine	7	8	7.5	7.5
Barbiturates	8	7	7.5	7.5
Beer	5	5	5.0	5
Cocaine	1	1	1.0	1
Hard liquor	6	6	6.0	6
Heroin	3	3	3.0	3
LSD	9	9	9.0	9
Marijuana	4	4	4.0	4
Speedball	2	2	2.0	2

Ratings

Factor analysis produced a complex structure that was difficult to interpret. The structure has relatively clear locations for all drugs except amphetamine (which does not load heavily on any factor) and heroin (which loads moderately on all factors). His description of amphetamine sounds like his own self-concept: dangerous, exciting, wrong, hazardous, fast, and pleasant — in a class by itself.

Barbiturates are also in a class by themselves. Tom definitely did not like them: dull, sick, dangerous, weak, negative, calm, and unpleasant.

Evidently, Tom did not regard heroin as distinctive from substances other than amphetamine; it shared the characteristics of all other substances.

Another factor is bipolar, representing a contrast between hard liquor and cocaine. In the following list, the first word of each pair applies to hard liquor, the second to cocaine (the contrasts reported were selected from a larger group in order to reflect the distinction Tom seemed to be trying to make):

Passive — Active
Trite — Creative
Tiny — Mighty
Wrong — Right
Dull — Bright
Slow — Fast

Cautious — Rash
Unsuccessful — Successful

The final factor contrasts drugs-in-general plus LSD, on the one hand, with beer and marijuana on the other. The former are: bad, dangerous, wrong, and hazardous. The latter: good, safe, right, and slow. Interestingly, Tom placed speedball in the same class as beer and marijuana (which he seemed to regard as about as dangerous as Pepsi-Cola); they produce a smoother and less harsh reaction than cocaine alone. It is consistent for Tom to consider such a substance not to be a drug at all.

Pattern of Use

Social Context

Tom used cocaine for almost eight years, during the last four or five on a daily basis. He snorted cocaine "off and on" over this period, but was primarily a shooter. "I do some snorting with broads when we are into sex, but hell, it is not at all the same as shooting." Tom was introduced to intravenous cocaine use when he was about twenty: "We were at a party. Some friends asked me if I wanted to try shooting some cocaine. I thought what the hell, why not? So I did it. I have never been afraid of the needle."

Commenting on the first time he used intravenous cocaine, Tom stated, "I thought, Jesus Christ! I never felt anything so good in my life! Wow! It was such a damn ego trip! I felt nine feet tall and like I could literally bite through steel. I thought, shit, this is how Superman must feel. Wow! I have never forgotten it."

Tom said cocaine was his drug because "it makes me feel so damn good. Damn near anything can get me off into coke; anything that bothers me can get me started — for example, people that let me down. I am down in the dumps a lot. Coke will lift me out quick. I am afraid of depression. Coke perks you right up. Of course, sheer boredom can set me off, too; I have a low boredom tolerance."

Tom stated that probably 40 percent of his cocaine usage was alone. "I will shoot alone pretty often, but I never do snorting alone." About 10 percent was with one other person, snorting if he was with a woman or shooting if with a male friend. "I like to snort some with broads, but I never have fired cocaine with broads. Broads are afraid of the needle; they don't like the sight of blood, the jacking-off with the needle and stuff. I worry that a broad might overdose on cocaine." Tom estimated that 50 percent of his cocaine usage was with two other male friends. "If I am shooting, I like to be with two friends of mine. I get paranoid as hell firing cocaine, so I don't like shooting with more than two friends; more than two people means just that many more people I figure will be plotting against me."

Tom's typical level of cocaine consumption until last year was two or three grams per day. "If I do over three-and-a-half grams of high-grade coke I get crazy as hell! I had plenty of cocaine most of the time. My friends and I would have cutting parties; we would cut it, sell it within a week or ten days, make our money and a profit. I had to cut back after I had the trouble with my heart. Now, I only do two grams a day or as much as I think I can handle — then I break the syringe. I hate to do that, but otherwise I might be dead."

Tom preferred one-or two-day cocaine runs. "Hell, my friends and I would do runs. They were short, hard runs for a couple of days. We wouldn't sleep much, just fire up, lay around, visit, and fire up again. The coke high is fantastic but brief, so within fifteen or twenty minutes you have to fire up again to get the rush. I must have done a hundred or more runs over the years. I'll shoot when I deal or cop too. Most guys are afraid to shoot when they are copping, but shit, it helps me! It keeps me up and on my toes. However, I'll only do about a gram while I am dealing; I don't want to get all fucked up, but I want to be on my toes then."

Tom described a clear daily pattern in his cocaine usage. "Most of my cocaine I do at night, unless I am on a run — runs usually start at night, though. During the day I was out hustling, man.

"In the last year or so, when the money I could put my hands on hasn't been so good, I was hustling to get my money together to buy so I could sell that night. A lot of dudes like to sell at night; it's safer that way. I have worked New York and Miami getting coke; the blacks in New York can be mean, but they're like pussy cats compared with those fucking Cubans in Miami! They're animals! They will take your money and your life! I lost more than $40,000 down there last year — I was never so scared in my life! If I ever catch those mother fuckers out of Miami, I will waste them, those dirty bastards!"

Tom reported that 20 percent of his total cocaine usage was street cocaine — "It leaves a lot to be desired!" He tried pharmaceutical cocaine only two or three times but didn't like it — "It has a lot of drive, but it made me edgy." Although he had also tried liquid cocaine once or twice he didn't like that either. He stated 80 percent of his total usage was rock-crystal cocaine — "In my opinion, that's the finest coke in the world!"

When asked how he determines the difference between street and high-grade cocaine, he stated, "Quality is partly determined by who you are getting it from, but I never rely on that alone. I have a laboratory I use when I am buying kilos, but if I was buying locally I would use Clorox. You dump a little cocaine in the Clorox; if it turns red or dark red, it is procaine or cut with procaine. Most people, if showed procaine and cocaine, would choose procaine; it has a rush of its own. Cocaine is one of the easiest drugs in the world to camouflage. Benzocaine does not really have a rush, but it will numb the shit out of you! If I was buying locally I would look at the rocks. I'd try it with Clorox. I'd put it in a spoon and run water over it. I might burn some of it in a spoon. If it has a heavy alcoholic smell and breaks down easily in water without stirring, it may be good. If I was making a *big* buy I would shoot a tenth of a gram; that's how I would really tell.

"However, if you're buying no more than a gram you have to depend on the person selling, because he is not going to let you shoot out of a bag that small. If you know the difference in reactions to procaine, benzocaine, and cocaine, firing it up is best but you have to be ready to make big purchases."

Tom reported that he did develop a temporary tolerance to cocaine. "When I first fire up, I am using a tenth of a gram and get a fantastic rush. Everything else after that is to try to get back to that first rush. You never do, but you always try. Before the night is out, it is easy to be shooting a quarter gram of rock crystal at a whack, but you never get back to that first rush." It was Tom's opinion that tolerance to cocaine never lasts much longer than forty-eight hours. "You get some sleep, and in forty-eight hours you can run again and get off good."

Tom reported that withdrawal from cocaine was very difficult. "There is nothing in the world worse than running out of coke! When I do coke I am not violent at all; however, when I run out I could be violent very easy. If I was trying to put money together to finish a run, and some son of a bitch got in my way, he would have trouble on his hands. You are tired, worn-out, and beat after a two- or three-day run, you're physically worn-out, but hell, you can't relax; your head aches from the cut and you are wired so much your mind and body are still going like hell! The only way to come off is to do some heroin or Dilaudid, or if you don't have anything better, tranquilizers or even alcohol. That's how you get hooked on heroin, trying to get off cocaine."

Reactions to Cocaine

Physiological Reactions

Table 5.5 indicates that for Tom, with his intravenous, daily, high-dosage use, physiological reactions associated with stimulation of the central nervous system and sensitization of the autonomic nervous system always occurred with cocaine usage. The sympathomimetic signs included (100 percent) elevation of heart, respiration, and pulse rates, sweating, tightness in the chest, dryness of the mouth and throat, accelerated mental activity, and loss of sensations of fatigue. Tom also reported that dizziness, a ringing in the ears with the rush, muscle spasms ("If I do over two grams"), and a compulsion to do more cocaine were regularly associated with use. He asserted that weight loss was also a correlate of daily use because "you simply don't eat!"

A second clustering of physiological responses occurring about 75 percent of the time included diarrhea and loss of sensations of hunger. Tom reported that sensitivity to light and vomiting were irregular occurrences. He thought cocaine use was associated with development of cavities and tooth decay, but he attributed this to the lactose in the cut rather than the cocaine itself.

TABLE 5.5. Physiological Reactions to Cocaine Use and Abuse: Tom P.

Commonly Reported Reactions to Cocaine Use/Abuse	Reactions Observed Yes	Reactions Observed No	Percent/ Time Observed	Qualifying Comments and Observations
Dizziness — feeling of light-headedness	Yes		100	Crystal coke will make me feel light-headed every time.
Sweating — perspiration or increases in temperature	Yes		100	I sweat like hell, particularly in the summer.
Rhinorrhea — running nose		No		That goes with snorting coke.
Tremors — muscle spasms	Yes		100	After two grams, my muscles would twitch. I would also get that reaction coming down off a run.
Lacrimation — tears to eyes		No		It happens sometimes snorting.
Mydriasis — dilation of pupils, light sensitivity	Yes		30	Your eyes get sensitive to strong light. After two grams, everything would get hazy. I would blink a lot after I had been shooting awhile.
Gooseflesh		No		Not for me.
Emesis — vomiting	Yes		20	It makes me vomit some, but you feel nauseous right after the hit.
Reactive hyperemia — clogging of nasal airways		No		Only if you snort.
Anorexia — loss of appetite, sensation for hunger	Yes		75	You don't eat! Heavy cokers are always kinda skinny, if you do coke everyday.
Dryness of mouth and throat, lack of salivation	Yes		100	It's just dry, man!
Increased heart rate	Yes		100	Your heart pounds like hell after a big hit!
Tightness in chest or chest pains	Yes		100	It feels like you have a steel band around your chest.
Local anesthesia, numbness		No		You only get numb if you miss a vein. You can get bad burns with coke. I have only been burned a couple of times. It leaves bad scars if you miss a vein.
Nosebleed		No		Never.

Elevation of pulse rate	Yes	100	You're pulse pounds. You can feel it along your temple.
Increased respiration rate	Yes	100	You're breathing hard after a hit. It levels off some.
Cellulitis – inflammation following administration	No		That's with snorting.
Infection of nasal mucous membrane	No		Snorting.
Yawning	No		I never noticed it.
Hyperphrenia – excessive mental activity	Yes	100	Your mind is going like crazy. It is hard to keep it going in one direction sometimes.
Weight loss	Yes	100	You do a lot of runs, you're going to lose a lot of weight because you don't eat.
Fainting	No		I never fainted. The room got dark a couple of times, but I never passed out.
Increased sensitivity to allergies	No		Not for me.
Diarrhea or explosive bowel movements	Yes	75	Hell, at first I thought coke must be a laxative, but later I learned it just stimulates your whole system. It stimulates your kidneys, too.
Hepatitis or liver infections	No		That you get when you don't use new spikes.
Headaches	Yes	50	If the coke is cut with crap you can get bad headaches coming down off a run.
Loss of fatigue	Yes	100	You don't feel tired at all, man. You feel like you could go on forever.
Ringing in the ears	Yes	100	If it is good coke.
Convulsions	No		I have seen one or two guys go into convulsions on a long, hard run.
Cavities	Yes	20	I think it's the lactose they use in the cut.
Compulsion	Yes	100	You get this crazy compulsion that you have to have more coke after 4–5 hits. It's crazy.

161

162

TABLE 5.6. Psychological Reactions to Cocaine Use and Abuse: Tom P.

Commonly Reported Reactions to Cocaine Use/Abuse	Reactions Observed Yes	Reactions Observed No	Percent/ Time Observed	Qualifying Comments and Observations
Increased feelings of self-control	Yes		75	It makes me feel like I could do anything. I am on top of my act on coke.
Increased optimism, courage	Yes		75	I felt like I could do anything, anything at all.
Increased activity, restlessness, excitement	Yes		100	You are restless, excited, and feel like movin'.
Feeling of increased physical strength or ability to do physical work	Yes		100	There is no way to describe it. You feel like you could gnaw through steel.
Intensified feelings of well-being, euphoria, "floating," etc.	Yes		100	You don't feel like you are floating, but you are euphoric as hell. You are on top of the world. It's fantastic, but it only lasts about 15 minutes.
Feeling that everything is perfect	Yes		100	It is as perfect as the world will ever be!
An exquisite "don't care about the world" attitude	Yes		100	That's how coke made me feel.
A physical orgasm in the "rush"		No		I never had any shit like that.
Increased thinking power and imagination	Yes		100	Your mind is going like crazy.
Feeling that the mind is quicker than normal, the feeling that one is smarter than everyone else	Yes		100	You think you can outwit anyone.
More talkative than usual, a stream of talk	Yes		100	You just rattle on and on.
Indifference to pain	Yes		100	After two grams, you don't notice much pain.
Decreased interest in work, failure of ambition, loss of ambition for useful work	Yes		65	You're only interested in the high of that next hit, not work.
Insomnia	Yes		100	You get so "wired" you have to use heroin or tranquilizers to get off the coke.
Depression		No		You don't get depressed doing coke. I get depressed as hell when it's all gone, if I run out of coke. There is nothing worse than running out of coke.

Anxiety	Yes	100	I get anxious as hell, though, after a couple of grams of coke.
Prolonged sexual intercourse	No		Shooting coke, you're not interested in sex. The "rush" is all you are after.
An aphrodisiac or sexual stimulant	No		You are not interested in sex. It is an aphrodisiac for women though. I have never seen a woman turn down coke.
Better orgasm on coke	No		Like I said, you are not interested in sex.
Irrational fears	Yes	100	You get paranoid as hell, you misinterpret what happens. You have all kinds of paranoid ideas.
Terror or panic	Yes	50	I have been so paranoid and crazy about 40 percent of the time that I would "split" and get away from people.
Tactile hallucinations — the feeling that insects are crawling on or under the skin (particularly fingertips, palms of hands, etc.)	No		I never had that reaction on coke. I've seen guys get it with amphetamines.
Changes in reality or the way a room or objects look — the wall waving or in motion, etc.	Yes	75	The room begins to look hazy and blurry after I do two grams. You don't see too well.
Paranoid ideas — the feeling that people are after you. You believe you are being watched, talked about or threatened, a wife or girlfriend is unfaithful, untrustworthy, etc.	Yes	100	Everytime I do about two grams, I can bank on being paranoid as hell. Something happens, a sound, you misinterpret it, think the police will be coming in any moment.
Causes one to carry a gun or run from imaginary enemies	Yes		Shit, we all carried guns anyway. It was part of the scene. There is always some dude who will try to break in and get your cash or your coke. I shot three or four of the bastards. I didn't try to kill them.
Visual hallucinations	Yes	50	I've seen things that weren't there. Lots of times I would stack all the furniture against the door. I thought I saw cops out the window.

163

TABLE 5.6. Psychological Reactions to Cocaine Use and Abuse: Tom P. *(Continued)*

Commonly Reported Reactions to Cocaine Use/Abuse	Reactions Observed Yes	Reactions Observed No	Percent/ Time Observed	Qualifying Comments and Observations
Auditory hallucinations — hearing voices talking about you, threatening, etc.	Yes		50	You misinterpret normal sounds. Shit, a guy turned on the water faucet in the bathroom. I thought it was a snake. I jumped up with my gun to kill the son-of-a-bitch.
Olfactory hallucinations — new odors, smells, etc.		No		But your sense of smell is keener, you are more sensitive to odors.
A trigger for violence		No		Shit man, you are paranoid out of your mind. The last thing you want is violence. I don't even want to open the door when I am doing coke.

In Tom's experience shooting cocaine was not associated with infections or hepatitis, gooseflesh, numbness, allergic reactions, fainting, convulsions, or the physiological reactions commonly associated with snorting (rhinorrhea, cellulitis, tears, running nose, etc.).

Psychological Reactions

Table 5.6 indicates that Tom's use of cocaine propelled him into both satisfying and painful emotional states. His usage was always associated with intensified feelings of well-being and euphoria ("but it's so brief!"); the feeling that his mind was quicker, he was on top of the world, and everything was perfect; a don't-give-a-damn attitude toward the world; increased physical strength, imagination, thinking power, restlessness, excitement, talkativeness, and indifference to pain. Although these positive reactions always occurred with his cocaine usage, it was also always associated with intense anxiety, insomnia, irrational fears, paranoid ideation, and depression ("when I come off cocaine").

A second cluster of psychological responses, occurring 50–70 percent of the time, included a polyglot of positive and negative psychological states: increased self-confidence and optimism, terror and panic, increased feelings of self-control ("I felt like I could do anything"), loss of ambition for work, visual anomalies ("everything would get fuzzy and hazy"), and visual hallucinations ("I kept thinking I was seeing cops outside").

Cocaine usage was not associated with tactile or olfactory hallucinations, nor did Tom feel that cocaine was an aphrodisiac for men, prolonged sexual intercourse, or induced better orgasms. He never experienced an orgasm with the rush. Since Tom avoided shooting cocaine with women, he had no information concerning the effects of intravenous use on sexual performance. The general impression he left, in fact, is that sexual intercourse itself is relatively pale and insignificant compared with the "fantastic" reactions obtained by shooting cocaine.

Integration

Cocaine performed several crucial functions in Tom's adjustment. First, regular use helped him ward off or abort the depression and dysphoria permeating his existence.

Second, it provided Tom with that rare experience of being on "top of his act." His self-doubts and feelings of inadequacy vanished temporarily and he felt supremely self-confident and self-assured, able to outwit anyone, powerful, superhuman. Tom was a formidable adversary on any occasion; however, when using cocaine he felt invincible and unbeatable. These feelings were in such striking contrast to his normal psychological state that he was more than willing to pay the price, to endure the irrational fears, anxieties, and paranoia accompanying use of the drug. It may be that cocaine contributed to Tom's survival in his chosen occupation, for most people would understandably avoid direct confrontation with a quick, decisive, and violent man acting with boldness and authority.

Third, cocaine helped this hypersensitive man to either ignore or react more quickly to the slights and rebuffs from other people which otherwise would be a source of ruminative worry to him.

Finally, Tom's use of cocaine helped him survive in that it enabled him to keep his explosive anger, rage, and violence under control. Tom once tried to stop using cocaine for a week. During this period his judgment faltered, he misinterpreted situations with other drug abusers that he normally would have grasped quickly, became depressed and despondent, and reported his life was hopeless. When he returned to regular use of cocaine, these symptoms vanished. Tom's cocaine use may have served to prevent the outbreak of a full-blown psychosis.

LIFE ACTIVITIES AND EXPERIENCES

No life activities and experiences are reported for Tom. One day he missed a scheduled interview session, not an uncommon occurrence with our men. Two weeks later his intermediary reported Tom had been shot and killed in a coastal city. His body was sent to Santa Fe for burial.

6

George B.

LIFE THEMES

George B. is strong, self-reliant, and well-disciplined. Though only in his twenties, he has been a highly successful salesman. Systematically and deliberately, George has tried to construct a fortress-like self impregnable to any assault by any force from any direction. During the last year, however, he found his fortress breached — from within.

The central themes in George's life are:

- If I show any sign of weakness, women will destroy me by emasculation and men will destroy me by aggression.
- Consequently, I must be stronger and more aggressive than anyone I meet, and I must become entirely self-sufficient.
- But the laws of my existence have been shattered by drugs; therefore, I must now make a new life.

Cocaine Use in Relation to Life Themes

George B. used cocaine intravenously, daily, and at high-dosage levels. It was his drug of choice because it

- made him feel self-confident and potent,
- gave him energy and stamina for his work as a salesman,

• allowed him to turn his body into a "machine" (by obliterating the malaise, shocks, and pains of existence it enabled him to maintain a high performance level for long, grueling hours),
• helped him to be gregarious and eased his relationships with others, and
• helped him to fill his lonely existence yet avoid being dependent upon any other human being.

EVOLUTION OF LIFE STYLE

Introduction

George is a handsome, well-built, twenty-eight-year-old Caucasian male. He dresses tastefully in the young adult style — custom slacks, tailored shirts, leather jacket, and loafers. He wears his hair in a natural, curly style.

On the surface George appears relaxed but reserved. His poise is deceptive, however; he experiences more tension than he betrays. His tendency to act independently was shown when, without notifying anyone, he withdrew from this research after the initial assessment session. Quite by accident, one of the investigators later saw him in a hospital. George was in considerable physical and mental pain; he was seeking admission to a methadone maintenance program because he had become addicted to opiates while using them to control the adverse effects of cocaine. The investigator visited with him briefly. Later, George said, "I decided to quit the project, but you sat down with me at the hospital and asked if there was anything you could do to help me. You were interested in me, so I came back." Another reason for continuing, he said, was his hope that someone might benefit from his experiences.

Developmental Experiences

George was born in rural Oklahoma, the younger of two children in an oil well rigger's family. He has an older sister thirty-three years of age. His parents were divorced when George was one year old; despite this, he has maintained a reasonably close relationship with his biological father, a fifty-six-year-old mid-management supervisor in the oil-processing and petrochemical industry. His father is a person George feels he can still rely on when he needs help: "I guess I am as close as you can get with a divorced father; we have worked together and gone on vacations together. He had a farm. When I was growing up, I would go out there and work for him in the summertime." He says there is very little he would change about the man.

George is not sure why his parents divorced. "I guess my father was pretty wild like me. He was a hell-raiser and I guess he didn't want to accept the responsibilities then. I am sure he regrets it now." When asked how he felt about his parents' divorce, George replied abruptly that he was very young when his father "pulled out" and he really didn't think much about it one way or another.

The most significant person for George in his family was his mother. He described her as a tiny fifty-eight-year-old woman who had managed and supported the family alone for several years, a friendly, gentle woman who nevertheless fought for her children. "She had a terrible time disciplining me. She would never use physical discipline; she would try to talk me into doing things, but it was no good because she couldn't control me. She would tell me to do a certain thing and I would ask why; she would tell me again, and if I refused she would just cry. I know she loves me very much. She would do anything for me. In fact, now she loves to do things for me I don't even need done."

His mother was stronger than she appeared. "She worked as a credit manager and ran our family alone for seven or eight years. She had a hard time, but she is a deceptive little woman: When she is faced with crisis, she appears weak, and you think she may come unwrapped; however, as a problem goes along she gets stronger."

His mother remarried when he was thirteen years old; his stepfather was supervisor for an oil company. "He was strict. However, if he tried to correct me my mother would step in and protect me. I guess he tried to develop a relationship with me during my teens, but I didn't care to have a relationship with him. He bothered me because he would never look at me when he talked to me. We fought a lot; he would shout and holler at me and I would shout back at him. He and my mother had a lot of arguments over my sister and I. If he had any influence at all on me, I guess it was negative." In the last three to four years George and his stepfather have become closer: "We are both mellowing out, from bad to better. We have a fairly decent relationship now."

George's older sister Loretta "wasn't a wild hell-raiser like me. She was an A student, she stayed close to home and never caused any trouble. We were real close; she felt the same way I did about my stepfather. In fact, most of the feelings I had about him I got from her." George and his sister still visit each other regularly, though they live several hundred miles apart.

George indicates that his parents' divorce and the appearance of his stepfather were the most important crises during his developmental years. He feels his family had an average middle-class income and home: "We didn't lack things we needed. There were things we wanted, but by and large our basic needs were met."

During his early years — until he was thirteen — George lived in rural Oklahoma, but when his mother remarried the family moved to Kansas City. "I would stay out late every night running around with my friends. I didn't get into any real trouble. We did break into a pop machine once; that's about all. I was pretty independent and rebellious even then; I didn't want to go with the crowd. I don't let many people get close."

"My stepfather and my mother said they would pay for my clothes, feed me, and give me a home, but if I wanted anything else I had to work for it. So as a teenager I worked! I washed dishes in a restaurant, worked in a janitorial service for a while, worked in a car-wash place, worked as a waiter, you name it. I learned how to work and earn my own spending money!"

George made Bs in most subjects until he was in high school. "Then I got to playing around with girls, wouldn't study, and my grades fell. So my parents decided I should go to military school to learn some self-discipline. My first six months in military school made me realize I didn't want to stay there, so the second six months I made good grades! I didn't like it, but it taught me self-discipline and I am grateful for that. It was actually a rich boys' reformatory school. At Christmas the second year I told my parents I wasn't going back; they said okay. I picked up in school and did well, I was highly motivated. Since that time I have been able to excel in anything I really want to do."

George never allowed women to get close to him emotionally. "In high school I didn't want to get married like most other guys. I didn't think it was for me; I just wanted to be free to do what I wanted to do. If I wanted to take a trip to Mexico, I wanted to take it and not worry about how I was going to finance it. I didn't want to be a 'Freddie Lunch-Bucket!' Life is too short. I have made my own way since I got out of high school, and I have done very well."

George attended a university for one semester. "I got bored by it and enlisted in the Marine Corps. I was going to go over and help clean up that mess in Viet Nam. Besides, all I did in school was party anyway."

George served in Viet Nam for fifteen months, during eleven of which he was in heavy combat. "I liked it. I was highly motivated. I lost some of my buddies, but was only wounded once, and not too seriously. I was scared, but it was exciting. It may sound crazy, but I did my first drugs in Nam: I smoked some pot and opium; it gave me a real jolt because I didn't know what it was. I did well in the service; I was a sergeant before I was discharged and could have gone to platoon leaders' school. I would have made it as an officer, but I decided I wanted out."

Following his return from Viet Nam, George held a variety of jobs. He worked in the roofing and construction business, as a cement finisher on commercial buildings, as a long distance truck driver, selling advertising, and operating a successful business of his own. "I made good money, but the business was boring, so I sold it."

At twenty-three George became a salesman. He has sold cars, real estate, air-conditioning, and home security systems. "I work strictly in commission sales; your best salesmen are always commission salesmen. Besides that, I am pretty much my own boss. The income I make depends entirely on me and I like that. Besides, I am moving, meeting people, and doing things. The only time I have ever been fired was when I worked on salary-plus-commission: My boss tried to tell me how to do my job, we got into an argument, and he fired me. That was okay with me; a good salesman can always find a job. I am no organization man, I like to be in charge of my own act and be held accountable for doing it."

At age twenty-two, George began sporadically using amphetamine to increase his energy and drive. Although he had snorted cocaine socially from age twenty-three to twenty-six, he did not use hard drugs heavily until he was twenty-six. Cocaine was the first drug George took intravenously. "I'd fire up in the moring before I went to work, and again then during the day if I needed it. I could run circles around the other salesmen — I was able to do three times as much as the rest of them and I enjoyed outrunning them all!

"Good salesmen make good money, but you live under tremendous pressures. You are always pushing your limits. A lot of older salesmen use alcohol to help them deal with their jobs. I guess I was from the new generation, because I didn't use alcohol; I was using cocaine, and I performed fantastically for a couple of years, until I lost control of the coke."

Major crises have occurred in George's life in the last two years. "I didn't have any financial problems until the last year or so, I have always had money in the bank. Coke ended all of that. Breaking out of the drug scene has been hell; it is not only breaking away from the drug — which was hard — but I have to break away from all those old relationships — and that has been hard, too, because they don't want to see a guy break away. After I quit, they kept coming by the house trying to give me free stuff. They would give it to me free because they wanted me back in. They even sent good-looking hookers by to deliver the stuff and throw in free sex, too. It tore me up to turn all of that down — I did, though, and they have given up on it. They had my mouth watering a couple of times, though; it has been very hard."

Despite his heavy use of cocaine, he has had no difficulties with the police or drug enforcement personnel — "I don't want any problems with them either." He has been arrested five times in his life; three times for traffic violations, once on a misdemeanor charge for "disturbing the peace," and once for possession of marijuana. He pleaded guilty to both misdemeanor offenses and was placed on parole.

George's fear of being caught was one of the reasons he broke from drugs. "A year ago I had $10,000 in the bank and I was making about $125 a day. It all went — on coke and Demerol, morphine, stuff like that. I had reached a point in my life where I had to decide what was going to become of me. I decided I would have to either get into the drug thing full-time and make all the money I could, but face the likelihood of getting killed or caught and going to prison, or get completely out, turn my life around, and go the other way. I enjoyed the drugs, but I decided to get out, and I have."

George indicates that by and large his health was very good. However, he had anemia for a while, which he thought was related to his drug use.

Although George has been sexually active, he did state proudly that he never let any women gét close. However, he had been living with a woman, Darlene, for nearly three years, and after he decided to withdraw from drugs they married. He describes her as a self-sufficient, well-organized woman who holds a position of responsibility in a national sales organization.

George said that he had not been a religious person; he had attended church only four times during the last year. But George's attitudes toward church and religion changed abruptly; his decision to break away from drugs precipitated a major upheaval. George experienced religious conversion, joined a fundamentalist Protestant church and was baptized. The church soon became one of his mainstays in his efforts to reorganize his life.

George has no political interests. "I am not a conservative, liberal, or anything else, and I don't want to have anything to do with politics. They are all crooks, the way I figure it."

During his last interview, George was asked about his goals in life. "I want to be self-contained. I just want to be my own man, be on top of my thing, and lead my own life. That may mean I'll stay in sales, maybe not, but whatever I do, I want to be my own man."

Interpretive Integration

At least nine conditions or critical events during George's developmental years have formed his life style. These included experiences associated with the following:

- Abandonment at age one by a perhaps irresponsible father
- Possible development in George of guilt that he was responsible for his parents' divorce
- A difficult period of several years during which his mother assumed responsibility for the support and management of the family
- A warm, affectionate mother who lacked the toughness to control a willful son, but who in her own way was a skillful manipulator
- At a critical period in George's life (early puberty), the intrusion into the family of a stepfather who was insensitive to the needs of a teenage boy and was seen by George as a poor substitute for his biological father
- Apparent success by the mother in blocking the stepfather's efforts to assume a meaningful role in the training of the children
- Essentially middle-class experiences during his developmental years with reasonable financial and emotional security
- Sustained but premature efforts to develop self-sufficiency
- A painful but rewarding experience in military school where George learned how to "become his own man"

Because he was reared in this kind of environment, George developed a life style with the following characteristics:

- Denial or suppression of anger; resentful respect for authority

- General acceptance of societal values; basic honesty and integrity in relationships with people
- A set of life decisions which included (1) the conclusion that most people are insensitive, calloused, and exploitive, (2) the conclusion that those who are sensitive, who express needs for affection and dependency, can be hurt and are vulnerable to being laughed at and embarrassed, (3) a decision, therefore, to become self-sufficient so he would never be dependent upon anyone, (4) the related decision to be his own man and let no one get close to him, and (5) a vow to achieve and succeed
- Development of the skills and discipline to make such a life pattern workable
- Gravitation to a career which maximized opportunities for personal control over his fate and income with little control from supervisors and authority
- Development of a sense of alienation, malaise, and low-grade but enduring depression and dysphoria

George's life has been arranged around deliberate efforts to become independent and self-sufficient and to avoid intimacy and closeness with others. When asked what kind of animal he would like to be, George stated, "I would want nothing to do with people; I'd be in the wild. I'd be a cat, a tiger. No one messes with a tiger. They're graceful and self-sufficient to a maximum degree." When asked what kind of car he would be George said, "I would be a Maserati. They're expensive, fast — they outrun everything — and they are graceful."

A fear of intimacy pervades his sex life. Although he said, "I have bedded well over a hundred women and lived with some of them," George actually fears women. He feels safe with them only if he keeps them from getting close to him. George's fear suggests that his mother was stronger and, in her own way, more emasculating than he realized. He equates intimacy with being controlled, manipulated, and rejected. Consequently, he has attempted to eradicate intimacy and dependency from his life. He would rather tolerate isolation than risk being hurt or disappointed by others.

George is not introspective. Even after extended inquiry, he showed little awareness of how certain painful experiences and events have forced him to grasp for a lonely way of life. All he verbalized was that he has to live this way.

He has attempted to create a world where he can achieve peace and tranquility. He would like his epitaph to be "Here lies a man in peace." When asked what kind of flag he would fly on the antenna of his car to depict himself as a unique person, George said, "I'd leave it blank. I wouldn't need a symbol to prove what I am — no, I would put a black dove on a white field. The white field and the dove would symbolize that I wanted to be peaceful. I would make the dove black to tell everyone that even though I was peaceful, I am not going to take any shit from anyone either."

There is little doubt that George is resourceful and disciplined, a fierce competitor. By age twenty-eight he had achieved status and financial success in a highly competitive field. By his own choice George underwent "cold turkey" withdrawal from methadone, because he resented both the disruptions in his life made by required daily trips to the clinic and the notion that he was dependent upon anything. "I was sick with cramps. I was nauseous, sweated like hell, and thought I would die for a while. But after the first week or two it began to ease off. For several weeks I had these burning sensations in my arm, these weird involuntary reflexes; my arms would snap out violently all by themselves, they would hit anything in the way. They were pretty bruised and scraped up for a while. It doesn't happen so much now. They don't burn and tingle like they did either."

George's self-rehabilitation also included marriage, conversion, "rebirth," and a radical job change. "I am getting pretty good at it [his new job as a drafts-man]. I'll stay six to eight months or maybe even a year, if I have to, until I get my act together again. It's a routine job, but I'll stay with it until I am ready to go back into sales. It's not the pressure I am worried about, it's the traveling. I am not sure I can go to St. Louis, Chicago, or Dallas, and be certain that I wouldn't try to contact people who would turn me back into drugs, so I'll wait till I feel ready."

Concerning his self-rehabilitation, George stated, "I treat myself like an ex-alcoholic. As long as I don't touch drugs I'll be okay. I know that the first time I do drugs again, the whole thing will start all over. Hell, I am even afraid to take aspirins."

It has been extremely difficult for George to break out of the drug scene. "It has been the hardest thing I have ever done in my life. During the period when I had just gotten into the methadone program, I was sitting home one night talking with Darlene. All of a sudden, I started sobbing; I just sobbed and cried my heart out. Darlene held me and I just sobbed and sobbed, I couldn't stop. It was the first time I've cried since I was just a kid. I have always tried to stay on top and be in control of my act. It was tearing me apart. I had to do something to get back in control."

FORMAL PSYCHOLOGICAL ASSESSMENT

Dimensional Test Findings

Intelligence Tests

George functions in the Bright Normal intellectual range. With his driving ambition, George could undoubtedly have completed a college degree had he decided it was necessary.

MMPI

George's MMPI shows a depressed and irritable individual with a high level of inner tension, anxiety, and frustration (figure 6.1). Although George is preoccupied and ruminative, there is no evidence of a serious thinking disorder. The Validity scores indicate that he attempted to follow the test instructions and answer questions honestly.

The test shows George to be reserved, inner-directed, somewhat taciturn, and frequently uncomfortable with others. Though socially perceptive and sensitive, he maintains distance and may be seen by others as rather aloof. Despite his reserve, he is articulate and able to communicate ideas clearly.

It is important to him that he see himself and be seen by others as a masculine, potent individual. These masculine strivings cover strong but unacceptable passive-dependent needs. At this point George is also experiencing difficulty controlling feelings of resentment and hostility; consistent with his image of masculine self-sufficiency, he tends to deny or repress any emotional distress.

Clinically, the picture is that of a neurotic individual who relies on denial and repression to maintain control and does not have insight into his own behavior. Under prolonged stress he may respond with psycho-physiological symptoms: headaches, bodily aches, and gastrointestinal complaints. This would be particularly the case if for some reason George were limited in physical mobility; for work, action, and physical activity are major outlets for much of the anxiety and frustration he feels.

Sixteen PF

The pattern of scores in table 6.1 is congruent with other data concerning George's life style. The Sixteen PF depicts him as strong, assertive, resourceful, and driven to achieve and succeed. Stubborn, competitive, and self-assured, he shows no hesitancy to fight for what he wants. George is not a warm, gregarious, or cheerful man and he does not have strong needs to be with other people; rather, he is a serious and somber warlord who insists on remaining in his fortress of self-sufficiency.

The Sixteen PF aptly depicts George's wish to live a kind of "John Wayne" existence characterized by manliness, independence, autonomy, self-sufficiency, and — as shown by his cold-turkey withdrawal from methadone — true grit. The test also captures the other pole of a major life conflict: strong but unacceptable needs for affection, intimacy, closeness, care and nurture.

Generally, George accepts societal values as guides for his behavior. (However, he will do what he feels is appropriate whether or not it meets with social approval.) He may not always like the people he works or socializes with, but maintains a basic honesty in his relationships and will not take unfair advantage. He practices a live-and-let-live philosophy as long as others do not attempt to "rip him off" — or get close.

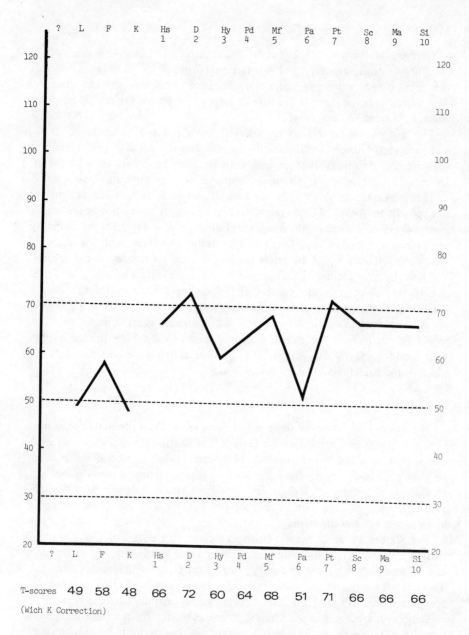

T-scores	49	58	48	66	72	60	64	68	51	71	66	66	66

(Wich K Correction)

FIGURE 6.1. MMPI Profile: George B. *Reproduced from the Minnesota Multiphasic Personality Inventory Profile and Case Summary form, by permission. Copyright 1948 by the Psychological Corporation, New York, N.Y. All rights reserved.*

George is not at ease with himself. Rather, he is a person with a high level of ergic tension, only part of which can be dissipated through work. The rest churns in his gut and creates frustration and discontent, adding to the driven quality of his life.

Surprisingly, the Sixteen PF Test suggests that George is not a shrewd judge of others; he frequently misinterprets their motives and intentions. This may account in part for his need to maintain social distance. It also suggests that on some occasions when he has reached out to others he was embarrassed, hurt, or taken advantage of. George is sensitive; being let down would intensify his efforts to avoid closeness, reinforcing his conviction that he must maintain his solitary way of life.

Other Dimensional Measures

George obtained consistently low scores on all variables measured by the Sensation-Seeking Scales. These data indicate that this practical, hard-driving person has less need for the kinds of experiences these scales tap than the normative population of young male adults. Although George is restless, action-oriented, and easily becomes bored, one could hardly describe him as impulsive; rather, he is serious-minded and well-controlled, and chooses experiences critically, not in terms of thrill and excitement but in terms of their contribution to success, achievement (money), and independence.

In general, George's scores on the Novelty Experiencing Scales are comparable with scores obtained by normative groups. There is one exception: His scores on Internal Sensation are more than one standard deviation below the mean for airmen and nearly two standard deviations below that for college men. His scores on most subscales were relatively stable across testing intervals; his scores on Internal Sensation, however, fell from 12 at the first session to 4 at the second to 1 at the third. The Internal Sensation scale measures the tendency to like unusual dreams and fantasies and internally generated sensations in general. Given the experiences, personality upheaval, and efforts at reorganization of life style which George has recently undergone, the decline on this variable may reflect an attempt to control himself by suppressing his inner life.

George obtained a score of 41 on the Change Seeker Index. This score compares with mean scores of 43.30 for army males and of 49.06 obtained from college males. These results substantiate findings on other scales, and indicate that George has no greater need for stimulation and change than comparable adult male groups.

George obtained scores of 3, 15, and 1 on the Extraversion, Neuroticism and Lie Scales of the Eysenck Personality Questionnaire. These scores compare with normative scores at the fifth, eighty-seventh, and twenty-third percentile for male adult industrial subjects. Standard interpretation suggests that George is

TABLE 6.1. Cattell 16PF Profile: George B

Standard Score	Low Score Description	Factor	Standard Ten Score (Sten)	High Score Description
5	Reserved, detached, critical, cool, aloof, stiff, precise, objective	A	5	Outgoing, warm-hearted, easygoing, trustful, good-natured, participating
6	Less intelligent, concretistic thinking, less well-organized, poor judgment	B	6	More intelligent, abstract thinking, bright, insightful, fast-learning, better judgment
4	Affected by feelings, emotionally less stable, worrying, easily upset, changeable	C	4	Emotionally stable, mature, unruffled, faces reality, calm (higher ego strength)
9	Humble, mild, easily led, docile, accommodating, submissive, conforming	E	9	Assertive, aggressive, stubborn, headstrong, competitive, dominant, rebellious
1	Sober, taciturn, serious, introspective, reflective, slow, cautious	F	1	Happy-go-lucky, enthusiastic, talkative, cheerful, frank, quick, alert
6	Expedient, disregards rules, social conventions and obligations to people (weaker superego strength)	G	6	Conscientious, persistent, moralistic, persevering, well-disciplined (stronger superego strength)
5	Shy, timid, withdrawn, threat-sensitive	H	5	Venturesome, uninhibited, socially bold, active, impulsive
8	Tough-minded, self-reliant, cynical, realistic	I	8	Tender-minded, sensitive, dependent, seeking help and sympathy
2	Trusting, accepting conditions, understanding, tolerant, permissive	L	2	Suspicious, hard to fool, dogmatic

178

Score	Low	Factor	High
9	Practical, "down-to-earth" concerns, guided by objective reality	L	Imaginative, bohemian, absent-minded, unconventional, easily seduced from practical judgment
5	Forthright, unpretentious, genuine, spontaneous, natural, artless, socially clumsy	M	Astute, polished, socially aware, shrewd, smart, "cuts corners"
4	Self-assured, placid, secure, self-confident, complacent, serene	N	Apprehensive, self-reproaching, insecure, worrying, troubled, guilt-prone
8	Conservative, respectful of established, traditional ideas	O	Experimenting, liberal, free-thinking, non-moralistic, experiments with problem-solutions
10	Group-dependent, depends on social approval, a "joiner" and sound follower	Q_1	Self-sufficient, resourceful, prefers to make own decisions
4	Undisciplined self-conflict, lax, follows own urges, careless of social rules	Q_2	Controlled, exacting willpower, socially precise, compulsive, persistent, foresighted
8	Relaxed, tranquil, torpid, unfrustrated, composed, low ergic tension	Q_3	Tense, frustrated, driven, overwrought, high ergic tension
		Q_4	

Average

shy and introverted with crippling neurotic problems. Introversion and success as a salesperson may seem incompatible; but George's life style has been constructed in such a way that he does not become close to anyone, even when appearing relaxed and at ease in sales situations. George is not certain he even likes people.

Integration

Data from the dimensional measures can only be construed as substantiating in every respect the conclusions drawn from the review of this man's developmental experiences. The data show George to be a superficially successful man who achieves a great deal by sheer energy and hard work and constantly tries to deceive himself into believing that he is, or can be, entirely self-sufficient, independent, and invulnerable. However, the data also show that George is not basically at ease with or sensitive to himself or others. He worries excessively, yet his worrying is unproductive. He fears personal impotence, weakness, dependence, and softness. To escape self-awareness he turns to vigorous, even exhausting, physical action. As much as he wants to keep control of his own life, George fears that he will not be able to do so. And he can imagine no fate worse than that.

Findings from Morphogenic Measures

Overview

George's morphogenic data show the impact of his recent initiation of a process that could produce a profound change in his personality. George's progressive dissatisfaction with his current self is clearly expressed, as are the changes taking place in his value system and conception of the kind of person he would like to be. George seems to attribute all his problems to his use of cocaine; consequently he seems to feel that if only he could stop using drugs his troubles would be over and his newer, better self would emerge automatically. It is too early to tell whether George's program of self-change can produce the deepseated alterations in his self-concept necessary for successful long-range readjustment.

The Q-Sort data show George's growing dissatisfaction with himself, and identify the source of his dissatisfaction as a change in values and ideals rather than in basic self-concept. The data also show that, as indicated in the preceding paragraph, George blames his problems primarily on cocaine. The picture George presented was of a driving, ambitious, independent, dominant person. Implied in his self-presentation also is the connection between his drive for success and his cocaine use, which he felt gave him a competitive edge. The data indicate that George took cocaine not because he gained pleasure from it, but in order to maintain the highest possible level of excitement for the longest period of time. This he needed to support his conception of himself as a powerful, achieving, sexually active person. Nevertheless, George also expressed a wish to slow down and seek peace, happiness, and self-satisfaction. The data lead to the explanatory hypothesis that George must have had to struggle hard to overcome feelings of impotence, weakness, and dependency.

The Rep Test reveals George's ambivalence about financial success — the dominant goal of his life. He divides successful people into two groups. Some are kind and helpful; George would like to associate with these people, but they are connected with drug use and he will incur their dislike by giving up cocaine. There are also successful people who are stubborn, selfish, and hard to get along with; this is the group George fears he will be forced to associate with in the future, and he does not like the prospect. The problem is that George wants to change in every way *except* in his need to be socially dominant and financially successful.

Q-Sorts

Standard Items

George used the standard Q-Sort items rather consistently. The median correlation between his descriptions of his usual self was .870 within sessions and .775 between sessions, for an overall median close to .800 — a very high value. Remarkable for its deviation from his typical performance was George's description of his ideal self. This changed abruptly at the time of the first reassessment. The nature of the change and its probable meaning are described below under *Factor analysis*.

Partly due to the change in George's conception of his ideal self, the correlations between his descriptions of his usual self and his ideal self decreased steadily from a median of $r = .830$ at the first assessment period to $r = .439$ at the second reassessment period. Clearly, George was becoming less self-satisfied as the research progressed.

The correlation between George's descriptions of his usual self and the typical cocaine user held steady and positive around a median value of .631. However, the correlation between his descriptions of his ideal self and the typical cocaine user dropped precipitously from .836 in the first assessment session to .112 at the first reassessment and -.011 at the second. In other words, George found the identification of himself as a typical cocaine user (which description did not change) less and less attractive. These findings imply that George is undergoing progressive loss of self-esteem, and that the loss is due not to a change in his conception of his usual self but to a shift of ideals prompting him to devalue his usual self.

Factor analysis. George's sortings of the standard items yield two factors. The first is a strong, general factor reflecting an overall consistency in George's sortings, regardless of instructions or assessment period. This factor is identified as a self-concept.

The second factor is associated almost exclusively with the descriptions of his ideal self that George provided in the two reassessment sessions. This factor is called the *new ideal;* it is this ideal that has provoked George's lessening satisfaction with his usual self.

The standard items associated with the highest and lowest loadings in Factor I show that George described his most general self as anxious, excitable, independent, and devoted to achievement. He rejected items that described signs of weakness, revealed a fear of being shamed or laughed at, strongly rejected the idea that he might have problems with sexual potency, and denied humility. Finally, but perhaps most important, he appeared to be struggling against the underlying pressure of sadness, depression or despair.

George's new ideal (Factor II) shows a reduction in the emphasis on excitement and an increase in the desire to feel at peace, be more humble, gain wisdom, and reduce negative anxiety, negative excitement (explosiveness, impulsiveness, violence), stubbornness, and self-centeredness. There was also evidence that George felt it desirable to increase his willingness to be dependent and become faithful sexually. These findings indicate that George has clear ideas about what sorts of changes he wants to bring about. Apparently, he is not just wishing for things to be different; he has given thought to what an improved state will be like.

Individualized Items

With two exceptions, George's sortings of his individualized items (table 6.2) were stable and consistent, both within and between sessions. The first exception was his description of his own bad self, which was quite different at the first reassessment than at either of the other two sessions. The second exception was his descriptions of most nonusers of drugs; these were unreliable at all assessment periods.

The correlations between George's descriptions of his ideal self and his usual self were fairly high and consistent (median $r = .630$) when he used individualized Q-Sort items. Of course, George changed the wording of two-thirds of the items, so it is possible that he modified the individualized Q-Sort items so as to avoid the necessity of describing his conflict. All other findings point to a change taking place in George's thinking at the time of the first reassessment, a change involving a considerable shake-up in beliefs. Significantly, however, it involved values rather than actualities; his self-concept did not change markedly.

Factor analysis. Four factors have been extracted from the data. The first factor is called a *drug self,* because its highest loadings are on all descriptions of himself during a cocaine high and an amphetamine high. George's descriptions of his usual self and his bad self also achieved modest loadings on this factor, but only during the first reassessment session.

TABLE 6.2.   Individualized Q-Sort Items: George B.

Achievement
Positive
*1. Reaching a goal
*2. Become successful
Negative
*3. Wearing your body down to get what you want
*4. Stepping on someone else to get what you want

Affect
Positive
5. Rushing
6. High
Negative
7. Intense sadness
8. Hurting (in your feelings)

Anxiety Level
Positive
9. Down
10. Easy
Negative
11. Needles and pins
12. Wired

Chastity
Positive
13. Not stepping out (sexually)
*14. Faithful (sexually)
Negative
*15. Sexually impotent
*16. Afraid of chicks

Dependence
Positive
17. Needs others
18. Relies on others
Negative
19. Parasite
20. Mooch

Dominance
Positive
21. Powerful
*22. Strong
Negative
23. Has no control over self, others
*24. Feeble

Excitement
Positive
25. Energetic
26. Racing
Negative
27. Short fuse
28. Ready to explode

Humility
Positive
*29. Humble
*30. Modest
Negative
*31. Often ignored
*32. Lonely

Independence
Positive
*33. Independent
34. Free
Negative
35. Stuck on himself
*36. Self-centered

Knowledge
Positive
*37. Wise
38. Smart
Negative
39. Stupid
40. Dumb

Restraint
Positive
41. Has good will-power
42. Good self-control
Negative
*43. Dragging
44. Misses the boat all the time

Self-satisfaction (Stasis)
Positive
45. Happy with what he is doing
46. Enjoys where he is at
Negative
*47. Lazy
48. Lacks ambition

Sexuality
Positive
*49. Romantic
50. Likes to get it on
Negative
51. Makes love to animals
52. "Prostitute"

Interpersonal Relations
Positive
*53. Kind
54. Courteous
Negative
*55. Cruel
56. Deceitful

Social Recognition
Positive
57. Known as a good guy
*58. Well-known
Negative
59. Turkey
60. Fool

Note: Items marked with an asterisk are not significantly altered from their original (standard) wording.

The second factor is called an *ideal self* because its heaviest positive loadings are on all descriptions of the ideal self, while its heaviest negative loadings are on descriptions of the bad self provided at the first and second reassessment sessions.

The third factor, though small, is specifically associated with *wanting cocaine*. Evidently this is a psychological state George finds distinctive.

The fourth factor is also small but distinctive. Its highest loading is on the description (provided during the critical first reassessment period) of most nonusers of drugs.

Significantly, George's descriptions of himself as he usually is are not consistently identified with any single factor. This finding is a product of George's doubts about his own identity.

The items with high scores on Factor I (drug self) reflect George's emotional orientation and his desire to rush, to be high, excited, energetic, and racing. George also strongly endorsed items conveying his desire for independence and dominance (which are, for George, much the same). Despite this emphasis on energy and excitement, George does not appear to have explosive tendencies. Periodic outbursts are not his style; he wants to move at top speed all the time.

There is nothing aesthetic, sensuous, or pleasurable in his use of drugs; they simply gave him a way of keeping psychological energy flowing at its maximum. George appears to be fighting off a pull into depression and to be strongly denying a desire for peace, quiet, and inactivity. He seems to regard any appearance of these tendencies as a sign of weakness; their arousal stimulates the need to become hyperactive in compensation.

Factor II is bipolar: On the one hand, it represents his best or ideal self, what he would like to be; on the other, simply reversing the factor provides a good picture of his bad self, what he is at his worst. His ideal self wants self-satisfaction — which, as has been shown, George does not now possess — wisdom, restraint (that is, self-control), achievement, and positive social regard. At his worst George suffers deep hurt and sadness and is cruel and deceitful, lazy and a parasite; this is a painful state, one which he has in the past always escaped — with the help of drugs — through driving activity and the pursuit of ambitious goals.

Factor III describes George's discomfort on feeling the need for cocaine. This condition is tied to his ambition to achieve. Further, it is associated not only with tension (negative anxiety: needles and pins) but also with doing anything to get what he wants and the threat of uncontrolled explosion. Possibly, George took cocaine to avoid explosive behavior; it may have helped him regulate energy expenditure in a way not otherwise possible when he is tense and on edge. With drugs, he could keep driving steadily, instead of blowing up catastrophically. Factor III also indicates that George may fear sexual impotence, and took cocaine as a way of avoiding that possibility. His rejection when he wants cocaine of thoughts of impotence and fear of women suggests that he uses sexual activity to reinforce his concept of himself as a powerful, achieving person.

Factor IV would not ordinarily merit interpretation because it accounts for so little variance in the data. However, it does give some indication of how George sees other people — from whom he feels quite different — and it gains significance from the fact that it reflects his feelings during the first reassessment session, when he was undergoing a personal crisis. Though other people seem self-satisfied and happy, to George they are dependent and feeble — traits George would naturally despise — and lack control over their own destinies. They are not kind or courteous; they are ambitious. Of course, unlike George, they are not supercharged by drugs. George once considered that this gave him a distinct advantage, but he is no longer certain that the game is worth the candle.

Rep Test

Role Groups

In general, George's descriptions of important people in his life were consistent from one assessment period to the next. On two such descriptions (mother and father) his responses were identical every time. His least reliable conceptions: a liked employer, the person who needs you most, and yourself when on cocaine. These are perhaps understandable, since George likes employers only if they leave him alone, free to work independently; rejects dependence and probably refuses to associate with people he regards as needy or dependent; and was undergoing a reevaluation of himself in relation to cocaine usage.

The constructs George generated was as follows:

Interpersonal Constructs

1. Trying to be good
2. Loved by me
3. Stubborn
4. Respected by others
5. Kind
6. Straight
7. Not intelligent
8. Successful
9. Hard to get along with
10. No sense of right or wrong (don't care)
11. A close friend
12. Comfortable to be around
13. Has a dislike for me
14. Wants to be pitied
15. *Wants* to be self-controlled

Factor analysis. Although five factors have been identified, only the first three are sufficiently strong to justify interpretation. The first is bipolar and seems to represent a simple like–dislike dimension in George's mind: People who are positive on this factor are trying to be good; they are kind, straight, comfortable to be around, and strong. Those negative on this factor are selfish and weak, want to be pitied, and have a dislike for George.

Factors II and III both contain people who are straight and successful, but people in the second factor are kind and helpful, while people in the third are stubborn, selfish, and hard to get along with. A peculiarity of these factors is that George says people belonging to the second factor dislike him, while he dislikes people in the third factor (the disliked employer is the main member of this group). It seems that George has divided successful people into two groups. One contains nice people, but they do not like George. (Because at least one member of this group is a friend with whom George has taken cocaine, it is possible that the dislike stems from his efforts to quit drugs.) The other group contains unpleasant people, and George dislikes them. George apparently sees himself as a past member of the first group (Factor II), but is ambivalent about becoming a member of the second (Factor III), which contains people he does not like. It appears that while he is willing to try giving up cocaine, he is not willing to give up success and achievement.

Construct groups

Factor analysis produced five groups of constructs in George's descriptions of people. Of the five groups, four are interpretable; the fifth is too small to justify further consideration.

Three easily interpreted factors (Factors II, III, and IV) reflect George's tendencies to judge people in terms of three basic questions: How much do I love this person? How good and kind is this person? How successful and socially respected is this person?

Factor I is more difficult to understand. It is identified mainly by characteristics with negative loadings: not mean, do not dislike George, do not want to be pitied, and not unintelligent. The only positive things George says of people possessing this trait is that they "*want* to be self-controlled" – George emphasized the word "want" to indicate that as yet the effort is not successful. One suspects that the people possessing this trait are a group who do not use drugs or are in the process of being rehabilitated from drug use. George does not wish to ascribe negative attributes to them, but he does not know them or like them well enough to say much that is positive.

Setting Survey

If one were to judge only by the number of hours per week George spends in each environmental setting, one would call his behavior pattern stable. Consistency is evident primarily because George continues to spend most of his time at work. With respect to the variety of settings entered, the picture is somewhat different. Two important changes in George's behavior pattern were that he began to go to church and to spend time in settings devoted to treatment of physical health. Both changes appeared at the time of the first reassessment session.

Another change taking place at about this time was a decrease of penetration into the work setting, including a reduction of contacts with financial institutions. This indicates that, while George continued to appear at work, his participation in independent vocational activities diminished. Perhaps he only marked time for several weeks while getting himself reorganized.

The first reassessment session also saw George engaging in social-recreational activities for the only time. What these activities were is not known, but they, too, may have been connected with his religious conversion and start at rehabilitation.

Despite his problems, George has kept up a level of activity that shows an effort to cope with his problems and maintain well-organized patterns of behavior. Furthermore, his satisfaction levels have remained generally high. The most interesting values are those indicating relatively high satisfaction both with church and financial activities; apparently George enjoys both the material and spiritual impartially. At the other end of the scale is his dissatisfaction with work. This value was neutral at the time of the first assessment session, shifted at the first reassessment session to indicate a feeling of being "mostly dissatisfied," and stayed at this value during the second reassessment. One therefore suspects that George will change career patterns rather than reconcile himself to his present occupation.

Integration

One of the main features of George's morphogenic data is its characterization of him as a driving, energetic, and ambitious person. A major theme is that he feels he must make himself self-sufficient by becoming so strong and successful that his psychological position will be unassailable. Clearly, his drive, energy, and ambition are integral with this aggressive, competitive, and self-centered approach to life.

Morphogenic data of the kind collected in this research are more sensitive to reactions to the current situation than to feelings about the past: George did not reveal the origins of his belief that he must go at top speed to achieve the dominance and independence he wants. But the data do suggest that an underlying fear of sexual impotence and a fierce rejection of wishes to be passive and dependent drive him to demonstrate his virility and superiority. Sexuality accomplishes for his relationships with women what competitiveness accomplishes in his relationships with men: Both prove that George is not to be dominated. Of course, there would be no necessity for him to prove this if he were not troubled by serious doubts of its truth. When George deals aggressively or sexually with someone, he is trying to conquer himself.

For a long time George thought of drugs as weapons giving him the advantage in his struggle to gain self-sufficiency and make his fortress impregnable. That drugs are powerful and dangerous only made them more exciting; he was sure he could conquer them as he had conquered all other opposition. The morphogenic data do not reveal what happened to provoke the crisis that followed. But at some point George realized that he had finally encountered something stronger than himself, that drugs — and the people involved with them — were dominating him, not he them. At that moment his world must have shattered; George had violated the basic law of his existence by losing control of his fate. Significantly, he did not try to escape responsibility, but placed the blame and the obligation to change directly upon himself. Thus, his first step was to put himself back in control of the situation. It was probably George's turning to religion that gave him the strength to do this; he must believe that God is stronger than any drug.

George is starting to make a new life in which he will again be in charge of his own destiny. Significantly, he is not working to change his basic personality or long-range goals — only to give up drugs. He still wants to achieve social recognition, but he wants to restore his self-control and accomplish his purposes in more restrained ways. In spite of his emotional distance from others, George is capable of love, and he is starting to learn that it need not imply passivity, dependency, or loss of masculine vitality, as he always feared it would. There is hope for George, but as long as he cannot endure the relaxed intimacy and trust that love — divine or human — implies, his troubles will continue.

STYLE OF DRUG USE

General Pattern

George's pattern of drug use was unique in some respects. First, George was twenty-six years of age before he began any heavy use of hard drugs. Second, the range of substances he experimented with was narrow: Aside from marijuana, which he stopped using at about age twenty-four, and methadone, which he has taken for rehabilitative purposes, the only drugs George took on any regular basis were cocaine, heroin, and other opiates. And third, George showed a pattern of "turning on and off" to various drugs: It is almost as if he was engaged in a search, and after a period of experimentation with a drug would conclude, "No, this is not the one."

Table 6.3 shows that alcohol was the drug George used most frequently during his adolescent years. However, regular use of alcohol ended at about age seventeen — "I quit because I got an ulcer." At present, George considers himself a teetotaler — "I'll only drink an occasional glass of wine at parties or when people come to dinner."

From ages nineteen to twenty-four, George used marijuana regularly (several times a week) and tranquilizers on an intermittent basis. He first used marijuana while in Viet Nam. He gave it up at age twenty-four "because I found I really didn't like grass." He reported that he only used tranquilizers intermittently for relaxation.

George began taking amphetamine (diet pills, mini-whites, and crystal) at about age twenty-two. "I ate them. I was just starting in saleswork and I used them – I'd get them fifty to a hundred at a whack – to keep up my drive, energy, and stamina. After a while I said to hell with them because they made me edgy all the time, and I didn't like the speed feeling."

George snorted cocaine off and on socially for two or three years and began intravenous use of it – his first of any drug – at age twenty-six. With daily use of cocaine, George almost immediately began using heroin and other opiates (morphine, Demerol, Dilaudid) to counteract the high. At this time he also had his first brief period of experimentation with hallucinogens. As he said, "Hell, after I started using the needle at twenty-six, I was ready to try anything."

Cocaine seemed to help George in his work as a salesman. "It worked great for a couple of years: I would buy a quarter ounce of coke, use it every day, and it would last me two to three weeks. However, in the last year or so it got out of hand because I was using a quarter ounce a day. That's when I got strung out on heroin; the more cocaine I used, the more opiates I needed to get off the coke high. At the last, I bought a case of a thousand Demerol to sell, but hell, I used them all myself. It got to the point where I couldn't do without it – I was hooked."

George's pattern of increasing cocaine and heroin use continued until he became involved in a "hard run" where he used an ounce of pharmaceutical cocaine in a continuous two-day session. After this terrifying experience, he abruptly stopped using cocaine – but found himself addicted to heroin. He then entered a methadone maintenance program. Concerning this period George remarked, "It was all crazy as hell. I got into coke so I could keep my drive up to sell. I got into heroin to get off the cocaine. Now, I am taking methadone to handle the heroin habit. It's all crazy."

George remained in methadone maintenance for approximately two months. "I got to the point where I even liked the stuff; it took the edge off of everything. I was much easier to get along with and much more comfortable with people." However, he became angry about the required daily trips to the clinic – they disrupted his life. He also became angry that he had become dependent upon methadone. As a result, he precipitously quit the program, underwent "cold-turkey" withdrawal from methadone, and then set about developing a program to rebuild his life.

George states that during the last two to three years his drug use cost him from $100 to $125 per day, approximately. He does not regard this cost as prohibitive. He states he overused cocaine on numerous occasions but never over-

TABLE 6.3. Genealogy and Pattern of Drug Use and Abuse: George B.

Drug Substances	Age (12–30)	Frequency of Drug Usage	Comments
1. Alcohol	(age ~13–30)	Rare	I never really drink now, only an occasional glass of wine.
2. Marijuana	(age ~19–24)	Regular	I did it regular for a while but found I really didn't like it.
3. Psychotropics (Librium, Valium, etc.)	(age ~19–25)	Intermittent	I used them to relax but never on a regular basis.
4. Amphetamine	(age ~22–25)	Intermittent	I ate them but found that I don't like the speed feeling at all.
5. Cocaine	(age ~24–30)	Daily	I snorted socially for two or three years, but once I used the needle with coke, I was really into it.
6. Heroin	(age ~27–30)	Daily	I used it to "come off" coke. I didn't need it till recently. Then I was "hooked".

			Frequency	Comments
7.	Other opiates Demerol Dilaudid morphine	↕ ↕ ↕	Daily	I used Dilaudid and Demerol when heroin was not available to "come off" coke.
8.	Polydrug (cocaine/heroin)	↕	Daily	I used them daily for three years.
9.	Hallucinogens (psychedelics)	↕ (dashed)	Rare	I tried them for a year or so but didn't like it, the "tripping."
10.	Barbiturates		Never	I tried them once and didn't like it.
11.	Illegal methadone		Never	I have enough trouble on legal methadone.
12.	Inhalants		Never	I think some kids do it.
13.	Non-prescription, over-the-counter drugs		Never	I was never into it.
14.	Other			I really didn't use anything till I picked the needle with coke when I was 26, then I got into the opiates, too.

Legend
—— Denotes regular usage
- - - Denotes intermittent usage

191

dosed, blacked out, went into convulsions, or suffered serious medical effects from the drug. He indicates that from the time he "picked up the needle" he had not stopped drug use even for a single day. George says, "A man who breaks completely out of the drug scene by himself would have to be one strong dude."

Preference Rankings

Table 6.4 shows George's strong preference for speedball — cocaine buffered with heroin. Amphetamine occupies the intermediate preference range, being second in preference to cocaine and heroin. Marijuana, barbiturates, and LSD occupy the low intermediate preference range, while hard liquor and beer are the least preferred.

TABLE 6.4. Drug Preference Rankings: George B.

Substance	First Assessment	First Reassessment	Second Reassessment	Mean	Composite Rank
Amphetamine	4	4	4	4.0	4
Barbiturates	6	6	6	6.0	6
Beer	8	9	8	8.3	9
Cocaine	3	2	2	2.3	2
Hard liquor	7	8	9	8.0	8
Heroin	2	3	3	2.7	3
LSD	9	7	7	7.7	7
Marijuana	5	5	5	5.0	5
Speedball	1	1	1	1.0	1

Ratings

Mathematical procedures yield three factors from the semantic differential ratings provided by George. For Factor I he linked cocaine, amphetamine, and speedball (barbiturates had a high negative loading on this factor — meaning that to him they are the *opposite* of the factor members). Drugs positive in this factor were characterized as: strong, beautiful, secure, mighty, refreshed, valuable, clean, healthy, vigorous, and successful. It is consistent with his personality that barbiturates, with their sedative and quieting effects, would constitute a strong negative example of the drugs in this group, for George rejects anything that reduces energy levels. That apparently includes beer and hard liquor, for both also have moderately negative loadings on Factor I.

Factor II contains only drugs-in-general and marijuana. It is a weak factor, describing these as: good, positive, passive, and cautious.

Heroin is not localized in a specific factor; it appears with moderate strength in both the first and second factors.

Factor III is also weak, primarily containing LSD and a slightly negative loading on heroin. George sees LSD as: dangerous, hazardous, loud, bright, hard, fast, rash, strong, and bad.

Pattern of Use

Social Context

George's first experiences with cocaine (snorting it at parties at the age of twenty-three) were positive. "It made me feel good — I liked it because it made me feel powerful, strong, creative. I thought coke was a good party high. I went to parties where there might be as many as ten couples together getting a snorting high." Three years later George began his intravenous use of cocaine: A friend brought some by and asked him if he wanted to try it with the needle, saying it was much better shooting it than snorting. George tried it. "It was a total surprise! I felt so fantastic, I couldn't believe it. I felt like a million dollars. There is no way to describe it. Wow! From that first hit of coke, I never snorted coke from that point on! That may give you some idea of the difference in effects between snorting and shooting."

Most of George's cocaine was taken alone (60 percent) or with one other person (35 to 38 percent). (The remainder [2-5 percent] was taken at parties at the time he first began to use it intravenously.) "I did some coke at parties. There were usually two rooms, like a living room for the snorters and a bedroom or bathroom for the shooters. Women like to snort cocaine, but very few like shooting; they are afraid of the needle and they don't like the blood, so the shooters were usually guys."

The reason George gave for his solitary pattern was, "I just got too damn paranoid!" (Even snorting a gram of pharmaceutical cocaine would generate a mild paranoia.) "After shooting two grams of coke I would start getting paranoid. I would get afraid something was going to happen. You feel like someone is reading your thoughts, that people are out to get you, that the police are going to break the door down any minute. In fact, the quickest way to get paranoid is to live alone and do coke, because you misinterpret the normal noises and sounds in a building; you get to thinking you hear people whispering about you. Besides that, you get deceitful, scheming thoughts and ideas as well: You think about things like how you might get even with someone who has been unfair with you. You get obscene thoughts like dreaming up an orgy, or how you might do a sex orgy with one individual. It is pretty damn scary, so when I had used up to two grams of coke, I went to my place or I would be with one other person I trusted. A lot of the time, however, I would drive out in the country where I could be outside, be by myself, and get unwired."

George did not feel cocaine was an aphrodisiac. "I thought it was, at first, but not now. It only prolongs intercourse and the climax; it gives you stamina to last longer. Now I really think you do better when you're normal. People don't realize it, but you're pretty numb; after two grams, I would be so numb that all I would get shooting was the rush and the ringing in my ears. I really don't see how it is possible to have a greater climax on cocaine after you get so numb." Though George did not feel intravenous cocaine was an aphrodisiac for men, he thought snorting might be an aphrodisiac for women.

For the past two years George used intravenous pharmaceutical cocaine on a daily, three-grams-per-day basis. "I have done six grams a day, but I was a bumbling idiot." The largest amount he ever used was an ounce of pharmaceutical cocaine during a two-day run, an experience so terrifying that he gave up cocaine immediately afterward.

When cocaine was available in substantial quantities George would take it in runs. "If it's there and available in quantities, you get started. Once you get started, you don't stop until it is all gone." Over a two-year period he did about twelve or fifteen cocaine runs. These were of two kinds: short ("hard") runs of one or two days' duration, without sleep (using from two to four grams of cocaine per day), and long runs of one or two week's duration (also using from two to four grams per day), "crashing" or "mellowing out" at night with heroin or other opiates — he would have a fix waiting in the morning and then start all over again. His longest run was of two months' duration. The only circumstance needed to trigger a run was the availability of cocaine. However, he reported a typical daily pattern in his use of the drug: "I'd fire up before I went to work in the morning, then I would go out and be with people. I would fire up again during the day if I needed it."

George stated that 90 percent of the cocaine he used was pharmaceutical, the remainder being rock crystal. "It came from the drugstore and was still in the jar. It costs more, but if you had the money and the contacts you could do pharmaceutical cocaine most of the time." Although George tried street cocaine, he generally avoided it — "the effects of street coke are a long way from the effects of pharmaceutical cocaine." The only way he could discriminate with certainty between pharmaceutical and street cocaine was to put it in his arm. "They will give you ten cents worth free. Good coke also has an alcoholic smell. The rush is different and the taste is different with street and pharmaceutical cocaine." George did not know if he could discriminate between cocaine and procaine: "I have been told the procaine rush or flash is more like an amphetamine rush, but I don't know. Maybe I have used some procaine or benzocaine; I don't think so, but if I did it was good."

It is George's opinion that one's body develops a *temporary* tolerance to cocaine. "I shot cocaine every day for two years. My guess is that I had to increase the size of the hit after about one-fifth gram; I would be shooting a half gram by the end of the day." It was necessary for him to wait two or three days after a run before he could get back to that first hit because "cocaine stays in your system approximately seventy-two hours."

The withdrawal reaction was always difficult for George. "You can't relax.

If you lay down, you're wide awake. You know you are not going to sleep or get any rest. You're depressed and anxious as hell that you have run out of coke. You're physically tired and worn out, but you're still hyper. Occasionally, I would get a headache coming off; also, a coke run makes me very thirsty. This is why I used heroin and other opiates or, if there was nothing better, tranquilizers to get down off the cocaine."

Reactions to Cocaine

Physiological Reactions

The physiological reactions that occurred every time George used cocaine (table 6.5) included: increased heart, respiration, and pulse rates, loss of sensations of hunger and fatigue, excessive and rapid mental activity, increased urination, tightness in the chest, increased light sensitivity, dizziness, and anesthesia. To him, these reactions indicated that his body was mobilized for action; he could work at a high level for long hours without respite.

A second cluster of physical reactions occurring with high frequency, but not complete regularity, included: weight loss, ringing in the ears, diarrhea or "dumping" bowel movements immediately after injection, and muscle spasms. George reported he vomited only once — "I thought it was the water I drank" — but that nausea was a common sequel to cocaine use — "I felt nauseous about 70 to 80 percent of the time."

George reported none of the other physiological reactions typically associated with snorting cocaine. He stated he had never fainted while using cocaine — "I came close once" — experienced gooseflesh or convulsions, or noticed any remarkable sweating or yawning. Although he developed serious abscesses or "burns" a few times, he never developed hepatitis — "If you use new needles, that doesn't happen."

Psychological Reactions

The psychological reactions George reported (table 6.6) were also remarkably consistent. The positive reactions occurring every time he used cocaine included: increased restlessness, excitement, self-confidence, optimism, and euphoria — "I felt like I was on top of the world and could do anything!" — the feeling that the world was perfect — "It was as perfect as it could be" — increased strength and motivation for work accompanied by greater ability to perform, increased thinking power, imagination, and talkativeness, indifference to pain — "I felt no pain at all. It was great!" — and the notion that his mind was quicker than others' and he could think faster than they could.

Along with the positive effects mentioned above, George reported a group of adverse reactions that always occurred with his cocaine use. These included: sleeplessness and insomnia, increased anxiety, irrational fears, and paranoia, auditory and olfactory hallucinations, and changes in perceived reality (which George attributed to lack of sleep and fatigue).

TABLE 6.5. Physiological Reactions to Cocaine Use and Abuse: George B.

Commonly Reported Reaction to Cocaine Use/Abuse	Reactions Observed Yes	No	Percent/ Time Observed	Qualifying Comments and Observations
Dizziness – feeling of light-headedness	Yes		90	You get a bit dizzy and light-headed with the rush.
Sweating – perspiration or increases in temperature		No		It may be, but I didn't notice it.
Rhinorrhea – running nose		No		Not shooting, but you get it snorting. You get to the point where you can't control your nose; it dribbles all the time. The only way to stop it is stop snorting.
Tremors – muscle spasms	Yes		40	I would get tremors during and coming off a long run. I couldn't stop them.
Lacrimation – tears to eyes		No		I don't remember that happening either snorting or shooting.
Mydriasis – dilation of pupils, light sensitivity	Yes		80	Your eyes become very sensitive to bright light. At times when you stare at something, it would get misty or hazy.
Gooseflesh		No		It didn't happen to me.
Emesis – vomiting		No		I only vomited once after a long hard drive. I think it was the water. You feel kind of nauseous during the rush about 80–90 percent of the time.
Reactive hyperemia – clogging of nasal airways		No		Not shooting. You get that about 75 percent of the time snorting though.
Anorexia – loss of appetite, sensation for hunger	Yes		100	Yes, two or three days after a run you get your appetite back, though.
Dryness of mouth and throat, lack of salivation	Yes		80	It happened pretty regular with me.
Increased heart rate	Yes		100	I didn't get it much at snorting, but every time I was shooting you could feel your heart pounding.
Tightness in chest or chest pains	Yes		100	It's a flexing of all the chest muscles. You just feel puffed up. It's tight, though.
Local anesthesia, numbness	Yes		100	I had it both snorting and shooting. Snorting, my nose, sinuses, teeth, gums, and lips would all get

				numb. It wouldn't happen right off the bat snorting, you wouldn't realize it. I was shooting so much I would be numb all over.
Nosebleed		No		Once in a while snorting.
Elevation of pulse rate	Yes		100	If it's good coke, every hit takes your breath away. You breathe hard.
Increased respiration rate	Yes		100	Your whole system is fired up.
Cellulitis – inflammation following administration		No		It happened two or three times snorting.
Infection of nasal mucous membrane		No		I used a nasal spray to rinse when I was snorting coke.
Yawning		No		Not that I remember.
Hyperphrenia – excessive mental activity	Yes		100	Your mind runs fast and so does your imagination.
Weight loss	Yes		50	If you stayed on a long run, you would lose weight because you don't eat. You would get back in four or five days after a two or three day run.
Fainting		No		I came close to fainting a couple of times, but I never did. I have seen other people black right out after a hit.
Increased sensitivity to allergies		No		I am not allergic to anything.
Diarrhea or explosive bowel movements	Yes		20	Sometimes I had to go take a dump right after I fired up.
Hepatitis or liver infections		No		I never did.
Headaches	Yes		20	I've had headaches during and coming off a run. I thought it was the cut. It didn't happen all the time.
Loss of fatigue	Yes		100	You just aren't tired at all. You feel great.
Ringing in the ears	Yes		60	With good coke they will ring.
Convulsions		No		I've been crazy as hell, but I never had convulsions.
Increased urination	Yes		100	You're whole body is stimulated.
Abscesses	Yes			I had them only two or three times. You can get them even when you hit the vein. They can come two or three weeks after shooting. They are hard to clear up.
Tooth Decay	Yes		50	Coke causes you to develop more cavities. It may be the cut, the lactose that does it.

TABLE 6.6. Psychological Reactions to Cocaine Use and Abuse: George B.

Commonly Reported Reactions to Cocaine Use/Abuse	Reactions Observed Yes	Reactions Observed No	Percent/ Time Observed	Qualifying Comments and Observations
Increased feelings of self-control	Yes		50	I felt like I had better control of myself at the time. However, it finally got to where the coke was controlling me.
Increased optimism, courage	Yes		100	I felt like I could do anything. I had this fantastic sense of self-confidence, like I was at the top of the world.
Increased activity, restlessness, excitement	Yes		100	You are hyper and restless as hell. Whatever you did you were really "into" it.
Feeling of increased physical strength or ability to do physical work	Yes		100	I not only felt like I could do more work, I did do more work! I ran circles around the other salesmen. You can go like hell on coke.
Intensified feelings of well-being, euphoria, "floating," etc.	Yes		100	Yes, it was fantastic how good you feel! I can't even describe it.
Feeling that everything is perfect	Yes		100	I didn't feel like everything was perfect, but I felt like things damned well were as perfect as they possibly could be.
An exquisite "don't care about the world" attitude	Yes		30	Occasionally. That's really more a heroin reaction.
A physical orgasm in the "rush"		No		No, that's rather absurd. The rush is good but not like that.
Increased thinking power and imagination	Yes		80	Your mind and imagination go like crazy. You get all kinds of crazy thoughts—deceitful schemes, obscene thoughts, too. You dream up a sex orgy or a plot against a person. It goes fast.
Feeling that the mind is quicker than normal, the feeling that one is smarter than everyone else	Yes		100	Your mind does move quicker, you're sharper, more on your toes. You feel like you can outwit the other guy.
More talkative than usual, a stream of talk	Yes		100	If you're with someone else, you're kind of goofy-acting. You just rattle on.

Indifference to pain	Yes	100	You don't notice it. It is not much bother to you.
Decreased interest in work, failure of ambition, loss of ambition for useful work	No		I always was able to do more work on coke unless I was on a run. Then the only thing you think of is that next hit. If I would fire up good coke in the morning, it would motivate me. I could triple what everyone else was doing.
Insomnia	Yes	100	It is very hard to go to sleep. You have to take tranquilizers, heroin, or something to "get down."
Depression, anxiety	Yes	100	I wouldn't get depressed as long as there was another hit. I would get depressed and anxious as hell if I ran out.
Prolonged sexual intercourse	Yes	100	You can stay longer. That's about all.
An aphrodisiac or sexual stimulant	No		Not for me, but it is for women. They are easier to bed. Coke takes their inhibitions away. They are ready for sex orgies. They will try anything.
Better orgasm on coke	No		No, all it did was prolong intercourse if you can "get up." If you do a lot of coke, I don't know how you could have a greater climax when you are numb all over. I never had a greater climax on coke in my life.
Irrational fears	Yes	100	It will happen every time but only with prolonged use.
Terror or panic	Yes	100	Every time with prolonged use. I freaked out and went crazy as hell a couple of times, but I was doing quarter-ounce hits at the end of a long, hard run.
Tactile hallucinations — the feeling that insects, bugs, ants are crawling on or under the skin (particularly fingertips, palms of hands, etc.)	Yes	30	Sometimes, you feel like something is crawling on you. I thought they were bugs. I tried to brush them off. It would only happen with prolonged use, though.
Changes, in reality or the way a room or objects look — the wall waving or in motion, etc.	Yes	100	If you are up past two days. I'm not sure it's the coke. I had the same problem in Nam, and I wasn't doing drugs at all. I think it was the lack of sleep, the mental fatigue.

TABLE 6.6. Psychological Reactions to Cocaine Use and Abuse: George B. (continued)

Commonly Reported Reactions to Cocaine Use/Abuse	Reactions Observed — Yes	Reactions Observed — No	Percent/ Time Observed	Qualifying Comments and Observations
Paranoid ideas — the feeling that people are after you. You believe you are being watched, talked about or threatened, a wife or girlfriend is unfaithful, untrustworthy, etc.	Yes		100	Two or three grams of coke and I get very paranoid. I couldn't trust anyone. You get to thinking people can read your mind, they are out to get you, the police will break in any minute, and things like that.
Causes one to carry a gun or run from imaginary enemies	Yes		10	I carried a gun for a while and did some running, too.
Visual hallucinations		No		I never did see things that weren't there. It was mostly sounds.
Auditory hallucinations — hearing voices talking about you, threatening, etc.	Yes		100	You misinterpret sounds on coke, you make something out of a sound. Someone turns on the water to wash their hands and everyone jumps up, pulls out their gun, and starts looking all around. It's scary as hell. You hear a little noise, and you misinterpret it: "Let's see if we can break the door down", — it sounds like whispers.
Olfactory hallucinations — new odors, smells, etc.	Yes		100	You don't really hallucinate odors. It's just that all your senses are heightened. You just notice odors more.
A trigger for violence		No		Not for me. I could see how after prolonged use it might be for some people. I never hit anyone. I once thought a guy was ripping me off; I confronted him, but there were no blows.

A second, small cluster of psychological reactions which were frequent but not unfailing occurrences included: increased feelings of self-control (50–60 percent), a "don't-give-a-damn" attitude toward the world (30 percent), and tactile hallucinations.

George reported that his cocaine use was never associated with a failure of ambition — "Hell, I was always able to go out and perform" — or a more spectacular sexual orgasm. He said that on two or three occasions he had "freaked out" on cocaine, carried a gun, and run in terror from imaginary enemies. However, he was ambivalent about whether he thought cocaine could trigger violence or antisocial behavior: "It didn't for me. I am not a violent person at all. I never struck anyone doing cocaine. I confronted or intimidated a guy once who I thought had ripped me off, but we never came to blows. However, I think that after prolonged use the potential for violence is there; I think the potential is there."

Integration

Of the several purposes cocaine served in George's life, a major one was its contribution to his success as a salesman. It "fired him up" and provided energy reserves for his work; he became a fast, efficient Maserati that could outperform the others.

George's typical usage was three grams of pharmaceutical cocaine per day. (He noted, however, that after two grams he only felt numb.)

Given his recurring references to the absence of pain with cocaine use, one gets the impression that George was attempting to obliterate all feelings except aggression. He sought and enjoyed the experience of being free of most negative feelings, feelings which are normal components of human experience. If he began to feel depressed, he could simply eradicate these feelings with cocaine and not have to deal with the question of what caused this emotional state. Similarly, if he became tense, anxious, or unable to relax at night, he could use opiates to help him fall into a drugged sleep, again without having to contend with the circumstances precipitating his anxiety. Thus, drugs permitted George to control his emotional states chemically, and avoid dealing in a reflective way with unpleasant aspects of his existence.

LIFE ACTIVITIES AND EXPERIENCES: IN GEORGE'S OWN WORDS

Overview

This section provides a detailed account of two days in George's life. The first day took place approximately one month after he had been through a shattering experience with cocaine, had married, joined the church, and entered a metha-done maintenance program for his addiction to opiates (developed through cocaine use). The second day occurred almost five months later.

At the time of the first day George was trying to stabilize on methadone and begin putting his life back together. George talks at length about his way of life, his view of himself, what has happened to him, and his plans for the future. He has not yet at this point mapped out the self-rehabilitation program that he ultimately will adopt. Later, on the second day, George tells how this rehabili-tation plan has gone and complains about the price he feels he is paying for it.

The first day begins with George taking his wife to work. After returning home George describes his last and final cocaine run, a terrifying experience; almost a month later, he is still frightened by it. He makes some business calls, then picks up his wife for lunch; George describes the characteristics of his wife which caused him, fiercely independent as he is, to marry her. Later he visits with his boss and closes a sale with a customer. George is reassured to learn that he is still able to sell; he had begun to fear that he might not be able to now that he had stopped using cocaine. George then drives to the clinic to get his methadone, describing his initial reactions to the drug, and picks up his wife at work. After supper they go to church. Afterward, they visit with a few couples on the church steps and then drive home.

The second day takes place in mid-July, almost five months after the first day. During the preceding months, George had instituted a "cold-turkey" with-drawal from methadone and, as part of his self-rehabilitation program, had left sales, taking employment as a draftsman-designer. (He had never done this before, but he is a versatile man and was doing the job well.) His plan was to stay in a "routine" job until early 1976; at the end of this period he would return to sales.

During this day George becomes increasingly restless and frustrated. He cannot understand how other workers stay on a job like this. He wonders about his future and toys with the idea of going back into sales. (Subsequently he did just that.) George works all day, then rushes to a night class, wondering on the way if it is worth it. After class, George goes home and ruminates on his dis-satisfaction. His rehabilitation plan is working, but he is paying a high price for it. He wants back into sales where he can make some money. For him, money is a measure of his competence.

Activity and Experience Audit

First Day: A Wednesday in January

7:30–8:00 a.m.

The alarm woke me up, I got up and got dressed. I also woke my wife, and she got ready to go to work.

8:00–10:30 a.m.

I drove Darlene to work, then came right back home; I have been taking her to work because her car is in the garage being worked on. As usual — since I have been on methadone — I didn't feel good. I didn't feel bad, I was just numb. I was thinking on the way home, What am I going to do when spring comes and the selling season starts? This can't go on!

I got home and fed my "buddies," my cats. Then I fixed myself some tea. (I usually don't eat breakfast.) I had the TV on, but wasn't paying attention to it because I was playing with my cats.

I was thinking about going to church tonight. My church and my religion have been a real help to me, trying to get out of drugs; you just don't worry about a lot of the things that used to bother you. I was never too religious till I got into this thing.

I get scared sometimes thinking about those days. When I was down talking with you that first day, it scared me just to talk about coke and what had happened to me; I almost didn't come back. I am not as scared now. I figure maybe some of this might help someone else.

I was crazy when I decided to quit. I was on that last run for two days, I just sat there on the bathroom stool firing one right after the other all day and night. My wife couldn't stop me. I know she tried! The longer I sat there, the crazier I got! She was at work the second morning and I was alone banging away. I was very paranoid; every time I heard a noise I would almost jump out of my skin! I didn't hallucinate, but I sure as hell was misinterpreting sounds — I thought the police were going to break in any minute. I began to get terrified, so I called some friends and begged them to come and help me. They got there and knocked on the door — I panicked! I flushed all the stuff down the stool, grabbed my car keys, went out the porch door, jumped in my car, and drove off as fast as I could go. I drove and drove till I was way out in the country. I kept watching my rear-view mirror to make sure the police weren't following me. It was pouring down rain; it was a wonder I didn't wreck the car! I found a big, wooded hill where you could see in all directions, hid my car, and ran up that hill stumbling and falling — running for my life! I finally got to the top and sat down there in the rain, watching all around, constantly looking and watching anything that moved. I sat out there almost all day in the pouring rain getting myself together.

I was in Nam for almost a year, my marine unit was in combat most of the time, and I was scared every time we went into action — but I have never been as terrified as I was out there in the rain. There is really no way to describe how I felt, just sheer terror! That run broke it; shortly after that I gave my life to God and asked Him to help me.

10:30–11:30 a.m.

I got on the phone and called three different businessmen. I was still feeling numb; that really gets me.

Then I went in the bathroom and soaked my infected arm in epsom salts to reduce the pain. The arm was not quite as swollen as the day before, but it has settled down to a dull throb now; the doctor said it would take a few days to get the infection under control. The pain pills help, but it still hurts. However, I am still feeling just numb — I was thinking I must be getting too much methadone.

11:30 a.m.–1:00 p.m.

I drove out to pick up my wife for lunch. She was waiting for me. I was sure glad to see her. She has stood by me through all of this. I don't like to lean on anyone; however, I depend on her, and she never lets me down. She is not like most women. She never crowds me, nor tries to tell me what to do, but she is always there when I need her. One thing I like about my wife is that she is a strong and very capable woman, she can stand on her own feet.

We drove home, fixed lunch, and ate it. She asked how I was feeling and how my arm was. We chatted and looked through the mail. I felt good, numb like before. About 12:50, I drove Darlene back to work. We didn't talk much.

1:00–2:30 p.m.

I drove on to where I work, and chatted with my boss. He said I looked pale. I told him I had been sick; it should have been obvious because my arm was in a sling. I like working for the guy; he doesn't crowd me, and as long as I do my job we don't have any problems. I guess there is no reason we should, because I am paid for what I deliver! I like it that way.

We did some planning on some sales coming up this spring. He told me to take good care of my arm; I said I would, and left. I enjoyed our visit; he is a very successful salesman, and I respect competence.

Next, I drove over to close a sale with a customer. The guy and I closed the deal and wrapped it up. We had been working on it for a while. It wasn't a big sale, and I didn't make a lot of money, but I was glad to know I could still sell something despite all the things that have happened to me. It was reassuring to me.

2:30–4:30 p.m.

I drove on down to the clinic to get my methadone. I don't like to go there; I try to go early, get my medicine, and get out. I don't talk much to the other people, except the nurse. I don't know if it's that I am ashamed to go there or what. It sure doesn't help my self-confidence to do it, but I need it now. When I got there, I chatted briefly with the nurse, took my methadone, and left.

I drove on back home from the clinic. I was first thinking I wished I didn't have to be on the stuff. Doing it every day breaks up an afternoon with the drive back and forth and all, but I don't need to be sick now.

I got home, turned on the stereo, sat down, and started working on our income taxes. I worked pretty steady at it and got part of it done. I was feeling numb again, neither happy nor sad; the methadone had taken effect. I thought, well, at least you're doing something constructive. Right after I first started on it the methadone hit me so hard I could hardly get out of the house. The nurse had told me I had to accept the fact that I was coming off of being on something every day, too. Before, if I felt down, depressed or anything, I would pop something. I figured my body had to readjust to being without all of that stuff, too.

4:30–5:30 p.m.
I drove out and picked up my wife at work. She was tired, but in a good mood. She was relieved that my arm had started to get a bit better. We stopped at the grocery store again and bought a few things. It was good to be with my wife, although I don't enjoy shopping. Maybe that's not quite right; I don't mind the shopping, I just hate to put out the money to pay for it. Our finances haven't been so hot since I got all strung out. That's one reason I wanted to get our income taxes done so we could get our refund back.
I drove on home. My wife was chatting about what had happened at work. I felt good to have her with me.

5:30–7:00 p.m.
We fixed supper and ate. I was eating and watching the "Star Trek" program; it's good and I like it. I also like a program, "Nova," that comes on educational TV. They are both good.
Darlene cleaned up the dishes. When the program was over, I went upstairs, took a shower, and dressed for church. (Darlene was already dressed.)

7:00–9:00 p.m.
We drove down to the church.
There was a good crowd. There was the usual thing; singing, the sermon, and all. Darlene and I do not know too many of the people very well yet, but it gives me some peace inside to be there. We said hello to three or four couples we have gotten acquainted with since we started going. They were about our age. We just chatted about the sermon and things. I enjoyed the evening, of course; church has to be a positive experience, doesn't it?

9:00–11:00 p.m.
Darlene and I went home. She was saying we should invite one or two of them over sometime. I agreed, but really I am not so sure I am ready for much of that yet; I would like to be more on top of my thing before we do a lot of socializing. The mess I got into had knocked my self-confidence down a bit. You know, I guess it's maybe the first thing I got into where I couldn't keep control of myself. I want that confidence back!
We got home, got our clothes off, turned the TV on, and just relaxed. I don't even know what we watched; I was just relaxing, sitting next to my wife. We didn't even talk much.

Finally I turned the TV off — it was not very good, whatever was on — went upstairs and got ready for bed. I was pretty tired, so I went right to sleep.

The Day: A pretty good day.

Second Day: A Wednesday in July

6:00—7:00 a.m.

I woke up with the alarm. I got up, shaved, and cleaned up. I was feeling pretty good, I guess.

I went downstairs and fed my buddies, my cats. I had some tea. Then I went out and got the paper. I was thinking it was a nice day; it was not too hot yet. I got ready and left for work. I didn't wake Darlene, she had her alarm set for herself.

I drove to work. I was thinking how nice it would be to go on vacation. I left a little early to stop and get some cigarettes at a 7-11 store; I didn't say anything to the clerk — to hell with him. I got in my car and drove on to work.

I am back thinking about vacations. I have been working long hours, twelve to fourteen hours a day since early May. I wanted to get away from it all for a while and go to the mountains where it is cool and secluded. Hell, I would get away from everyone except the animals. I have been thinking about moving to the mountains some place. I want to change my environment and get away from this screwed-up world. I haven't been able to figure out what I would do, though; I would have to be close enough to a city where I could make some money — I have to work.

7:00 a.m.—12:00 n.

I went in and got me a coke out of the machine; I filled the coke machine. Bill, the engineer and vice president, came in. Jim, the owner, was not there. It's unlike Jim not to be at work; it's his business and he's a "workaholic." He has worked us all twelve to fourteen hours a day for two months. Now he's not here. I thought well, maybe he is sick or something.

I said hi to Bill, then went in and sat down at my drafting board. It's a helluva way to start your day, but I was there because I wanted to be, I guess. I sat there about fifteen minutes trying to figure out how to make this part I was drawing move. My job is okay, I guess, but it is temporary. I like outside work where I am out part of the time, at least; this is a drag. I keep telling myself I can take it till next spring, then I will go back to sales. I have been giving serious thoughts to what I am doing, like working where I am as opposed to other work. This job is getting on my nerves. I can always get back on selling cars on weekends. It's all commission work. The owner is a friend of mine, he knows what I can do. Besides, he takes no risk; I only get paid for what I sell —that's fair. I'll still look around. I am doing okay, but it is very frustrating. The hours bother me — no, it's not that either: I am doing the same thing every damn day! That's what gets me! Every day is the same! Some of the guys out there in the shop do the same thing all their lives; I don't know how they stand it. It's not that I don't appreciate having the job, but it runs against the grain for me. I have no real mental involvement in my job! It's no challenge for me! I feel like I am not getting anywhere. I was thinking how I was making three or four thousand dollars at a whack instead of what I am making now. I don't know if business will be good next spring when I want to go back or whether it will be a bust; they say things are getting better, but I don't know. Maybe next year will be too late.

After a while, I went back out in the shop and talked with Bill about this damn part. He thought I was trying to make something complicated out of something simple. Hell, I have never been a draftsman before, but I do the job well; I learn anything quick when I want to, and I have done a good job for Jim and Bill, Anyway, I like Bill; he is easy to get along with, he kids a lot. We have a conference about the damn part. We decided to use a lever-and-button arrangement. That settled my problem, more or less. I went back and started to draw the part.

The secretary told me Jim was staying home today. He's not feeling too well.

I know some guys spend their lives sitting at drafting boards, but I don't really know how they do it.

I wondered if the part would work after it was put together.

I took a break and went outside and had a cigarette. It kind of bugs me, this routine. I kept thinking I know what I am going to do all next week! It bothered me. After I had my cigarette, I went back to work. It was not boring work, just frustrating. I was thinking that if a person is bored it's his own fault; I think you can make anything interesting if you set your mind to it.

I had Bill come in and look at the design. He said he thought it would work. I didn't think it would work, but he knows more about this than I do. At least I tried to check it out with him. I went back to drawing again, thinking that for something so damn simple this damn part is awfully hard to lay out and draw.

Right before lunch, Jim, the owner, came in. He wanted to know how I was doing; I told him okay. He got on the phone for awhile. (When I got back from lunch he was still there talking.)

12:00 n.–12:30 p.m.

I drove to a store and bought myself some hard-boiled eggs, a sausage, some milk, and a candy bar, then I drove back to work. I sat down under a tree by the office to eat lunch. Bill came out, sat down, and ate his lunch with me. We chatted. It was cool there under the tree.

12:30–5:00 p.m.

I went back to the damn board. I get disgusted with the board sometimes; I have to just walk away from it. I guess a lot of my problem is that I just won't look at my job in any permanent perspective. I don't intend to stay there, thank God, I don't! I don't think I could do it year after year.

I worked at the damn board all afternoon. I am looking forward to leaving. I was thinking I would be glad to see 5:00 p.m. come.

5:00–6:00 p.m.

I left work and drove home. I was thinking I have to get organized so I can get to school on time. (I usually work till 5:30, but it's a school night and I leave at 5:00 p.m. so I will be able to get there.) I drove home, not thinking much about anything except getting to class on time.

At home, I drank a quick glass of iced tea, showered, and changed my clothes. Darlene came home; she fixed me a sandwich. I took my tea, my sandwich and books, and left for school. I drove. I was wondering on the way if it was really worth it. I was learning things in one class, my philosophy class. The other class is a business class; I think it is a bummer! I was thinking, when all of this rushing around was done I would probably not be any better off than I was before. I have always been a person who figures to make my time work for me.

6:00–9:00 p.m.

I got to class and sat down. It's a usual-size evening class, maybe thirty people. The guy was talking about Oedipus Rex, the king, and his tragic flaw; he gave me the feeling he was interested in the subject. I only know one person in the class, and he's not here tonight; I don't even know the leader, whoever he is. I always sit by myself. There are big tables placed around the room; there is plenty of space. I am a loner, I guess. I am thinking the instructor is a pretty good teacher, he stayed with the subject pretty well.

9:00–11:00 p.m.

I get in my car and go home. It's strange, when I think about it: I go to that class and I only know one person.

I got home. Darlene was upstairs washing her hair and taking a shower and changing her clothes. She can take all night at that when she gets started at it.

I got some tea, and went out on the patio and sat down. I just sat there mulling over what has been going on the last few weeks — my job, school, and things. I concluded, my rehabilitation plan is working but I am paying a high price for it; it is causing frustration and duress for me. It is not bothering my wife, she is happy with the way things are going. I am not very satisfied with it at all. I want to go back to selling. I had decided to stay out of sales till the first of the year, to give me time to get myself together, but I have been thinking I want to find a job that is not so routine! There is definitely no excitement in it for me.

I guess the main thing I have been worried about is the cash flow. I am not making the money I was making three to four months ago. For a salesman, money is a measure of how good he is. By that standard I am not doing very well now. I told my wife maybe I am getting to be afraid to take a gamble, a risk; I find myself, instead of going out and buying something we need, I let it ride.

I was thinking about this. Darlene came out and asked me if I wanted some tea; I told her no — she went back in the house to dry her hair.

It is beginning to scare me a little. I don't want to be a "Freddie Lunch Bucket"; I can see it sort of developing. We are going to have to have a new car before long. Everything adds up to problems. I can only get in debt so far, I don't want to always be in debt, and you have to work to pay all of that off whether you like it or not. It is all kind of scary. I am not going to live that way!

11:00 p.m.

I went in the house, locked up, went upstairs, and went to bed. Darlene was still messing with her hair. I went right to sleep — I don't remember when Darlene came to bed.

The Day: The day was uneventful, just an indifferent day. I am getting too many of those lately. I can't live that way!

7

Al G.

LIFE THEMES

Al G. is a black street hustler in the ghetto. He is a gentle man with a physical disability, and was described by an acquaintance as a grape: He has a thin skin and is soft inside. He is a man who has lived in a world of hustlers, whores, addicts, and dealers, where violence is commonplace and death may wait in the shadows. Although Al has never achieved much in life, he has continued to try. The dominant themes in his life are these:

- I live in a world where everything seems designed to hurt me.
- I can't survive by fighting like others do, because I am weak and frail.
- The only way I can survive is by getting along—tricking people but being careful, not making enemies, and avoiding danger.
- All I really want is peace, contentment, and safety.

Cocaine Use in Relation to Life Themes

Al was a daily, intravenous, low-dosage user of speedball mixtures of cocaine and heroin. These drugs helped him feel less impotent in a predatory world. More specifically, they

- helped Al feel more self-assured and assertive,
- accelerated his mental activity, abolished fatigue, and made him more alert to events and the intentions of others,

- made him more at ease in situations in which he otherwise would have felt apprehensive,
- reduced the confusion that pervaded his existence, and
- neutralized the adverse effects of each drug taken separately, minimizing the likelihood that he would overdose with either.

EVOLUTION OF LIFE STYLE

Introduction

Al G. is a thirty-five-year-old Negro male. He is thin, hunchbacked, and walks with a distinct limp. Usually he wears an elevated shoe on one foot; sometimes he uses a cane. Al's dress is casual but somewhat disheveled: He usually wears a long-sleeve shirt, crumpled slacks, scuffed brown shoes, and a white waist-length athletic jacket with red trim. In cold weather he wears a scarf and knee-length coat over the same jacket, with a stocking cap pulled down over his ears. In warm weather he replaces the stocking cap with a black, wide-brimmed hat with a chrome-silver hatband.

Al's face is long and angular. He has a thin mustache and a wispy goatee. His large, limpid eyes are bright, alert, and restless. Al has proved to be a gentle but insecure and cynical man. His demeanor is that of a person who had just been in a fight and lost. Al is somewhat suspicious and alert to changes in social situations. Initially, he was tense at our interviews and would hardly do more than answer direct questions. However, as he became more comfortable, he relaxed and was more at ease — in fact, he relished the opportunity to talk about his life as an addict and street hustler. This does not mean that Al was entirely honest. If he felt the discussion was turning to dangerous topics, he would lie, change the subject, or scowl. On occasion Al obviously exaggerated, but we accepted his statements, though we tried not to allow his exaggerations to distort our assessment of his typical behavior.

Al stated that this was the first time in his life anyone had indicated that his ideas were worth anything, much less paid for them. He said that if his story might help people understand addicts or help some kid stay away from drugs, he would be very pleased. Though Al has made his living through subterfuge and dissimulation, we believed him when he said this.

Developmental Experiences

Al was the oldest child in a black ghetto family. He had a younger sister, a younger stepbrother, and a stepsister. "We was real poor. I never met my real father. Shit, I thought my stepdad was my real father till I was about nine or ten years old. A kid in school told me my father wasn't my real father — we had a fight right there! When I got home that night I asked my dad if he was my real dad; he said no, but he told me that he loved me as much as if I were his real son. I was really upset. The next year, he legally adopted me. It was sure as hell confusin' at school because I had one name in school already, and I had to change it to another one after my stepdad adopted me. Some of the kids harassed me about my names; I had some fights over it, but I lost most of 'em. I was born with a bad back and I could never get around as fast as the other kids.

"My stepdad was just like a typical father. He looked after his family even though it was a big one. He only went to the third or fourth grade, but he worked every day. He was a good carpenter and jack-of-all-trades; he could do most anything. He was also a part-time minister. He was a quiet, easygoin' man. I guess we were pretty close. We worked together around the house, buildin' things. He was a strict disciplinarian, though. Shit, he'd grab the nearest tree limb or a belt and give me a whippin', but I don't think I ever got a whippin' from him that I didn't deserve. My stepdad died when I was twelve or thirteen. He was close to seventy then, was in retirement, and was drawin' his old age pension. He just died in his sleep one night. I missed him after he was gone; he was a good stepdad."

When asked if there was anything he would change about his stepfather if he could live his life over, Al said, "No, I would just have him be my real father, that's all." When asked what were the most important lessons he learned from his stepfather Al stated, "I guess I learned to accept things the way they are, whatever it is."

"My mother was a heck of a lady. She was overly protective of me, though. She was a cripple, too, but she'd come runnin' if I was in a scuffle; she'd make me go back in and fight. It was scary as hell, 'cause I ain't no fighter. Shit, she'd have me fighting kids and she'd be fighting with their mothers over me. She said you had to fight even if you lose, 'cause that way them kids won't pick on you anymore. I guess she was right, but I didn't like it worth a shit.

"My mother ran everything in our house, includin' my stepdad. He would just laugh at her, but he'd do what the hell ever she told him. Shit, us kids wouldn't have had nothin' 'cept for her. She only went to the sixth grade, but she knew how to make a little bit go a long way. She worked as a nursin' aide in a hospital — did housework for some rich white people — was a waitress — did day work in a factory. We was never on welfare, my mom was too proud for that."

"My mom was very affectionate. Even though she was crippled, she'd get out in the yard and play with us kids. I could talk to my mother when I had problems. I wouldn't talk to my dad 'cause he was in the study, readin' or gettin' ready for his sermons on Sunday.

"My mom was a good mom, but she was very strict, too. I'd rather my old man whip me any time than my mom. She'd get mad quick and grab anything she could get her hands on and bust you with it. She expected her kids to mind and we did.

"I guess I was my mom's favorite — that's what my sister and stepbrother and stepsister always said. I don't know, but she always looked after me, gave me money and all for movies and things. Maybe I was the favorite."

When asked what he would do to change his mother if he had his life to live over, Al said, "I wouldn't change her at all except I would want things to be easier for her." When asked what lessons he had learned from his mother, Al stated, "She said I had to fight, and I did some, but the fact is I ain't no fighter and I could get all busted up tryin' to be one! I am too skinny and have a fucked up back, and I am supposed to fight? I would be annihilated. She never understood that. I don't like to fight; maybe I'm more of a lover than a damn fighter!"

When asked about his relationships with his sister, stepbrother, and stepsister, Al stated, "I was kinda close to my sister, but we don't get along too good now. I don't get along with her husband neither! She married another woman! He's a weak, passive man — I don't respect that. By the time my sister was thirty years old she was an alcoholic; That bug-juice took over her whole life, she just sits and drinks. I'm sorry about that, but that's how it is. I was never really very close to my stepbrother or stepsister; they was just little kids when I was in high school."

In describing himself as a child, Al stated, "I guess maybe I was sort of a bad kid. I did everything my parents told me not to do. My friends and I'd sneak off and go swimmin', we'd steal stuff from a foundry, steal vegetables, and stuff like that."

"I was small for my age and I was sick a lot. My mom told me I was sick when I was born; the doctors told her I was supposed to die, but I didn't. When I was small I was always catchin' colds, though. I was smart and made good grades in grade school — mostly Bs — when I could be there, but I was sick a lot and missed quite a bit of school."

"Despite all of that, I never did let it get me down. I won me some awards in grade school; my mother was proud of me. I was not a bad athlete in grade school; I didn't play football because I was kinda scrawny, but I played some basketball. When I was in high school, my back got worse and I walked all humped over. The doctor said it could be corrected surgically, but we didn't have the money. It really bothered me. No one made fun of me, but I got to be sort of an introvert and lost some of the spunk I had. My back is still a problem, as you can see; I still can't do nothin' strenuous, and I can't stay in one position too long. I got along okay with kids even though my back was funny. I even got along with those kids I had fights with."

"My body's pretty boogered up by now. I have been in a lotta car wrecks. When I was about ten, some friends and I were stealin' lettuce off a movin' truck. The truck stopped real quick and it threw me out on my head. I woke up in the hospital. I'd been unconscious for two days; I had a fractured skull.

Then, when I was thirteen or fourteen, I was ridin' with a friend in his car —
He was drivin' like a maniac! He lost control of it, and the car turned over
three or four times and ran into a fire station. I was all cut up and bruised;
You can still see some of the scars on my face. When I was about seventeen or
eighteen, I was ridin' with this girl out in the country. She was drivin' like
hell, too! We'd all been drinkin'. She broadsided another car. It threw me from
the back seat through the windshield. It fractured my skull, messed up my
neck and back, and broke my collarbone and a leg; I woke up in the hospital
again. They didn't set my leg right so I am stuck with this damned limp — one-
leg is shorter than the other one now. Then when I was twenty, I was ridin'
with a friend. We was comin' out of a service station, and some guy swerved
around the corner and into the station and broadsided my friend's car. The
jolt threw me out on my head! I woke up in the hospital with my back hurt
again, and I had a concussion. My back started burnin' and stingin'. Shit, they
were gonna operate on me! I got up, got dressed, and got the hell out of there!
Finally, when I was drivin' a cab, a cop broadsided my cab; he totally demolish-
ed the cab, but I didn't get hurt much in that one, just some bruises. Shit, I
began to think I was jinxed! The whole damn mess had made me very cautious
about who I ride with, particularly women drivers. If people start goin' too
fast, I ask them to stop and I get out. I don't want any more of those damned
wrecks."

"Well, anyway, I had this problem with my back in high school. I kinda
felt like a freak, but then I started meetin' girls that accepted me for me, and
I got okay again after a while. All I have now is a bad back and one leg shorter
than the other one. Course my eyes are bad and I got bad teeth, too!"

Al didn't like high school, but stayed until the tenth grade for his mother's
sake. "My head was fucked up part of the time because of my back. I really
wasn't too interested in school neither: I didn't like the teachers; they were
lousy. They went too fast and they wouldn't stop to explain somethin' if you
didn't understand. I just stopped askin' questions, and finally I just quit goin'
in the middle of my sophomore year."

"After I quit high school I left home and have been out ever since. A friend
and I decided to go to California. We hopped a freight train. Next morning we
slid out of the boxcar and walked downtown. Shit man, we were in Memphis,
Tennessee! We made our way back to Kansas City in a week or so; we felt
stupid as hell. After I got back I met a friend who was goin' to Denver. We
went out there and robbed and stole till I got on my feet financially.

Then I ran into a gal who introduced me to a group of guys who were a
religious singin' group. They traveled around singin' at churches all over the
country. I sang in our choir at church when I was a kid; I joined them and
traveled with them for five or six years. I didn't make much money, but I did
get to see the country and met a lot of people doin' a lot of hustles."

"When I was about twenty-four I came on back to Kansas City. I got me a
job as a porter in this hotel. Shit, I was addicted to heroin and was speedballin'

heroin and cocaine even then. I was doin' a little dealin' in the hotel to get by. It was nothin' big — I don't want to have nothin' to do with no big drug dealin'! I don't want to get killed and I don't know if I could take doin' time in the penitentiary, so I have always stayed on the edge of all that shit."

"Well, I had this job and I had a couple girls hustlin' for me. They weren't exactly workin' for me, they were livin' with me and tryin' to catch me as a man. That's when I met my first wife, Jean. I married her. I don't know why; she could cook real good, she had a nice body, and I guess I was lonesome. Well, anyway she moved in with me and the two girls. They all three worked the streets. Jean was kinda wild and acted kind of crazy. Sometimes she would fight me! It didn't bother me none, though; she and the other two girls was bringin' in the money. Jean and I was real close. We had two kids, a boy that's ten now and a girl that's eight. I am very fond of both of them."

"The women made a lot of money, but we never lived well. I was an addict, and you don't live well as an addict because you shoot up all your money. The two girls finally said they were leavin' because I was spendin' all they made on drugs. Some other gals would come and live with us for a while; they'd play for two or three months, then they'd leave too. A hustlin' broad has to respect her man — if he has that, no other man can take his women. It's the women who do the choosin', though. I guess I just didn't give my hustlin' broads what they needed, 'cause they all pulled out and it was just me, Jean, and the kids left.

"After that I lost my job as a porter and got another job as a clerk in a little store. I was doin' some gamblin' on the side. My wife started being bitchy as hell — she said I was runnin' around on her and threatened to kill me. Shit, I didn't know what she was talkin' about. She just wanted more than she could get — a house, a car, new furniture, NOW! Finally she just up and left and went to Detroit. She left our children with me and just took off. I didn't know what the hell to do, so my kids and I went back to my mother's place. My mother loved the kids."

"I started hustlin' on the streets, gamblin' with cards, dice, dominoes, pool, you name it. I drove a cab so I could prove I had legal employment, but I got robbed three or four times. The last time, a dude put a cannon right up against my head! Shit, I gave him everything I had. I was scared to death. I drove back to the cab office and quit on the spot!"

"My children and I are very close. My boy is affectionate, kind of bad and mischievous like I was, but very smart. Several years after she left, his mother suddenly divorced me and took the boy to Detroit; she wouldn't allow me to see him. My daughter stayed here with her grandmother, we are very close. Neither of my kids respect their mother, but she just wants to keep them away from me.

"I had known my second wife, Margaret, for about twelve years, and after Jean left me I was with Margaret a lot. She loved my kids and was good for my daughter. We got married four or five years ago. She accepts anything from me.

She's a very strong woman, like my mother. She has a good job working in a hospital. She takes good care of me. I am very affectionate with her. If I get angry with her, she cries; if I get angry enough, I knock the hell out of her — but she doesn't crowd me often. She talked me into goin' into the methadone program; it is the best thing that ever happened to me. She has stayed with me through a lot of shit. She wants a child by me; we tried, but it was miscarried. I told her we'd try again when she gets back in shape.

"I guess I am doin' okay; this is the first time in my life, since I have been on methadone, that I ever had anything. But I don't know — in some ways, life is not goin' too well. Maybe I should go back on the road. But hell, I'm married and settled down. We're buyin' a house, all of that stuff! Sometimes I think it was the stupidest thing I ever did, gettin' married! It's not that I don't care about my wife, she is good to me, but you're tied, man! Everyone knows me here; I get a game set up with a chump and the guys say to him, 'Don't you know he's a hustler?' and the chump quits. I'm fabulous with dice, but shit, no one will play me now. ('Course, I cheat, too, but a chump can't see that.) I'm pretty good at hustlin' at pool too, but everyone knows me. When you're on the road you can slip into a town and in a few days make some money; then you go on to a new place."

"I used to have a woman hustlin' for me but the dykes, the lesbians, have cornered all the prostitutes. I don't know why, but they get most of the young gals. I don't want a gal under twenty-one; I don't want no trouble with the law. The police have arrested me maybe twenty to thirty times, usually when I am just visitin' with hustlin' broads. They haul me in with the broads, but they let me go 'cause I ain't done nothin'. I usually have only one woman hustle for me; if you have more than that the broads get to fightin' and there is too damn much confusion. I don't know what I should do — just stay at what I'm doin', I guess. I don't have too many choices."

Interpretive Integration

At least eight modal events and circumstances provide the base for the evolution of Al's life style:

- An insecure childhood in a ghetto family
- Limited economic resources in a family that was barely able to make ends meet, although both parents worked full-time
- A physical disability which made Al look different from other children and limited his mobility as well as opportunities to develop self-confidence and competitiveness
- A childhood filled with frequent bouts of illness during which he was cared for by a resourceful and affectionate mother who herself had a crippling condition
- Loss of the only father he knew at the beginning of puberty

• Embarrassment about his physical disability which became more pronounced in mid- to late adolescence
• Intensified physical problems and new disabilities due to injuries in a series of auto accidents
• Lack of success at most of the things he has tried

Reared with these stresses, Al has developed a pattern of adjustment characterized by the following:

• Sensitivity to changes in bodily functioning which most people would ignore and ruminative concern as to the integrity of his body; a decision not to press his physical limits
• Rejection of competitiveness and aggressiveness and a decision to survive by being cautious, friendly, pleasant, and unassuming
• Diminished self-confidence, self-respect, and personal pride
• Avoidance of conflict, confrontation, and disagreements with other people, for fear of retribution or physical harm
• Enduring low-grade depression and dysphoria which he denies but attempts to dissipate through restless and at times aimless physical activity
• Difficulties in pursuing goals in the face of opposition
• Feelings of personal inadequacy; a feeling that he has little control over his fate
• Self-defeating behavior which reaffirms his inferior status and repeats the patterns of his childhood
• A search for a woman who could be exploited but would nonetheless look after and care for him (reinstatement of the maternal relationship)

In terms of the standards of larger society, Al is not a successful man. In fact, he has failed at most of the things he attempted. He could not compete with his peers as a child and was unable to redirect his energies to activities that do not require physical attractiveness or strength. He dropped out of school in the tenth grade. He enjoyed modest success in the traveling singing group, but gave it up. He failed as a porter, a drygoods clerk, pimp, and cab-driver. His first marriage failed. He attained only modest success as a street hustler.

Al may have acquired the nimbleness with cards, dice, and other gambling devices needed to beat the "chump." However, he lacked the toughness, glibness, and self-assurance needed to be a successful cardsharp or con man. In addition, Al recognized that if he misjudged his mark the chump could call the law or beat him severely; consequently, Al selected only harmless chumps or novices as targets for his manipulations, thus restricting his clientele.

Al stated that he would like to become a hair stylist, but made no effort to obtain information about how to attain such a goal. Al has found his inability to move toward goals frustrating. He once stated, "I am qualified and sharp enough to be doin' better than I am, but I'm not, and sometimes it bothers me. I don't do nothin' about it, though."

Despite his limitations Al was successful in achieving one goal: He was able to find and marry a strong but tolerant woman (Margaret) who has worked and supported him, providing him with some of the care, attention, and stability he needs. In his second marriage Al has reinstated the nurturant relationship that he had enjoyed with his mother.

In some ways Al was a successful manipulator of people; he manipulated them from a position of weakness and powerlessness. He made it clear that he was a harmless man who posed no real threat. Al placed himself in a position of defenselessness so that no one wanted to harm him. Al maintained this "belly-up" approach at some cost in self-esteem. However, he had taken his stepfather's advice to heart and was trying to "accept things the way they were."

When asked what kind of animal he would be if he had the choice, he stated, "I'd be a horse, man. I'd be a beautiful race horse, one of them Arabian stallions. They run. They perform! They're graceful when they move. I'd love to be one of them!" When asked what kind of car he would be, Al stated, "I'd be a Chevy. They're durable and steady and always perform well. You never have to make much repairs on them. Hell, if my body was durable as a Chevy, I wouldn't be livin' like I am."

FORMAL PSYCHOLOGICAL ASSESSMENT

Dimensional Test Findings

Intelligence Tests

Al functions in the Normal range of intelligence; he evinced as much ability for abstract reasoning, grasping and understanding problems, and acquiring new learning as the average man. While these measures may not be relevant to an individual's ability to survive in a ghetto street-culture — we know of none that are — this estimate probably provides a reasonable index of the level of Al's intellectual resources.

MMPI

A distinguishing feature of Al's personality as shown by the MMPI (figure 7.1) is his manipulative life orientation. Also noteworthy are tendencies on the one hand to bind up anxieties in vague somatic complaints, and on the other to discharge tension in restless, aimless activity. In stressful situations Al becomes frightened, confused, even immobilized. He is nonreflective and denies emotional problems. Results showed no evidence of a serious emotional disorder. The low scores on the Validity Scales indicate that Al answered test questions reasonably honestly.

The MMPI suggests that Al is a manipulative man who has an ability to

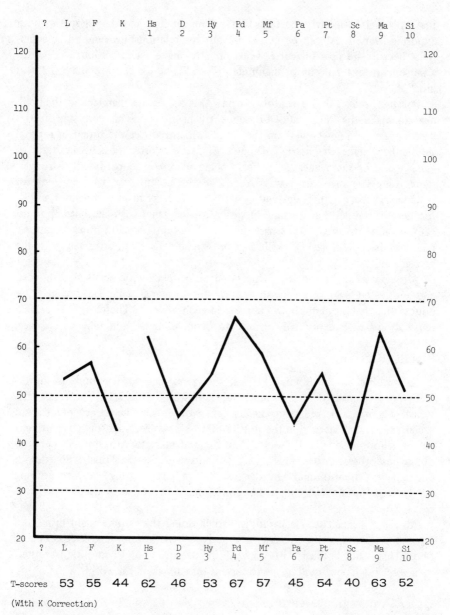

"size up" and adjust to rapidly changing social situations. He is likely to be seen by others as warm, friendly, likeable, nonthreatening, and perhaps ineffectual. Al's social sensitivity protects him; he can get close to other people without exposing himself. Al can be empathic, but his relationships tend to be superficial because he uses his social skills only to make such decisions as, "Is this a person whom I can con or manipulate?" or "Is he likely to retaliate if I beat him?"

Because he lives in a predatory world, Al is a cautious man lacking the boldness to make the "big play." Consequently he practices his cons and hustles with novices and newcomers on the street, which reduces the threat of reprisal should he "make the mark." Though Al sees opportunities, he hesitates to grasp many of them because he fears being placed in jeopardy with stronger, more aggressive men. In a way Al is like the hermit crab who depends for sustenance on what the tides and currents of life carry his way; however, unlike the hermit crab, Al has no shell in which to find sanctuary. He relies upon his caution and his ability to sense and assess potentially dangerous situations, maintain friendly relations with bigger fish, and fade unobtrusively into the background.

Al's view of the world is a cynical one; all people are hypocritical, dishonest, and motivated primarily by self-interest and personal gain. He is nagged by doubts that he is adequate to compete in such a world. Therefore, he feels he must always be exceptionally careful to "cop his bets" and take no chances.

Sixteen PF

Al's profile on the Sixteen PF test shows no marked deviations from normality or evidence of severe emotional pathology (table 7.1). The results describe a gentle, reserved man, an insecure worrier who needs acceptance and social approval. This is not the profile of an aggressive, bold, or self-confident person who knows what he wants from life and takes it. Al is not a leader who dominates others; rather, he is a careful and cautious individual who tries to understand a situation and consider his options before acting. Al takes nothing for granted; he is socially alert, has considerable street knowledge, and is difficult to fool.

Al is not moralistic. He carefully avoids doing things that might bring him into confrontation with the law, but he pays little attention to social conventions. This is not because Al is unaware of social rules and conventions; rather, he ignores them because they are irrelevant for survival in his world.

Other Dimensional Measures

Scores on the Sensation-Seeking Scales showed Al to have less need for sensation-seeking activities than comparison group populations; only one of his scores (Experience-Seeking) exceeded even the fifteenth percentile. His scores are consistent with a careful and cautious pattern of adjustment in a man who has wanted to quiet the waves in his life, not increase them. Data from the Novelty Experiencing Scales partially confirm the findings on the Zuckerman Scales. Al's External Sensation Scale scores are almost two standard deviations below the means for the comparison groups, and his Internal Sensation Scale scores are almost one standard deviation below the means for these groups. Clearly, Al is not a man who requires intense stimulation; on the contrary, he searches for ways to reduce stimulus input in his life.

Scores on the External and Internal Cognitive Scales reveal an unexpected orientation to the world, but one that is consistent with Al's life style: His scores on both these scales are substantially higher than mean scores for comparison groups. Thus, Al is a man who diligently tries to figure out things in the world about him, the ghetto street environment. It is not surprising to find such a pattern in a gambler and hustler who lives by his wits. Being able to grasp quickly the significant elements in a situation and the intentions of others is necessary in Al's occupation and can mean the difference between "making the mark" and going to jail, being beaten, or killed.

Al's Change Seeker Index score is almost one standard deviation above the means for college and army males. This result is somewhat difficult to interpret. Perhaps it only reflects Al's long-standing preference for leading a wandering, restless life.

Al G. obtained Extroversion, Neuroticism, and Lie scores of 4, 9, and 3 on the Eysenck Personality Inventory. These fall into the ninth, fifty-third, and sixty-fourth percentiles when compared with adult industrial norms. These data suggest that Al is highly introverted. His low neuroticism score suggests, however, that Al is reasonably comfortable, and is no more bound up in neurotic concerns and preoccupations than most normal adults. The L-Scale score, while within normal limits, does suggest that Al was capable of dissimulation and self-misrepresentation — a skill which has survival value in his occupation.

Integration

The formal dimensional test findings support and confirm findings reported in Al's developmental experiences. In his own unique way Al reveals himself to be a consistent individual: He is a man of average intelligence who is socially skillful but nonreflective. He experiences considerable tension and anxiety, but makes no effort to understand them or change his life. In a predatory world he survives by being unassertive and avoiding conflict. Yet, he makes his living as a hustler and con man who relies on his skill at deception and subterfuge; he knows how dangerous this mode of adjustment is, but has little reason to believe anything else would work better for him.

Findings From Morphogenic Measures

Overview

Al has tried to present himself as a person who is well integrated, happy, and getting along well. Closer analysis reveals that Al lives a marginal psychological existence; he is a person who tries to make the best of a bad situation. Though

TABLE 7.1. Cattell 16PF Profile: Al G.

Standard Score	Low Score Description	Standard Ten Score (Sten)	High Score Description
4	Reserved, detached, critical, cool, aloof, stiff, precise, objective	A	Outgoing, warm-hearted, easygoing, trustful, good-natured, participating
3	Less intelligent, concretistic thinking, less well-organized, poor judgment	B	More intelligent, abstract thinking, bright, insightful, fast-learning, better judgment
4	Affected by feelings, emotionally less stable, worrying, easily upset, changeable	C	Emotionally stable, mature, unruffled, faces reality, calm (higher ego strength)
4	Humble, mild, easily led, docile, accommodating, submissive, conforming	E	Assertive, aggressive, stubborn, headstrong, competitive, dominant, rebellious
6	Sober, taciturn, serious, introspective, reflective, slow, cautious	F	Happy-go-lucky, enthusiastic, talkative, cheerful, frank, quick, alert
6	Expedient, disregards rules, social conventions and obligations to people (weaker superego strength)	G	Conscientious, persistent, moralistic, persevering, well-disciplined (stronger superego strength)
6	Shy, timid, withdrawn, threat-sensitive	H	Venturesome, uninhibited, socially bold, active, impulsive
6	Tough-minded, self-reliant, cynical, realistic	I	Tender-minded, sensitive, dependent, seeking help and sympathy
7	Trusting, accepting conditions, understanding, tolerant, permissive	L	Suspicious, hard to fool, dogmatic

Standard Ten Score (Sten) scale: 1 2 3 4 5 6 7 8 9 10

	Average	
Practical, "down-to-earth" concerns, guided by objective reality	5 (L)	Imaginative, bohemian, absent-minded, unconventional, easily seduced from practical judgment
Forthright, unpretentious, genuine, spontaneous, natural, artless, socially clumsy	8 (M)	Astute, polished, socially aware, shrewd, smart, "cuts corners"
Self-assured, placid, secure, self-confident, complacent, serene	7 (N)	Apprehensive, self-reproaching, insecure, worrying, troubled, guilt-prone
Conservative, respectful of established, traditional ideas	7 (O)	Experimenting, liberal, free-thinking, non-moralistic, experiments problem-solutions
Group-dependent, depends on social approval, a "joiner" and sound follower	4 (Q)	Self-sufficient, resourceful, prefers to make own decisions
Undisciplined and self-conflict, lax, follows own urges, careless of social rules	5 (Q)	Controlled, exacting willpower, socially precise, compulsive, persistent, foresighted
Relaxed, tranquil, torpid, unfrustrated, composed, low ergic tension	6 (Q)	Tense, frustrated, driven, overwrought, high ergic tension

not well endowed with the capacities needed for high-level achievement, Al must find ways to get along in the hard world of the street. He does so to the limits of his abilities, but apparently he is frequently victimized and must constantly contend with the knowledge that others are out to take him for all they can get — just as he takes from others to insure his own existence.

Al has characterized himself as a hustler, but he is probably not very successful at it; as often as not, it is probably he who gets hustled. Through it all Al tries to maintain his image of himself as a joyful and contented person. Not surprisingly, the persistent problem that speaks out through Al's morphogenic data is his struggle with feelings of impotence, incompetence, passivity, and dependency.

On the Q-Sorts it appeared that Al used cocaine to accomplish either or both of two objectives: The first is to generate self-assertiveness (perhaps enough to stimulate or make sexual activity possible), the second to bring about a sense of peace and contentment.

On the Rep Test Al's interpersonal constructs revealed a relatively simple organization of social contacts. He described his world as consisting of people he likes (he himself is among them), people he dislikes and fears, and people who can be further classified into the successful and unsuccessful (Al admires the former but has direct dealings only with the latter).

In summary, the morphogenic data convey the impression of Al as a person with modest endowments who lives a constricted life and tries to stay cheerful in a threatening life situation. He uses cocaine and heroin to make his existence endurable, but the drugs are not wholly successful in this and the situation is complicated by the fact that in order to get drugs Al must expose himself to victimization. His overall life situation is stagnant, and, though it can certainly hurt him, there is nothing he can or will do to change it.

Q-Sorts

Standard Items

Correlations among sortings provided in response to identical instructions give the impression that Al's data possess reasonable internal consistency. The median correlations among his descriptions of his usual self were .660 within sessions and .634 between them. His descriptions of his ideal self and of himself during a cocaine high reached comparable levels of consistency.

Al's description of the typical cocaine user was less consistent than his other sortings (median $r = .351$). The pattern of reliability values associated with these sortings indicates that a revision took place at the first reassessment. This revision had effects on the outcome of the factor analytic procedure, discussed below.

Al's data showed high similarity between descriptions of his usual and ideal self (median $r = .713$). The cautious interpretation of this is that Al wished the investigators to believe that he is satisfied with himself. Whether he is so in fact can be decided only on close examination of other data.

The correlations between his descriptions of his usual self, on the one hand, and his descriptions of the typical cocaine user, on the other, produced contradictory results. If one looked only at data from the first session and the second reassessment session, one would conclude that Al identifies himself as a typical cocaine user. However, if one looked only at data from the first reassessment session, it would seem that Al sees little in common between the typical cocaine user and himself; the difference arises because Al changed his description of the typical cocaine user at the first reassessment session. Qualitative analysis showed that, as described by Al in the first assessment session and second reassessment session, the typical cocaine user is happy, pleasant, mellow, and peaceful — but also anxious and nervous. Al rejected the ideas that such a person might be hostile, cruel, sad, or depressed. At the first reassessment Al's description of the typical cocaine user also stressed being happy, pleasant, anxious, and nervous; however, instead of characterizing him as mellow and peaceful — indeed, at this time Al said that he is definitely *not* mellow and peaceful — Al said this person is stubborn, self-centered, and determined to get his own way. In this sorting, the characteristics most strongly rejected as being similar to the typical cocaine user were sexual impotence, being responsive to others, putting others ahead of yourself, and accepting help gracefully.

Comparison of the two descriptions suggests that Al experiences ambivalence about cocaine itself. He seems to be unsure whether it makes people feel good or bad — perhaps it does both. Or it may be that cocaine serves different purposes at different times: When it makes him feel good he thinks of himself as a user. When it makes him into someone he does not like — someone stubborn and self-centered — and when he no longer feels mellow and peaceful, he wants nothing to do with it. Possibly, Al sometimes takes cocaine mainly to make him feel mellow and at peace. At other times he may use it more to aid him in being self-assertive, so that he can overcome passivity, dependency, and perhaps sexual impotence. Probably, for Al cocaine is only partly successful at accomplishing any single objective — it always makes the user anxious and nervous.

Factor analysis. Al's standard-item Q-Sorts did not yield an easily interpretable factor analytic outcome. Factor loadings were more clearly associated with the time of testing than with any other variable.

At the first assessment session, Al presented himself as a happy, pleasant, independent person who stands on his own two feet and is kind and friendly. He rejected the ideas that he might be hostile, cruel, foolish, unintelligent, sad, or depressed. His self-presentation at the first reassessment session showed almost no differences at the high-rank (similar) end of the descriptive array from his self-presentation at the first assessment session. The most noticeable change here was for Al to strongly reject all items dealing negatively with sexuality; he shifted from denying cruelty and lack of knowledge, as he did the first assessment session, to denying lovelessness, sexual impotence, and fear of sex. Several features of Al's data suggest that Al often feels impotent or incompetent, and that he struggles against these feelings sometimes by trying to escape into passive dependence, sometimes by trying to be self-assertive and independent. The former course may produce overt sexual failure and be threatening on that account. The latter course may produce failure of a different sort, for there is reason to doubt that Al has the personal resources his world requires for success.

Individualized Items

As was the case when he used the standard items, Al provided reliable descriptions of his usual self (median r between sessions = .772) and of his ideal self (median r = .655). Most of his other sortings showed some form of peculiarity in reliability. His description of himself when he wants to get high on cocaine changed markedly at the first reassessment session; then it returned to its original form at the second reassessment session. His description of himself after cocaine wears off shifted gradually to a point where the sorting he provided at the second reassessment session correlated slightly negativly with the first sorting he had provided. There was no description of himself when taking amphetamine because he claimed not to use it.

Correlations between Al's descriptions of his usual self and his ideal self were high and positive (median r = .662), as they were also when Al used the standard items. Correlations between Al's usual and ideal selves on the one hand and his descriptions of his bad self on the other, were appropriately negative; these values became steadily more negative on repeated assessments. Also fairly steady were the correlations between Al's descriptions of his usual self and his conception of most non-users of drugs; these coefficients do not vary markedly from their median of .653. Thus, it is clear that Al wanted to present himself as being self-satisfied and much like other people.

Factor analysis. Three factors were extracted from Al's data. The first was a general, self-presentation factor; it displayed heavy positive loadings on all descriptions of the usual self and ideal self, as well as on sortings depicting most non-users of drugs. Also included in this factor, but with high negative loadings, was Al's description of his bad self. The second factor consisted of a single sorting; it was Al's description, provided during the first testing session, of what he is like when on a cocaine high. Only three sortings had high loadings on the third factor; all were descriptions of Al without drugs, in either the state of wanting cocaine (one sorting) or the state after the effects of cocaine have worn off (one sorting). While Factor II is as near as Al gets to providing a description of himself when on drugs, Factor III describes what he is like when not on drugs.

In Factor I, Al described himself in favorable terms: relaxed and at ease, content and satisfied. Although he said he is overjoyed and exuberant, he also felt

TABLE 7.2. Individualized Q-Sort Items: Al G.

Achievement	Dependence	Independence	Sexuality
Positive	*Positive*	*Positive*	*Positive*
1. Get ahead	17. Needs help	33. Makes it on his own	49. Voluptuous
2. Getting your goals	18. Needs someone else	34. Doesn't want any help	*50. Sensuous
Negative	*Negative*	*Negative*	*Negative*
3. Breaking the law to get ahead	*19. Tied to someone's apron strings	*35. Stubborn	*51. Perform loveless sex
4. Robbing a bank	20. Mama's boy	36. Too proud	52. Cold, just doing sex because it's the thing
Affect	**Dominance**	**Knowledge**	**Interpersonal Relations**
Positive	*Positive*	*Positive*	*Positive*
5. Feel good	21. Powerful	*37. Wise	53. Listens
6. Enjoy	22. Dominant	38. Has knowledge	*54. Friendly
Negative	*Negative*	*Negative*	*Negative*
7. Hurt	23. Weak	*39. A fool	55. Hateful
8. Sick	24. Follower	40. Stupid	56. Cruel
Anxiety	**Excitement**	**Restraint**	**Social Recognition**
Positive	*Positive*	*Positive*	*Positive*
9. Relaxed	25. Overjoyed	41. Will power	*57. Respected
10. At ease	26. Exuberant	42. Self-controlled	58. Celebrity
Negative	*Negative*	*Negative*	*Negative*
11. Mad	27. Fighting	*43. Slow	*59. Shamed
*12. Nervous	28. Beating someone	44. Boring	60. Known as a bad man
Chastity	**Humility**	**Self-satisfaction (Stasis)**	
Positive	*Positive*	*Positive*	
13. Virgin	*29. Humble	45. Content	
14. Pure, clean	30. Wants no big fuss over himself	*46. Satisfied, at ease	
Negative	*Negative*	*Negative*	
15. Freak that doesn't involve himself in normal sex	*31. Ignored	*47. Lazy	
16. Some type of maniac, who has the desire, not the ability to do sex.	32. Snubbed	48. In a rut	

Note: Items marked with an asterisk (*) are not significantly altered from their original (standard) wording.

227

he has will power and self-control. He denied criminality, being a sexual freak or maniac and being loveless or sexually cold.

He said that when he is high on cocaine (Factor II) he no longer feels good; instead he becomes mad and nervous, weak, a follower, feels lazy and in a rut, hurt and sick. The only positive aspect of drug use he described is that it makes him friendly and willing to listen to others. Al's reaction to cocaine is far from what popular opinion leads one to expect. In Al the drug seems to activate a conflict between active hostility and passive dependence.

Al described his post-drug state (Factor III) in easygoing terms, almost as if it were the period immediately following sexual intercourse. Both positive and negative aspects of sexuality diminish to minimal significance; he feels content, satisfied, at ease; he is self-controlled and his will power is high; he is friendly and he listens. All in all, this sounds like a person from whom great inner tension has been removed.

The overall picture, then, is one in which Al appears not to take cocaine for the immediate effect it produces. He takes it for the after-effect, the relaxation and relief that follow. The data also suggest that cocaine permits him to function sexually; it helps him overcome his concern about adequacy and feel more self-assertive. Q-Sort data seem to point to a common conclusion: If Al could be sexually competent and self-assertive without cocaine, his need for the drug might diminish.

Rep Test

Role Groups

Apparently, Al's perceptions of people are none too clear or consistent, for many of his descriptions of them changed over time. The people he described reliably were: his own usual and ideal self, his wife or girlfriend, mother, father, and the person who needs him most. All these people turned up in the same group when factor analysis was performed on these data.

Al's responses to the Rep Test gave the impression that he is not sophisticated in interpersonal perception. Even the constructs he invented mentioned only superficial characteristics that are vaguely described:

Interpersonal Constructs

1. Considerate
2. Likes me
3. Hard worker
4. Smart about everyday living
5. Accomplishes things
6. Not sharp, phoney
7. Dog—bad attitude
8. Money hungry
9. Not respected
10. Wants to hurt me

11. Gets along with people
12. I can do without them
13. Can get a decent conversation from him (or her)
14. Feels like he can do it
15. Strong

There is no reason to believe that he was purposely lying — though he was trying to put up a good front. Nor did he seem to be in the coils of emotional conflicts clouding his thinking. Rather, his world of phenomena seems to become vague when he gets beyond the range of stimuli with which he is familiar in his home environment. In short, he is not accustomed to verbalizing his thoughts.

Factor analysis. Al's data yielded three person-groups or factors. People who loaded heavily on the first factor are all persons with whom Al is intimate and toward whom he has affectionate feelings: ideal and usual self, wife or girlfriend, mother, father, other-sex cocaine friend, interesting person, person who needs you most, person you feel sorry for, and self on cocaine. Al described these people as: considerate, strong, kind, helpful, wise, competent (feels like he can do it), and they all like Al.

By way of contrast, people who loaded heavily on the second factor are people Al dislikes, including his own worst self. He described these people as strong, but mean, selfish, and phoney. They want to hurt Al, and he could do quite well without them. Because the person from whom he gets cocaine is included in this group, it may be presumed that Al feels victimized as a result of his use of drugs.

Al's third factor seemed to imply a polarity of success and failure. At one end he placed successful people and likable employers; at the other, those who drink a lot of alcohol. Successful people have accomplished things and are strong, wise, and helpful. People at the other end of the continuum lack these characteristics and are also mean and selfish; unfortunately, they seem to like Al — a trait that probably makes Al's life uncomfortable from time to time. Significantly, this factor does not include Al himself at either pole.

Construct Groups

Factor analysis of Al's constructs produced a surprisingly complex array of five factors. Of these, the first three were strong and clear, the fourth was of uncertain meaning, and the fifth was weak, though specific.

Factor I was bipolar and grouped a great many unfavorable constructs together in such a way as to suggest that it reflects the degree to which Al experiences people as threats. This factor was also strong and general enough to indicate that it dominates Al's perceptions of others and is the first thing he assesses in them. Constructs at the positive end of this factor are: mean, selfish, wants to hurt me, I can do without them, not respected, dog—bad attitude, not sharp—phoney. Constructs with negative loadings here are: considerate, likes me, kind, helpful.

Factor II was an achievement cluster, containing the constructs: wise, hard worker, smart about everyday living, and accomplishes things.

Factor III contains two items concerning strength: strong, and feels he can do it.

Factor IV is identified by the strange combination of being money-hungry and providing good conversation. Constructs in this factor are applied to the person from whom Al get cocaine and to the friend of the same sex with whom Al takes cocaine. This factor may describe a smooth-talking con artist. The people to whom it applies may be those who take Al's money in exchange for drugs and good company.

Factor V consisted of the single construct: sexy. It was applied mainly to the roles: wife or girlfriend, and person of the other sex with whom you take cocaine.

Setting Survey

The record Al provided of his activities was consistent in some respects but inconsistent in others. The measures of penetration into settings and satisfaction with activities were reasonably reliable. However, his reports of times and hours per week for entering and occupying various settings were not reliable; the unreliability in these data was due to an anomaly in the first assessment period. This anomaly was that during the period covered by the first assessment session Al spent no time in social-recreational settings, while he reported entering them seven times at the first reassessment session and twenty-seven times at the second reassessment session. From zero hours spent in these settings, he went to thirty-five and sixteen hours. Al's actions are like his inner psychological life; they are characterized by their variability and cannot be represented by statistical averages.

Al did not report entering work settings; however, as a hustler, not a person who punches a time clock, he could scarcely be expected to appear in traditional employment settings. The appearance of church as a setting in which he spent time seemed unusual, for other data give little evidence that Al is a religious person. Perhaps he does seek solace in some sort of religious activity — at least, he reported that he finds it satisfying.

Integration

Al lives somewhat precariously in a world outside the experience of most middle-class Americans; it is a world of hustlers, whores, addicts, and violent people. Al provided a mixed picture of himself as one of this world's inhabitants: On the one hand he seems weak and vulnerable; his apparent impotence, lack of insight, and tendency to lose as often as he wins seem to show him as a person who should not be expected to survive. On the other hand, his friendly and easygoing manner, desire to enjoy life and get along with others, and continued search for contentment all suggest that he has found ways to survive reasonably effectively.

Al is not an introspective or a philosophical person; logical consistency is not important to him, and he becomes confused when required to think analytically. Nor does he concern himself with what is right or wrong. "Safe" and "dangerous" are the dimensions along which his life has been built. Success, in the sense of material or social achievement, is beyond reach, and he knows it, so immediate gratification has become all that matters. But even that would be given up were it necessary to insure his safety.

All in all, Al gives the impression of being a person convinced of the existence of serious personal deficiencies in himself, who has deliberately determined to get what satisfaction he can out of life in spite of them. Drugs give him a way to bolster his courage to face a frightening world and achieve the contentment and peace he needs to counterbalance his constant feeling of danger. On the surface, Al looks like a loser; he never made it big and was lucky to have made it at all. Yet even though drugs are needed to make it possible, Al's life has probably yielded as much personal satisfaction as anyone in his position could reasonably expect.

STYLE OF DRUG USE

General Pattern

Although he had tried three or four other substances, cocaine and the opiates were the only drugs Al used for any extended period of time (table 7.3).

The first drug he ever tried was marijuana, at about age fifteen. "I smoked weed off and on for two or three years, but I really don't like that damn alfalfa! It makes me drunk and dizzy and I don't like nothin' that makes me drunk!" At about age seventeen he tried inhalants but did not like them either: "I only did them (Velos) once and I don't know why anyone fucks around with shit like that." At eighteen, Al was introduced to heroin and Dilaudid: "This friend of mine asked me if I wanted to try some heroin. I was afraid of that damn needle, but I went ahead and did it anyway. It made me feel real good; it relaxed me. I am usually a tense guy. I was real mellow and relaxed, not uptight at all. My head felt together. After that I did a lot of Dilaudid 'cause I didn't have any good dealer contacts to get heroin regularly. I did some morphine and Demerol, but I don't like them as much as heroin or Dilaudid; I only did them when I couldn't get the others. When I was about twenty-two, travelin' with that singin' group, I got addicted to heroin. At about the same time I started speed-ballin' heroin and cocaine. When I got into the methadone program the first time — five or six years ago — all the other addicts was tellin' me how you could 'speed by' the methadone usin' cocaine. Shit, I had been speedballin'

TABLE 7.3. Genealogy and Pattern of Drug Use and Abuse: Al G.

Drug Substances	Age (13 14 15 16 17 18 19 20 21 22 23 24 25 26 27 28 29 30 31 32 33 34 35 36 37)	Frequency of Drug Usage	Comments
1. Marijuana	(dashed arrow ~16–18)	Rare	I don't like weed. It makes you drunk.
2. Inhalants	(short arrow ~17)	Rare	I tried "Velos" once. I didn't like it.
3. Heroin	(dashed arrow ~21–22 then solid arrow ~24–37)	Daily	I like heroin and coke. They make me very relaxed and settled down. I could mix all day and shoot all night.
4. Other opiates: Dilaudid, Morphine, Demerol, Dolophine	(arrows ~18–25, ~25–26, ~25–26, ~30–37)	Intermittent	I would use them when heroin was bad or not available. I take methadone, Dolophine, at the clinic.
5. Cocaine	(arrow ~24–37)	Daily	I don't like coke without heroin. It pumps your heart too fast; speeds me up too fast; makes me flighty, edgy, jumpy, and nervous.

232

6. Non-prescription, over-the-counter drugs (cough medicine)	Once	I bought some cough medicine once and drank it. It made me sick.
7. Illegal methadone	Never	Never. I don't want nothing to do with it.
8. Alcohol	Rare	I don't like to drink.
9. Barbiturates and other sedatives	Never	I don't like heavy drugs like barbiturates and amphetamine. I have seen the way it makes people act. It makes you paranoid and crazy.
10. Amphetamine	Never	Same as barbiturates and other sedatives.
11. Hallucinogens (psychedelics)	Never	I want to be on top of my act and know what is going on around me! I don't want to mess with anything where I don't have control of my senses.

233

TABLE 7.3. Genealogy and Pattern of Drug Use and Abuse: Al G. *(continued)*

Drug Substances	Age 13 14 15 16 17 18 19 20 21 22 23 24 25 26 27 28 29 30 31 32 33 34 35 36 37	Frequency of Drug Usage	Comments
12. Psychotropics-tranquilizers		Rare	I never use them since my car wreck.
13. Polydrug (heroin and cocaine)	←————————————→	Daily	They are good together.
14. Other			

Legend
———— Denotes regular usage
– – – – Denotes intermittent usage

234

heroin and cocaine for more than eight years by then. I've done quite a bit of girl (cocaine) too, to get high while I was on methadone, but their tellin' me about how good cocaine was, was nothin' new to me."

"I like heroin. I am an addict, but when I do heroin alone it lays me out; I can't do nothin' cause it makes me want to go to sleep. When I mix boy [heroin] and girl I am awake and on top of my thing. You get the best of both, speedballin'. It must be good 'cause I have been shootin' heroin and coke for fifteen years now. I still do some heroin once in a while, even though I am in the methadone program, but you don't get nothin' out of it — you have to shoot a hell of a lot of heroin to override the methadone and I can't afford that kind of money. I am just an addict. The money I have is the money I'll spend on drugs. I'm not crazy or nothin', I just like to get high. I am not hooked on the needle or any shit like that. I'm just hooked on the drugs, but I am not even hooked on that, now that I am on methadone. I never bothered no one and even though I am an addict I have my honor. I would never buy, get, or give heroin to anyone who didn't have the habit."

Al never wanted to have anything to do with alcohol — "I don't like alcohol. You don't find many old addicts, who are alive, who use alcohol. Heroin and alcohol can be lethal for an addict, man"; barbiturates — "Shit, man, them barbs make people mean, they make you do crazy things"; amphetamine — "No sir, they make you draw up. You get introverted and paranoid shootin' them damn amphetamines. They mess up your head"; hallucinogens — "Shit no! I don't want to take no trips"; or tranquilizers — "I took some of them when I was in the hospital, I don't use them anymore". The basic reason for the narrow range of drugs Al was willing to use was that he did not want to take "nothin' that puts me in a place where I don't have control of my senses. If it does that, I am not gonna mess with it and that's that! I want to be on top and know what's goin' on around me."

Al reports that being an addict has had no adverse effects upon his health. "I used to be sick a lot as a kid, but since I've been an addict my health has been better than it *ever* was before. I don't know if it's just 'cause I am older or if it has somethin' to do with using drugs, but my health's been good the last ten or twelve years."

Al finds it difficult to calculate the daily cost of his habit, because "it depends on my money situation. If I have $50, I'll shoot $50; if I have $200, I'll shoot $200. I'll shoot whatever money I have." When asked the longest period he had ever stopped drug use on his own, Al stated, "I stopped once for almost a year, but that's 'cause I was in the county jail and couldn't get any stuff. My ex-wife had me jailed for not payin' child support and they made me come off heroin 'cold-turkey.' I told them I was an addict and asked them for some meds, but they wouldn't do a damn thing for me! I was sick as hell. I could have gotten some heroin in the jail, but they wanted four or five times as much as you pay on the street and I didn't have the money, so I was sick." Al only overdosed twice: "The first time I was alone. I drank me some milk and went out on the street and kept walking — more like stumblin', I guess — till it wore off. People thought I was drunk. The second time I was with my woman. She shot some salt water in my vein, got some milk down me, and then just walked the hell out of me."

Preference Rankings

While Al's drug-preference rankings show modest variability (table 7.4), it is clear that heroin, cocaine, and speedball are his preference. Marijuana, beer, and hard liquor occupy the intermediate preference ranges while barbiturates, amphetamine, and LSD are the least preferred.

TABLE 7.4. Drug Preference Rankings: Al G.

Substance	First Assessment	First Reassessment	Second Reassessment	Mean	Composite Rank
Amphetamine	8	8	8	8.0	8
Barbiturates	7	7	5	6.3	7
Beer	5	5	7	5.7	5
Cocaine	3	2	2	2.3	2.5
Hard liquor	6	6	6	6.0	6
Heroin	2	1	1	1.3	1
LSD	9	9	9	9.0	9
Marijuana	4	4	4	4.0	4
Speedball	1	3	3	2.3	2.5

Ratings

On the rating scales Al did not provide a clear description of his attitude toward drugs in general. However, his descriptions of specific substances fell into two distinct clusters. The first factor contains heroin, cocaine, and their combination, the speedball. Al's attitude toward these substances is favorable; they are good, safe, positive, beautiful, pleasant, right, active, exciting, major, mighty, refreshed, soft, and healthy. Beer and hard liquor both had negative loadings on this factor, indicating that to Al they are the opposite of heroin, cocaine, and the speedball.

All drugs in the second factor are substances of which Al has an unfavorable opinion. This factor contains amphetamine and barbiturates primarily, although marijuana, hard liquor, and LSD also have moderate loadings. Besides being the opposite of substances in Factor I, the drugs in the second cluster are weak, trite, exposed, hazardous, unsuccessful, and worthless.

Pattern of Use

Social Context

Al reports that he was a shooter, not a snorter. "I wouldn't snort that stuff. I knew several guys who lost the inside of their nose doing that. I like my nose fine just the way it is. I don't like to do heroin alone, and I don't like to do coke without heroin, either. I have done coke alone since I have been on methadone, but it is kinda like doin' it with heroin. If I do coke alone without heroin it pumps my heart too fast; it speeds me up too fast and makes me flighty, edgy, and nervous as hell. I don't need nothin' to make me more nervous; hell, I'm a nervous enough guy as it is."

When asked how he was introduced to cocaine Al stated, "I got started on it with that singin' group. I was doin' some boy with two of the guys. They asked me if I had ever shot girl with boy. I told them no. They asked me if I wanted to try some. I wasn't sure what the hell it would do, so I said no. They shot up and seemed to enjoy it. It was six or seven months later before I tried it though, and I tried it alone." Regarding his reaction to the first time he used cocaine intravenously Al said, "I thought my heart was gonna stop, it was poundin' like hell. I didn't take much that first time, but shit, it gave me a helluva sudden jolt, WHAM! Then it eased off and I began to feel better. I thought for a minute, though, that I had done somethin' stupid."

Al estimates that about 30 percent of his total cocaine usage was when he was alone. "I'll shoot up alone if I am home, but usually my wife is in the other room." He estimates that 65 percent of his usage was with a male friend and about 5 percent with two, three, or four male friends. "I really don't want to shoot no drugs alone. That's why I wait for my wife to come home before I fix. I want someone there who can help me in case somethin' goes wrong. Mostly I do drugs with one other friend; I don't like too much of a crowd. You get three or four drug addicts together, and the next thing, you have the police on your ass. Besides that, it creates all kinds of hot-headed confusion. If you get four or five dudes doin' drugs, one guy is sure as hell gonna drop more than his share. That will make one of the other dudes mad, and the first thing you know there is a fight. Shit, if there are just a couple of guys who are friends, it doesn't make any difference if one guy drops more than his share."

Usually Al used cocaine daily. "I'll speedball every day. How much I do depends on my money. If I don't have any money I don't do any drugs; if I have made a lot gamblin', I'll buy a lot the next day. Usually it's no more than four or five pills of cocaine a day with the heroin. That's maybe a third of a gram of street coke. I'll do some boy first, then shoot some girl, then boy again to come off at the end; sometimes though I'll mix 'em before I shoot.

Mixin' and shootin' relaxes me, settles me down. Besides, it keeps me from doin' criminal stuff. Shit, I could mix and shoot all day and all night. Some dudes like to do speedballin' runs for a couple of days. I don't have enough money for that. I do drugs every day, but I don't do no runs."

Al knows of no particular life circumstances that would precipitate speed-balling heroin and cocaine. "Shit, man, I have done it for so long it's part of my life, like brushin' your teeth every morning or goin' to work every day if you are a square dude."

Al described a daily pattern in his drug use. "I will do drugs mostly at night. That's 'cause at night I am out hustlin'. That's when I make my money. I sleep during the daytime."

When asked the type of cocaine he has used Al stated, "Most of it is street coke. It's 7-12 percent pure. However, sometimes I can get cocaine that is as high as 20 percent pure depending on the dealer." Al estimates that 90-95 percent of his cocaine was street cocaine. Perhaps 5-10 percent of it has been pharmaceutical cocaine, but he added, "I try to stay away from that pharmaceutical cocaine. It gives me a strange type of feelin'; It makes me para-noid quick, and shit, I don't want to be paranoid, I want to relax and be mellow. That pharmaceutical stuff will put you in a funk, a paranoid funk! If I can get that 20 percent stuff, that's plenty good enough for me. You get your high right now, and you don't have to shoot near as much. With typical street stuff, you just get a flash. When you pull the needle, it's through!" Al never tried rock crystal, but said that if it was stronger than pharmaceutical cocaine he wanted nothing to do with it.

When asked how he determines the quality of cocaine Al states, "One way I tell is by lookin' at it. Some coke has got a little glassy look, other coke looks like powder. I can tell procaine when I shoot it, because it sets my teeth on edge and makes me edgy, too. I can't tell the difference between procaine and cocaine just by the looks, though, and tasting it is a waste of time. Mostly, I just buy four to five caps. I can tell later what I bought when I shoot it. If a dealer gives me procaine for cocaine, I won't make a fuss, I don't want to get in no fight with no dealer. I will just mind my own business, but buy from another dealer the next time."

Al felt he has not developed a tolerance for cocaine. "It ain't like boy. Boy builds up, but I don't have to build up on coke to get a high. If it is good coke you don't have to do a lot. If it's not good, you have to do a whole lot to get any high at all."

Al has not experienced withdrawal reactions. "Course, now I don't do a lot of coke, but I do feel tired and a little restless, I guess. I need to relax and get some sleep. Sometimes, I have a headache from the cut, but I go to bed and go right on to sleep."

Reactions to Cocaine Use

Physiological Reactions

Because Al G. is not particularly introspective or insightful, he did not provide entirely accurate reports. Futhermore, his responses — especially with respect to psychological reactions — show a heavy reliance on "professed power-lessness," possibly as his way of avoiding self-revelation. Al is a cautious man who does not like to take risks or chances. He does not enjoy intense reactions of any kind. Al has displayed the same pattern in his use of cocaine evident in other areas of his life: Thus, since he has used cocaine in modest dosages, buffering it with heroin, the reactions he reported were well-contained (table 7.5). The only regular physiological reactions to cocaine were: increased heart, pulse and respiration rates, accelerated mental activity, sensitivity to light, sweating, loss of sensations of fatigue, and headaches from the "cut." Al reported that occasionally he has experienced dizziness or sensations of light-headedness, gooseflesh, ringing sensations in his ears, and occasional numbness at the site of injection. Al reported none of the physiological reactions associated with snorting, nor did he report vomiting, muscle spasms, diarrhea, convulsions, and so on. Although he indicated that if a person used cocaine heavily he would lose weight, Al has not experienced loss of appetite.

Psychological Reactions

Al's psychological reactions were also relatively mild (table 7.6). The drugs regularly made him feel more restless and excited — "Sometimes I'll clean the hell out of the house" — and produced feelings of strength and the ability to perform physical work. They also made him feel his mind was quicker, made him more talkative, and made it more difficult for him to sleep unless he followed the cocaine with heroin. Al notes that occasionally cocaine would make him suspicious and paranoid, but that when such reactions occurred he would again eradicate them with heroin. He notes that if used in modest dosages cocaine could prolong sexual intercourse, but he does not feel the drug is an aphrodisiac or provides a better or more spectacular orgasm: "Coke affects different people in different ways. It will prolong sex sometimes but it don't make your dobber get up and it won't make it stay up! I've heard a lot of people say it does that for them; I think it's a lot of shit, because it doesn't do that for me. I've heard guys say too that they get an orgasm with the rush, but I never had nothin' like that happen to me. It would scare the hell out of me if it did!"

Al reported that cocaine has never made him feel optimistic, euphoric, nor has it increased his feelings of self-control. The drug has produced in him no visual, auditory, tactile or olfactory hallucinations, anxiety, panic reactions, or

TABLE 7.5. Physiological Reactions to Cocaine Use and Abuse: Al G.

Commonly Reported Reaction to Cocaine Use/Abuse	Reactions Observed Yes	No	Percent/Time Observed	Qualifying Comments and Observations
Dizziness — feeling of light-headedness	Yes		20	If I do too much coke it makes me giddy and kinda light-headed.
Sweating — perspiration or increases in temperature	Yes		100	I sweat like hell on coke.
Rhinorrhea — running nose		No		Hell no! I don't snort coke and I ain't gonna. I knew several guys who lost the inside of their nose that way.
Tremors — muscle spasms		No		Nothin' like that happened to me.
Lacrimation — tears to eyes		No		Nope!
Mydriasis — dilation of pupils, light sensitivity	Yes		100	It is harder for me to see clear on coke. Things are fuzzy. You don't realize it at first.
Gooseflesh	Yes		20	That happens if it is good, high quality coke.
Emesis — vomiting		No		I never vomited. Course, I don't do that much coke.
Reactive hyperemia — clogging of nasal air passages		No		Snorters have that.
Anorexia — loss of appetite, sensation of hunger		No		You're gonna lose weight if you shoot over a long period of time. You gotta burn off that energy if coke is pushing you.
Dryness of mouth and throat, lack of salivation		No		Not for me.
Increased heart rate	Yes		100	It makes your heart pump harder.
Tightness in chest or chest pains		No		Shit, I wouldn't do it if I got a reaction like that.
Local anesthesia, numbness	Yes		10	You will get numb wherever you're fixin' at if you miss a vein.
Nosebleed		No		Never!
Elevation of pulse rate	Yes		100	You can feel your pulse pounding.
Increased respiration rate	Yes		100	That too!
Cellulitis — inflammation following administration		No		Snorters have it. Like I told you, I ain't no snorter.

Infection of nasal mucous membrane	No		You can get damn bad abscesses shootin' coke, bad burns. They're hard to clear up, too.
Yawning	No		Not me.
Hyperphrenia — excessive mental activity	Yes	100	Your mind runs fast as hell on coke.
Weight loss	No		Not me, I can eat on coke, but, if you do a lot over a long period of time, you sure as hell will lose weight.
Fainting	No		I never fainted on coke. I have on heroin, though.
Increased sensitivity to allergies	No		I don't have no allergies that I know about.
Diarrhea or explosive bowel movements	No		I never had that.
Hepatitis or liver infections	No		You have to use new spikes. However, if you let it chill and coagulate some before you shoot, coke will make you sick.
Headaches	Yes	90	I get headaches comin' off coke. It's the cut.
Loss of fatigue	Yes	100	You just don't feel tired, or get tired.
Ringing in the ears	Yes	20	If it is high-grade coke your ears will ring with the hit.
Convulsions	No		Not me, I never had nothin' like that!

TABLE 7.6. Psychological Reactions to Cocaine Use and Abuse: Al G.

Commonly Reported Reactions to Cocaine Use/Abuse	Reactions Observed Yes	Reactions Observed No	Percent/ Time Observed	Qualifying Comments and Observations
Increased feelings of self-control		No		I don't feel no better control at all.
Increased optimism, courage		No		Nothin' like that. It don't make me feel like no hero.
Increased activity, restlessness, excitement	Yes		100	I just feel more restless. Sometimes, I will clean the hell out of the house on coke.
Feeling of increased physical strength or ability to do physical work	Yes		100	You feel you could do more, but when you're shootin' coke all you are interested in is shootin' coke.
Intensified feelings of well-being, euphoria, "floating," etc.		No		It doesn't do anything like that for me.
Feeling that everything is perfect		No		Hell, I never felt that way, even on heroin!
An exquisite "don't care about the world" attitude		No		You get that sometimes with heroin, but not with coke.
A physical orgasm in the "rush"		No		Hell no, man!
Increased thinking power and imagination		No		I don't get that.
Feeling that the mind is quicker than normal, the feeling that one is smarter than everyone else	Yes		100	I feel like my mind is quicker, but I don't feel smarter than no other dudes.
More talkative than usual, a stream of talk	Yes		100	It makes you talk and talk and talk. You just babble on. It's mostly nonsense though.
Indifference to pain		No		Not me.
Decreased interest in work, failure of ambition, loss of ambition for useful work		No		It's not that you couldn't work. You just don't want to do that!
Insomnia	Yes		100	I can't sleep on it. I use heroin to get off.
Depression, anxiety		No		I get depressed and feel bad sometimes coming off.
Prolonged sexual intercourse	Yes		20	It makes you last longer if you don't do too much.
An aphrodisiac or sexual stimulant		No		I don't want to be bothered with sex or anything else on coke.

Better orgasm on coke				Hell no!
Irrational fears	Yes	No	5	Too much coke will make you paranoid. You will get paranoid anytime you shoot too much!
Terror or panic		No		I've known guys who have done crazy things on coke, but not me.
Tactile hallucinations — the feeling that insects are crawling on or under the skin (particularly fingertips, palms of hands, etc.)		No		Hell no, man!
Changes in reality or the way a room or objects look — the wall waving or in motion, etc.		No		Nothin' like that happened to me. Sometimes you don't see too good.
Paranoid ideas — the feeling that people are after you. You believe you are being watched, talked about or threatened, a wife or girlfriend is unfaithful, untrustworthy, etc.	Yes	No	5	I have got paranoid some. I shot some heroin to stop that nonsense!
Causes one to carry a gun or run from imaginary enemies		No		I don't carry no gun. You carry a gun and you'll have the man on your ass, or end up usin' it.
Visual hallucinations		No		Not for me.
Auditory hallucinations — hearing voices talking about you, threatening, etc.		No		I never heard voices or shit like that doin' coke.
Olfactory hallucinations — new odors, smells, etc.		No		I never smelled nothin' either.
A trigger for violence		No		Not me, I'm not more aggressive. I am not aggressive, period!

changes in perceived reality; Al would have terminated his use of cocaine if it had produced such reactions. Further, he did not feel his use of cocaine ever made him more aggressive: "Hell, I am not a violent man and I don't take nothin' that makes me that way."

Integration

Al is a gentle and insecure man who lives with strong feelings of inadequacy. With his physical disability, limited vocational skills, and lack of achievement in life, he feels compelled to give the impression that he is "making it." He is basically a passive man who feels doubts, uncertainty, and even impotence. In a general sense, intravenous speedballing of cocaine and heroin help this insecure and introverted man feel less impotent in a dangerous and predatory world. More specifically, these drugs (1) help Al feel more self-assured and assertive, (2) accelerate his mental activity, abolish fatigue, and make him feel more alert to events and others' intentions, (3) help him at the same time relax and feel mellow and at ease in situations where he otherwise would feel nervous and apprehensive, (4) reduce the confusion and doubts pervading his existence, and (5) neutralize each other's adverse effects, thereby minimizing the likelihood that Al will precipitate an overdose with either.

LIFE ACTIVITIES AND EXPERIENCES: IN AL'S OWN WORDS

Overview

This section presents two days of Al's life. Notice that Al's daily pattern here is unusual: He slept during the day and worked the streets at night, usually going to bed at 4:00 or 5:00 a.m. As Al describes the events in his life, his friendliness and natural, childlike charm come through clearly, as do his cautious approach, cynicism, restless activity, and constant attempts to figure out the meaning of events going on around him; Al has survived by being alert to the nuances of social relationships.

A good storyteller, Al enjoyed talking about himself. It was the first time he had ever received any indication that the events in his life were important to anyone other than himself. Because of this unique opportunity, he may have exaggerated a bit on occasion.

There are three main characters in his life: Al, his wife, and his "lady." His wife, a strong but quiet woman, wakes Al when she comes home evenings from her work at the hospital. Al's "lady" is a female friend; as Al states, "She is

Number One after my wife." His lady has a car and provides Al with transportation, for he has none of his own.

On the first day, Al's lady drives him to the clinic to get his methadone. Al gets sick; the cause is unknown. Later he feels better and takes her on a tour of some of the bars, joints, pool halls, and so on, that are his normal habitat. Al tells how to make a buck "selling slum" and playing "Tonk" and "Kelly Pool." Late in the evening his lady states that another man wants to date her. Al tells her to go ahead; he angers her with his cold, impersonal attitude.

On the second day, Al is home with his wife and an addict who wants to stay the night; Al is trying to figure the man's motives. The addict "fixes" and leaves; Al is relieved. Then he and his wife go to bed. The next afternoon Al goes out to the streets, ending up with some "hustling broads" in a pool hall. He makes a few dollars playing pool and gets into comical trouble with one of the hustlers. His story about always beating at pool the man who manages this woman may be exaggerated, but Al does begin to think he had better be more cautious in the future; he decides it would be wise to go home before he gets into more difficulties. At his house, he finds a couple he doesn't like, but he puts up with them till they leave.

Activity and Experience Audits

First Day: A Wednesday in March

12:00 m.–4:00 p.m.
I was asleep. I had had a long day Monday, and Tuesday had not gone the way I had wanted it to go. I got into a couple of fights; I lost some money in a couple of games — it was bad. I went to bed Tuesday night at 10:00 p.m.

4:00–5:30 p.m.
My wife woke me. I was kinda hot, had slept so late. Yet I still had to go to the hospital and get my meds. I was tired, very tired, and depressed.

I got up, got dressed, pulled the window blind down so my lady would know to pick me up.

She arrived at five minutes after four. I wasn't quite dressed yet. She didn't say much, she was smokin' her weed. I finished gettin' dressed and we left. On the way to the hospital she was askin' me what was the matter. I was tired, didn't feel good, I wasn't sayin' nothin' to her; I was hopin' she would shut up.

I went in to get my meds and they were late! It pissed me! My lady went downstairs to visit. I sat there for ten minutes. I didn't say nothin' to no one. I was wonderin' where the hell the meds are. I don't feel good. I hoped no one had robbed them or somethin'. There was a crowd of people there because the meds were late; everyone was bitchin' and complainin'. They finally arrived.

I drank my meds and went downstairs. I stood there for about ten minutes looking at nothin'; I was feelin' funny, peculiar. I thought, well, maybe it's a reaction to the meds. I was kinda dizzy, lightheaded, and sick at my stomach. I went back upstairs; laid down on the couch. I felt sick, had chills, felt nauseous. I guess I went into a kind of sick sleep, because my lady came up in about an hour to wake me. She asked if I was okay; I said yeah, sat up, and got myself together. I never had a reaction like that — I was kinda scared. I decided we had better leave so I asked my lady to take me home.

5:30–7:30 p.m.

She drove me home. I tried to explain to her how I felt. I don't think she understood; of course, neither did I. I went in and laid down; I was still feelin' nauseous, light-headed like when you're sick. The meds had not taken effect yet.

My wife asked me what had happened. I told her as best I could. She got me some aspirins, and I went in and laid on the divan feelin' pretty rocky.

My lady had brought her daughter's coat over for my wife to fix. My wife sews and they were talkin' about that.

I laid there tryin' to figure out what had happened to me. I didn't hurt anywhere, but I felt funny as hell. Then I started sweatin'. It poured off me, so I got up, went to the bathroom, washed my face in cold water, then started feelin' better. In a few minutes I felt normal, I felt okay. I don't know what the hell could have caused that.

I went in and told my wife and lady that I felt okay. My wife was quite upset about it; she's been readin' on how the methadone programs have been usin' people as guinea pigs. She said I should start cuttin' down or something would be fucked up in my insides. I decided I wanted somethin' cold to drink.

We all drove up to a Dairy Queen. They were talkin' about what kind of ice cream they were wantin'. I was glad I was feelin' better. I got an ice cream float and drank it; they had sundaes.

On the way back we had to stop because I got sick. We pulled over. I leaned out the car and lost it all, it wouldn't stay down. Shit!

We went on back home. I was feelin' better, though, I was all right, not sick like before. However, there was nothin' in me.

7:30–8:00 p.m.

I sat at home debatin' whether I could eat anything, whether I could hold it down or not. My lady and wife went in the kitchen and fixed me some breakfast: bacon and eggs and toast. We ate it, watchin' TV. My wife and lady were talkin' 'bout how my lady's daughter tears up her clothes and that kind of thing. I am feelin' better again. I decided to go out, go lookin'.

8:00–10:00 p.m.

My lady drove me to another part of town. She wanted to know what was down there; I told her the gamblin' places, dice houses, whorehouses, an all-night restaurant, and all different kinds of places. She didn't believe me; she'd never been there. I told her it was a place where hustlers — guys and broads — make a little money. She was surprised; she is a very square gal, and I thought, this is gonna be an interestin' night in her education.

We went to the crap house first. I walked in and looked around; there were only four or five guys in there. I said hi to the owner and walked out. No action there!

We walked on down to a café and looked around. There was a pretty good crowd in there. I saw a couple of guys I shoot pool with; I asked 'em how things were goin' and they said it was slow as hell. Some girls were there playin' Tonk or Blackjack. I sat down at the tables and visited with them. I asked them were they makin' any money? They said it was slow, but it might pick up later. I was wonderin' if I should come back later; it looked pretty slack.

My lady and I went in and out of three or four places. I spoke to two or three guys I know; they said nothin' was happening. My lady and I went into the back rooms where the prostitutes are. They waved and hollered, "Hi Al," and I waved back. My lady got mad.

We drove over to a couple of other joints. My lady was surprised as hell at all the places and people there. We would just drive up, chat with a guy, and drive on. It was borin' as hell; it looked like there was not much goin' on down there.

We went into two more places and looked around. They was almost empty. It was a damn bad night!

My lady and I walked down to one other place. She's not sayin' much; still angry about me being known by those whores in the other place. I didn't say much either; I never told her I was no angel.

We went into the joint. I know the owner. There were four or five people sitting in a booth. The owner had two or three girls down at the end of the bar, teachin' them how to play Pill Box or Kelly Pool. You have this box with numbered balls in it; you shake it and turn it up and a ball falls out. People make bets on the number, usually twenty-five cents. On a good night you can make good money at it.

My lady and I sat watchin' them. I asked her if she'd like to be workin' the Pill Box or working for 'tricks.' The owner said a good gal workin' the Pill Box can make as much as the whores; there are ways you can influence what balls come out, and a number of people can bet at the same time. The quarters add up quick if you have four or five players! My lady didn't care for the place. She said we should go. She said the girls looked cheap. They didn't look cheap to me; they looked like prostitutes, but they didn't look cheap. I didn't tell her that. Shit! Why upset her?

10:00–10:30 p.m.

My lady drove me back to town. We came through the strip. We stopped the car and talked to two guys in front of a joint on the corner. I asked them if there was any action in the area; they said nothin' was movin'.

We drove to the bus stations, both of them. I was lookin' for a guy I know, he sells slum. He was not workin' the bus station. A guy said he had seen him in a nearby bar earlier.

In sellin' slum you go to a place I know and buy rings and watches: one-dollar, two-dollars, five-dollars at the most. The watches have expensive covers and faces — Rolex, Tissot, Auditron and stuff like that, but Mickey Mouse workings. The stuff looks good, very expensive; you clean it up and sell them to chumps in the bus station. I have sold fifty to seventy-five rings and watches that way. How much you sell depends on how gullible the chumps are. You tell the chump the watch was stolen and it's hot; you have to get across the fact that this is very hot merchandise. You tell the dude you're on the run and need the cash. You'll sell it to him cheap, but not unless he is leavin' town on the bus, because the police will catch both of us otherwise. You tell him you wouldn't sell it to him except you're up against it. He has to "hold it in" — not wear it for a week or two till the heat is off and the police quit lookin' for the stuff. It is surprisin' how people will jump at the chance to buy somethin' hot; you play on their greed. It's a con, a game, but it works. There are a lot of different ways to slum. I usually do it with a gal with me: We get to talkin' about me parting with the merchandise with the chump present where he can hear us. The woman pleads with me not to part with the goods; I tell her, "I gotta have the money." The chump drifts over and pretty soon you got him in. I like it better this way, because the chump comes to you and it makes the whole thing more plausible to him.

I finally found the guy. He's a little guy, a fast-talker, and beautiful at slum. I asked him how business was. He said rings were okay but watches were bad. He had gone into women's pendants and jewelry; it was going pretty good. I decided not to go slummin' for a while. It looks like he has got it all burned up down there now.

10:30—11:00 p.m.

My lady and I drove back to my end of town. She is wantin' to know if I know everyone in town personally. I tell her no, but over the years you sure as hell get to know a lot of people runnin' a lot of hustles. She said she didn't know all these things were goin' on.

I go back to the pool hall and look around; it is kinda slow, only two tables goin'. I go to the restaurant, to the joint, to the bar. There is nobody nowhere. I am wonderin' where the hell everyone was at.

I sat in the car with my lady a few minutes. She asked if I wanted to go anywhere else, 'cause she had to leave soon to go to work. I told her no (I wanted to go to some other places but they're out of the way). Things was slow everywhere that night, so we drove home.

She was talkin' about her workday. She said she hoped a certain man would not be there; she said he bothers her. She said he had asked her out, asked her to dances and things. I asked her why she didn't go with him. She got mad, she didn't like that too much. She told me I was cold and didn't care about nothin'. I didn't say anything.

11:00–12:00 p.m.

I got out of the car and went in the house. My wife was still up; she asked where I had been. I told her where, when, who, and what all I had done and who I had talked to. Everyone knows my wife, and had asked about her. I told her; she was pleased. She made me a sandwich and got out a new Monopoly game she had bought.

We sat up and played Monopoly till 3:00 or 4:00 in the morning. I lost.

The Day: An okay day. They happen like that. I was scared when I got sick earlier, I didn't know what the hell was happenin' to me. But later I got some fixes on action for the future.

Second Day: A Friday in May

12:00 p.m.–1:30 a.m.

I was at home, sittin' talkin' with my wife and a guy who wanted to stay at my house. He had come in about a half hour earlier. He was trying to weasel his way into my place. We was watching TV, talkin' about the weather and shit like that. I am tryin' to figure out what is going on, what he's goin' to do. He decided he wanted to shoot up there — he's an H dude. He fired up. The wife doesn't like it, but quietly accepts it. I knew she was mad. I felt all right, I don't mind him fixin' if he brings his own stuff. He fixed and left. He never did really say what he wanted. He got the feelin' we didn't want him, though.

We got comfortable after the dude left. My wife fixed me a sandwich and I ate and watched TV. I was feelin' okay, but thinkin' of nothin' in particular, except still thinkin' about that dude a bit.

Earlier in the week my wife had started her vacation. We had a rough time at a damn party and I got drunk and didn't like that at all.

We went to bed. I went right to sleep.

1:30 a.m.–3:00 p.m.

My wife woke me. She turned on the TV and started watchin' "General Hospital." I watched it, too. I had her give me my meds and drank half of it. I was feelin' pretty good.

I had a good night's sleep.

3:00–4:30 p.m.

I got up, went to the bathroom, and started gettin' myself together. I was gonna go out; I wanted to get some fresh air.

I walked up to the corner, feelin' good. I was thinkin' it was much colder than I thought, the wind was about to blow me down. I went up to a head shop. They sell weed pipes, records, pictures, psychedelic stuff, and things like that.

I visited with the owner a while. He's a nice guy — a big dude, but very friendly. He's about thirty-four or thirty-five and gets along well with everyone. He has a brother that helps work the place. The brother is a big, tall dude, but very moody. He shouldn't be there 'cause he drives customers away; he raises hell with customers and has a bad attitude. He gives people hell if they lean on the window. I don't have no problems with him, I have known him a long time. The first dude is cool — he's a player. The other brother is a square dude kinda hostile to everyone. He wants to make it with women, but no woman would put up with his shit. They have a nice business, have records, too; I listened to their music a while, then left. I don't know how long they will stay in business, though. I enjoyed visitin' with them and am glad to see they have a nice place.

I was gonna walk a little further, but a guy I know picked me up in his car. He drove four or five blocks with me. He's a workin' dude, construction is his game. He had some merchandise he wanted to show me, but he wanted too much money. He had some guns — big dudes, .38s and all. If he'd had a small one like a .25-caliber, I might have bought one for my wife. They were nice guns, if you like big ones, but he wanted too much for 'em. They were regular cannons!

Then I got out. What really made me get out was that a police car pulled up behind us. He told us to get movin', we was parked. I said, "I'll see you around!" Shit! He took off. The police wouldn't mess with a guy like that, though. He works every day, and had on one of those yellow construction hats.

4:30–5:00 p.m.

I went into a little restaurant and talked to two hustlin' gals who work up on the corner. I don't talk to many square ladies; my lady is not really square, even though she works every day. My lady doesn't want to be a hustlin' lady. However, it wouldn't bother me if she did, we could make some money at it. It doesn't hurt me or make me any difference. The gals were asking me where they could get some "Black Beauties," an amphetamine; they wanted something to keep up their drive. I told 'em where they could get it. They bought me a coke.

I talked with 'em about the short dresses they were wearing. I was freezin' to death with everything I had on, but these gals had on mini-skirts! The gals said they were just marketin' their merchandise. They said it had paid off for them last night, but there was no business, nothin' yet, tonight. Of course, it was early, too.

I went to a tavern, looked around, then walked right back out. There was nothin' but a bunch of juveniles in there, nobody I wanted to talk to.

5:00–10:00 p.m.

I went into a pool hall. It was very crowded; hell, I had to push through the door to get in. Every table was goin'! I was surprised to see all the people but they had it goin'! I stood and watched one game till it was finished, then got a seat.

I played a game of pool. My partner was a woman, a gal, a big tall gal, loud and very boisterous. She had been cut up real bad; she had long scars on her face and neck, she looked like she had been in a fight with a threshing machine. Whoever had cut her had tried to kill her. I would like to ask her about it, but she is very self-conscious about the scars. We won our game, so we changed from a "funny" game to "horse." Whoever losses has to drink a big plastic pitcher of water, you could say a bucket. I played six or seven games. I also drank a damn bucket of water! I saved a friend and damn if he didn't sock me with the bucket! I had to drink it. I enjoyed it, I won every game except that one. In horse, it's every man for himself.

I went over to the counter. The owner had a pool game goin'. Smith is a good dude, but I beat him out of seventeen dollars; he was playing my game, and I beat his ass. He wanted to play again, and I beat him again and took all he had. He borrowed a dollar back from me. He is a workin' dude, but he shoots every day. He must be used to losin', because he didn't get mad. I guess he felt the best player won.

I gave the house man five dollars for settin' up the game.

I wished he had had more money so I could have beaten him outta more! My mind was leanin' toward the fact that he didn't have much money. However, *he* raised the ante; he wouldn't stop, so I kept his nose to the grindstone and took all he had!

I went to a restaurant to get somethin' to eat. It wasn't crowded, and I ate alone. I was mad because I was sittin' too close to the damn jukebox! Some dude kept feedin' it, it was too loud. I didn't like it, but I didn't move. The same people was there when I left as when I came in. The restaurant is really a week-end restaurant, on Saturdays and Sundays you can hardly get in.

I left the restaurant. I had bought chicken but didn't eat it all, so I got me a doggy-bag and took some down to the guys at the pool hall. I sat down on the bar between two gals, two hustlers. One was a great big fat gal. The hustlers up there don't know how she does it, but shit, she makes a lot of money! Usually there are five or six people sittin' on the counter, but when she gets up there it only holds three! She has a badass dude who handles her. She's nice, she smiles all the time and laughs. She is always cryin', though, about how bad her man treats her. She likes me and doesn't like me, 'cause I beat her man at everything — pool, cards, and dominoes. She jokingly said she would quit him and be my woman 'cause I get all her money anyway.

He gave me a ring once and told me we were married! He said no one else could play me till he beat me. He beats the others, but the dude can't beat me. I harass him during the game. I even make him bow when he loses! Shit, he's three times bigger than me; one of these days he's gonna blow up and clean the pool hall up with me. Now that I'm thinkin' about it, I probably should ease off on the dude!

The other gal sittin' on the bar is a small gal with a beautiful body. She is very shy and quiet; she only turns a trick every six or seven months. She is not the type for hustlin'. Some guy comes up to talk to her and she hides her head and blushes. I haven't heard her say two or three words as long as I have known her. She's got some real bad teeth, maybe that's why she doesn't talk much. However, she's a favorite of the owner. He likes her and lets her stay. She doesn't have to work as long as she's out there and takes care of the owner.

I was sittin' there between these two gals, jokin' with them, pattin' them on the ass, and feelin' the big one. I was feelin' the halter on the back of the big one. I got the damn halter loose and her jillies fell out!

She knocked me off the bar on my ass! She forgot her jillies were out and jumped down after me. She was mad as hell! I ran around one of the tables.

Some dude found her halter and slung it over her chest; she looked like she had two coal sacks on her chest! She put her halter on and cussed me out. I felt sorry afterwards. I didn't think she'd hit me like she did! She really belted me! My ears was still ringin'. She started runnin' after me like a fool, till the guy gave her top back. I left! I had started enough shit!

9:00–10:00 p.m.

I walked out and started home, but the wind was so chilly I got a cab.

I got home and there were some people at the house, a guy and his wife. The guy, George, is an average guy, rather tall. I think he's got a bad disposition; he's jealous of his wife, jealous about everything she does. I've known him three or four years. He's twenty-eight or twenty-nine. He keeps his eye on his woman, and she turns everything around; he is jealous as hell, and she takes advantage of that. He's a fool! Being jealous like that makes her do things to make him more jealous. We sat down and talked about a club this couple and some other couple are startin'. They wanted to know if we wanted to get involved in it. I was against it, it would be nothin' but trouble. His wife kept crowdin'. He ought to bust her up the side of the head and make her sit down! He's always accusin' people. Then they decided they wanted to get some beer and play cards. I told them I was tired and was goin' to bed. They left.

10:00 p.m.–12:30 a.m.

I was sittin' there wonderin' what the hell my wife was doin' lettin' them in the house in the first place. She knows he is like he is, and that his wife goes out of her way to mess with guys. I don't trust him; I think the dude has got to be a little flaky to act that way. He doesn't act like he is crazy, but you never know when he might go off. I don't want the dude to go off around me, I'd just have to shoot him. I'd rather not be in his company at all.

I turned the TV on and started watchin' the news. My wife and I talked; I asked her why the hell she had let him in. She said it was an accident. She had gone to the window to peek out and see who it was, and they were lookin' right at her. She was stuck and had to let them in.

We fixed some toast and jelly and watched the TV — "Ironside" and "Perry Mason." I was thinkin' how silly the programs were, but there was nothin' else better to watch on the tube, so we watched those.

12:30–1:00 a.m.

I went to the bathroom, put my pajamas on, and went to bed. My wife was still watching TV. I didn't go right to sleep, I laid there and read a sports magazine. I laid there till she came in. I was almost asleep, was ready to go.

The Day: It was all right, satisfactory, a normal day.

8

John B.

LIFE THEMES

John B. is a hardworking, twenty-five-year-old blue-collar employee. He is unsure of himself and whether he will be accepted by others. His feelings are easily hurt by slights and rebuffs, and he suffers recurrent bouts of depression. Defining his life themes proved to be difficult because of his paradoxical nature. However, some themes that capture the cyclic qualities in his existence are the following:

- Cocaine takes me to a world where everything is fine. I would like to stay in that world, but when I take drugs for very long I begin to feel like a failure.
- That is because I desperately want to be accepted by successful people, and they don't like people who do drugs.
- To gain their acceptance I pay their "price" by giving up drugs, being good, and doing what they want.
- But no matter how hard I try they won't accept me.
- I start feeling worthless, and get confused about who I am.
- Then I want to go back where everything is fine, but before I do I also want to get even.
- I strike out against these people who have hurt me and then go back to taking drugs.

254

Cocaine Use in Relation to Life Themes

John has been a daily (whenever possible), intermediate-dosage, intravenous user of pharmaceutical cocaine. Cocaine is his drug of choice because it

- provides him an instant lift out of bouts of depression,
- buoys him up and eradicates his brooding worry, indecision, and doubts,
- helps him shake off and thus manage slights, hurts and disappointments, and
- gives him the euphoria which makes him feel more aggressive and self-confident.

EVOLUTION OF LIFE STYLE

Introduction

John is a twenty-five-year-old Caucasian male. He is tall, lean, and muscular. John wears his hair almost shoulder length, but it is neat and well-trimmed. Usually John dresses in workingman's clothes — blue jeans, a T-shirt, a short blue-jean tunic jacket, expensive high-top Frye Boots, and a bill cap. When John wore his Stetson — his dress hat — he looked like a cowboy in a cigarette ad: tall, lean, masculine, and rather handsome.

John is a paradox. Initially one is taken aback by the contrast between his size and his behavior; though large, he is gentle, timorous, and deferential. His comments are spiced or prefaced with a soft-spoken "Yes, Sir" or "No, Sir." He is also a man of radically alternating moods. During the first all-day assessment session he sat crumpled in his chair, his shoulders sagging, his arms lying limply in his lap. He stared vacantly at a spot on the floor between his outstretched legs. His hair was disheveled and his eyes bloodshot. He answered questions in an almost inaudible whisper; his responses were slow, halting, and hesitant. Finally, John stated that maybe his "hang-ups" were so bad that he should drop out of the research, and asked if he should do so. When told no, John completed the session, but the gloom and malaise continued. John never explained what had triggered this reaction; perhaps he did not know.

But as sessions progressed, his mood improved. Eventually the sad and dejected John was replaced by a bubbly and zestful John full of exuberance and optimism. This person smiled, joked about the interview tasks, and was filled with such restless energy that he had to get up and pace about the room as he talked. He stated he was not on drugs but on a "natural high."

John rarely missed a scheduled appointment. He said his promptness and regularity were partly selfish; he knew he had hang-ups and hoped the project might help him understand himself better.

Developmental Experiences

John was born in Kansas City, the third of four children. He has two older sisters, one age thirty, the other twenty-eight. He has a younger brother age twenty-one. "You couldn't say our family was poor, but we weren't rich either. We had plenty of food, clothes, and things. My father always drove a new car; my mother had a washer and dryer. My father was a salesman, a manufacturer's representative; he made good money. He should have, though, he worked all the time. I was not around him a lot. I was pretty much raised by my mother. He was only home on weekends, and when he *was* home he was generally puttering, fixing things around the house.

"I was never close to my father. He took me to a ball-game once, though, I remember that. He was not affectionate. I don't know even now if he really loves me. He never got to know me, either, he was too busy with his business. I guess he cheated me out of a lot of things I needed. By the time he was ready to give them to me, when I was a teenager, I wasn't ready to accept anything from him; it was too late. I am sorry it couldn't have been different for us. I am not really even angry about it, because being angry wouldn't undo it.

"My father was a relatively strict man — when he was home. He would discipline me with a belt. He was fair about it, but no joke, he would make that belt hurt. Now that we are older we are pretty good friends, I guess. He knows about my involvement with drugs; he offered me some help to get my life back together. I always feel lately like he is glad to see me. He told me he felt responsible for some of the things I have done. I told him I chose the routes I had taken just like he chose the routes he took. He never tried to tell me anything about his business; I have never told him much about the way I live or what I do. It's just that way."

When asked how he would change his father if he could live his life over, John stated, "I'd change him a lot. I wouldn't want him so preoccupied with 'bread.' I would rather we had less and he was home more. But money was important to him. His parents died when he was young, he had to quit school after high school and help raise his brothers and sisters. It was hard for him, I guess. I would want him to be more of a father, though, and do things with me, take me fishing, help me like myself more, but that's all just fantasy shit. Nothing can be done about it. I wish he had had enough bread not to be gone all the time. He earned money so the family could be comfortable. Building his business was first, then working on the house; that was it.

"My mom is fifty-seven. She is just the opposite of my father. She got us kids up, cooked our meals, packed our lunches, washed our clothes and ironed them, got us off to school and all. She is highly organized but very affectionate. She may weigh ninety pounds soaking wet but she always had a lot of energy. She was sick a couple of times when I was growing up, but she stayed on her feet through it all. Her motto was 'Life is not doing what you want to do but doing what you have to do.' She finished college and taught school for a while before she and my father were married. She was always concerned about what everybody thought, though; you know, our friends, our neighbors and all.

"I have always been very close to my mom. She is affectionate with me, compared with how she treated the rest of the kids. She was always hugging and kissing me. Of course, I needed attention; I didn't have much self-confidence. My mother couldn't discipline me after I was about twelve, because I was almost twice her size. She would yell at me some, though, if I really messed up. My mother raised us all by herself. My older sisters didn't always do right by her; they embarrassed her and hurt her feelings by the crazy things they did as teenagers. Both were married when they were fifteen or sixteen and had children. My mother is a very religious person; she is Presbyterian and goes to church almost every Sunday.

"When I was a teenager my folks bought a place on the Lake of the Ozarks. The family was always going down there on weekends in the summer. I would stay at someone's house, I wasn't interested in going with them. I was twelve or thirteen at the time, and was going through a stage where it was more fun to be with friends than with my family. Anyway, my mom liked the place in the Ozarks; she'd fish, cut grass, and relax. She still mows our yard at home.

"I am a lot more like my mom than my father. We both have a tendency to be really passive. I haven't raised a hand to anyone in years."

When asked how he might change his mother if he had his life to live over John stated, "I wouldn't change anything about her. I would want things to be easier for her, though. She deserves more than she got. She raised us kids; she had to do it all by herself."

When asked how his parents got along, John responded with some puzzlement. "Well, I assume they got along really well. They never fought in front of us. Of course, he wasn't around to fight much. My friends always said my father was a strange guy, with a droll, dry humor — but I didn't notice that so much."

John reported that he is closest to his older sister Rachel and his younger brother Marion. "Rachel was always good to me when I was a kid. My other sister Lana is stiff and hard to know. My younger brother Marion is still single; I like him very much and would really like to be able to see more of him."

When asked about his developmental years, John said, "Well, I guess I was average. I really liked baseball, I built model airplanes, stunt planes, ones with gas engines, I rode my bicycle a lot. I tried to stay away from fights. Hockey was my favorite sport, but I don't skate well enough to be a good hockey player.

"I have a difficult time describing myself. I was sort of uncertain, not shy, but not too aggressive. I made really good grades in grade school, except the teacher said I lacked self-control. She said I got upset about things. I was kind of shy, quiet and withdrawn; sometimes, I get that way even yet.

"When I was a teenager I couldn't get along with my father. I wouldn't fight him, I'd just leave. I ran away from home three or four times. My father would usually set it off. He was gone most of the time, but when he did come home he would try to exercise some control over me. I would just leave. If I had stayed I would have ended up fighting him with my fists; there was no sense in that.

"I guess maybe I was a lousy kid when I was fifteen or sixteen. They couldn't keep me in school. I always stayed out late. I drank a lot, and caused them a lot of concern. I started drinking when I was about fifteen or sixteen."

John stated his family was stable "but I never looked to them for help. The biggest problem I had growing up was the fights I had with my father."

"I did well in school. My grade average was a B-, but I had a hard time standing up in front of other people giving book reports or speeches. I lacked self-confidence; I guess I still do sometimes. Later I was sorry I quit school, but it was already done. I got my GED when I was in the service.

"After I quit school I got a job as a fry cook. I did farm work for awhile, then got a job as an assistant manager in a gas station. I got tired of it, and enlisted in the navy when I was seventeen. That's where I got turned on to drugs. I wanted to be a pilot, but my eyes were too bad, so I became a mechanic and crew chief on an aircraft carrier. I didn't like the navy. I didn't mind the work, but there was a lot of suckasses and they got the promotions; I thought it was damn unfair because I worked my ass off and my crew was one of the best. I decked three or four of the suckasses and ended up with a general discharge. The review later changed it to an honorable one. I was glad of that. I did quite a bit of drugs in the Navy: marijuana, LSD, cocaine, morphine, and stuff like that, but a lot of guys were doing drugs and I was never caught on it.

"When I came back from the service I got a job in construction, then in the roofing business. I married my first wife after I got out of the navy. We had a lot of trouble. She was very self-centered, she bought a lot of clothes. She worked, too; she felt her money was her money. She was always bitching because she couldn't do anything she wanted with 'her' money. Hell, I was going out and earning a living and taking care of myself to boot! I would end up doing the laundry, cooking the meals and everything. She was a lousy cook, so I cooked the meals. I had my own business and was making good money, but she didn't care anything about me. She took a second job so she wouldn't have to be around me. I tried to work things out with her, but I couldn't. I finally divorced her. I started doing a lot of dope then; I do more dope when I am under tension.

"The only time I was ever fired was when I was married to my first wife. I was doing a lot of dope and was late for work a week in a row. The foreman said if he couldn't depend on me he didn't want me there at all, so he fired me. I didn't blame him, it wasn't his fault.

"I started my own roofing business and did well at it for a year or so. I was on the verge of making it, but the other companies had more money behind them. I guess I just gave up. My mom says I am afraid of success; I have never felt that way, but maybe she is right.

"For a couple of years I didn't do much, I just did dope. Later, I took a job on the railroad. I ended up with my own crew and handled them well, I guess. I wanted to go to college, because I think I lack something. So I quit the railroad job and took the job I have now at this gas station. I make less money, but I have time for classes. I work all day and carry night classes at the university.

"For two years after my divorce I just lived with dopers and did drugs, mostly cocaine and heroin. I lived with this chick who was a cocaine dealer, so I always had all the coke I wanted. I became an expert in busting into drugstores with some other guys; we got a lot of dope that way. I learned how to beat the security systems they have. You may not know it, but they don't make a security system you can't beat, even the ones that are wired directly to the police station. The security you have here is lousy, it would be easy to beat — I noticed it.

"I have been arrested five or six times on drug charges. I 'skated' my first offense. I got arrested for having weed a couple of times. Then I had two or three burglary charges. I was lucky, I have never done time.

"I still do some dope. If I could, I would do nothing else but live in South America and do drugs. I know it would kill me, but I really love the stuff."

"I don't guess I am like most people. When I was younger and was doing psychedelics, I had this strange experience that left me with the conclusion that no matter what you do in life it doesn't make any real difference at all. That experience has stuck with me. The outcome of anything doesn't make any real difference in the end, no matter what you do."

John recently married again. "I married Susan. We have been living together awhile. She has a college degree and is a teacher. I love her very much. She is particular, clean, and much better organized than I am. Usually, she is a gentle, understanding gal, but if you cross her she can stand up for herself; she will yell at me and fight if she has to. She gives me attention, affection, and sex. The only conflict we have ever had is over my involvement with dope, and that's getting better; I tried to cut down on dope and straighten up my life. She gives me stability and drive, a willingness to work, and stuff. Without Susan I would be right back onto dope again, and shit, I don't need that life any more. I am trying to get out of the dope scene, but it isn't easy. Susan and I are trying to make some new friends, some straight friends, and that's not easy. It's hard to stay on the edge of the drug thing. It's too damn easy to get drawn back into it."

Interpretive Integration

At least seven modal factors during John's developmental years form the framework for the evolution of his life style:

- Reasonable economic security in a middle-class family
- An obtuse form of rejection by a father whose life was almost entirely invested in his business
- An evolving conflict between a stubborn son and an absentee father who either ignored his son or struggled with him to impose his will
- Open expressions of love, acceptance, encouragement, and support from a strong, devoted, and faithful mother
- Reasonable academic success; less success in interpersonal relationships, and failure in development of basic self-respect and confidence
- Adoption of middle-class values focusing on honesty, hard work, perseverance and consideration of the needs of others
- Continuation without open confrontation of the conflict between father and son, culminating at adolescence in a final act of rebellion — quitting school, moving away from home, and seeking independent employment
- An undercurrent of carefully contained resentment towards a strong but moralistic mother

Reared in such an environment, John developed a pattern of adjustment characterized by:

- A shy, introverted pattern of behavior
- A nagging fear that he was somehow responsible for the failure of his relationship with his father
- Lack of self-confidence and self-respect; ruminative self-doubts
- A tendency to become easily discouraged and disheartened by reversals
- Difficulties in managing relationships with people in positions of authority, particularly with those perceived to be unfair or unjust
- A well-developed conscience, with general acceptance of his mother's values
- Strong needs for acceptance by others accompanied by hostile reactions when they are perceived as withholding or withdrawing affection or taking unfair advantage
- Efforts to renounce anger as a response to differences between people
- As a consequence of the preceding, recurrent bouts of discouragement and depression

On the surface, John seems to be a conventional young man who has had somewhat more difficulty than the average person in attaining maturity. However, certain elements in his development are inconsistent with a picture of him as simply a middle-class but maladjusted young man who fell in with bad companions. For instance, John feels neither remorse nor regret over his being discharged from the navy for fighting with his superiors and then spending two years in the illegal occupation of thief and burglar.

Usually, John is introverted, pleasant, and accommodating, and seems to be accepting of middle-class values. However, he frequently feels inadequate and ineffectual. Despite his reversals — separation from the service, divorce from his first wife, the period of illegal drug involvement — John has been working to rebuild his life. He has secured legal employment, remarried, and begun attending night classes at the university.

John has been fortunate in his second marriage. Susan provides affection, support, and encouragement. John needs this because he is vulnerable to recurring bouts of depression. He is not certain he likes himself; he always anticipates rejection by others; consequently, he often finds it.

Rather than run the risk of being rejected, John tries to please and to deny all anger in day-to-day living. He finds it difficult to express even normal irritation with his wife because he needs her desperately. These feelings accumulate and ultimately intrude into his everyday life: In ruminating over perceived slights, John secretly becomes angry with others for not recognizing his plight and with himself for allowing others to take advantage of him. The more anger he feels, the more depressed he becomes. Ultimately, John reaches a point at which he must either deal with the situation directly or withdraw. His typical strategy has been withdrawal. Perhaps at this stage it is an appropriate one, because if and when John's long-suffering tolerance turns to rage he might hurt someone or jeopardize a needed relationship. He has done so in the past.

John would like the world to be a warm, supportive place where conflicts, disagreements, anger, resentment, and irritation do not exist. At the same time he knows it is not so. When asked on the Metaphors Test what kind of animal he would be if he had the choice, John stated, "I'd be a seal. They're graceful. They swim real graceful in the water. They take it easy, get along, never seem to have hassles with each other, and seem real mellow." When asked what kind of flag he would fly from the antenna of his car to convey his uniqueness to the world, he stated, "I don't know. I wouldn't have nothing on it. I don't know yet who I am. I would want it to be pastel blue. It's my favorite color."

FORMAL PSYCHOLOGICAL ASSESSMENT

Dimensional Test Findings

Intelligence Tests

John is currently functioning in the upper Bright Normal range of intelligence. He therefore has considerably more than average ability to take an abstract approach to tasks, acquire new learning, and handle the day-to-day problems of living. He can be a well-organized man, and he has the capacity to perseveringly follow tasks through to completion.

MMPI

The dominant features of John's MMPI profile include: easily mobilized depression, efforts to influence or manipulate others, and excessive brooding, rumination, and concern for an action-oriented person (figure 8.1). The MMPI also depicts an inhibited and insecure individual attempting to stave off depression and dysphoria. The relatively low Validity scores indicate that John understood the instructions and attempted to answer the questions honestly.

Figure 8.1 also depicts John as modest, unassuming, and conventional. In interpersonal relationships he is reserved, shy, and uncertain of himself. He tries to be responsible, do the "right" thing, and live by the rules of middle-class society. He can manage these rituals reasonably well, and most people probably find him pleasant and likeable. However, behind his social facade John is introverted and has strong feelings of personal inadequacy; he is an overly sensitive individual whose feelings are hurt by slights and rebuffs which others would ignore or disregard.

The MMPI does not portray John as remarkably aggressive or competitive. On the contrary, he seems to be a nonviolent individual who avoids confrontation. When things go wrong he contains his anger, privately fuming at the insensitivity of other people, for he fears rejection. Rather than risk that he berates himself. Consequently he becomes more depressed, self-deprecatory, and immobilized. He concludes that he is a "Caspar Milquetoast" who deserved what happened to him. On such occasions he feels useless and helpless, a failure. However, John has a high energy level and, when he finds himself ensnared in self-flagellation, attempts to block discouragement and depression by intensifying his work and general physical activity – and by turning to drugs.

John lives in a world he does not understand; he sees it as one in which people are selfish, dishonest, and motivated primarily by personal gain. With his need for acceptance and fear of rejection, John has difficulty getting along. He repeats a cyclic pattern of extending himself, trying to please, and becoming angry and depressed when he finds his efforts are ignored or not appreciated.

A second MMPI was obtained from John three months after the first. Prior to this first testing, his boss had failed to give John a promised raise and promotion. John waited six weeks, becoming more and more angry and depressed. After a long personal struggle, John finally confronted his superior. The promised raise was immediately provided. This next MMPI depicted a quite different side of John's personality: The depression, confusion, and immobilizing rumination, worry, and concern had vanished. He had become more aggressive, extroverted, and openly manipulative, hardly a person who would let others take advantage of him. This is a flashy and flamboyant John, a man who has expansive and optimistic hopes. This may be the kind of person John seeks to become when he uses cocaine: strong, ebullient, free of immobilizing self-doubt, worry, and concern, selfish and manipulative, but a man who can get things done.

Sixteen PF

John's profile on the Sixteen PF (table 8.1) is consistent with findings on the MMPI. That is, it depicts him as a reserved, gentle, mild-mannered man with a conventional life orientation, unsure of himself and avoiding confronta-

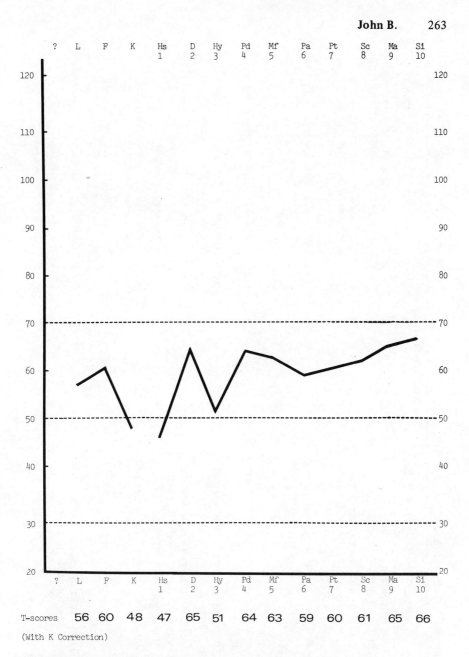

	?	L	F	K	Hs 1	D 2	Hy 3	Pd 4	Mf 5	Pa 6	Pt 7	Sc 8	Ma 9	Si 10
T-scores	56	60	48	47	65	51	64	63	59	60	61	65	66	

(With K Correction)

FIGURE 8.1. MMPI Profile: John B. *Reproduced from the Minnesota Multi-phasic Personality Inventory Profile and Case Summary form, by permission. Copyright 1948 by the Psychological Corporation, New York, N.Y. All rights reserved.*

tion with others. It does not depict him as a willful, stubborn, or competitive person. Rather, he is unpretentious, insecure, and always trying to get along with other people without friction or animosity.

TABLE 8.1. Cattell 16PF Profile: John B.

Standard Score	Low Score Description	Standard Ten Score (Sten) 1 2 3 4 5 6 7 8 9 10	High Score Description
3	Reserved, detached, critical, cool, aloof, stiff, precise, objective	A (3)	Outgoing, warm-hearted, easygoing, trustful, good-natured, participating
8	Less intelligent, concretistic thinking, less well-organized, poor judgment	B (8)	More intelligent, abstract thinking, bright, insightful, fast-learning, better judgment
7	Affected by feelings, emotionally less stable, worrying, easily upset, changeable	C (7)	Emotionally stable, mature, unruffled, faces reality, calm (higher ego strength)
3	Humble, mild, easily led, docile, accommodating, submissive, conforming	E (3)	Assertive, aggressive, stubborn, headstrong, competitive, dominant, rebellious
6	Sober, taciturn, serious, introspective, reflective, slow, cautious	F (6)	Happy-go-lucky, enthusiastic, talkative, cheerful, frank, quick, alert
8	Expedient, disregards rules, social conventions and obligations to people (weaker superego strength)	G (8)	Conscientious, persistent, moralistic, persevering, well-disciplined (stronger superego strength)
6	Shy, timid, withdrawn, threat-sensitive	H (6)	Venturesome, uninhibited, socially bold, active, impulsive
7	Tough-minded, self-reliant, cynical, realistic	I (7)	Tender-minded, sensitive, dependent, seeking help and sympathy
5	Trusting, accepting conditions, understanding, tolerant, permissive	L (5)	Suspicious, hard to fool, dogmatic

Factor	Score	Low description		High description
M	8	Practical, "down-to-earth" concerns, guided by objective reality		Imaginative, bohemian, absent-minded, unconventional, easily seduced from practical judgment
N	3	Forthright, unpretentious, genuine, spontaneous, natural, artless, socially clumsy		Astute, polished, socially aware, shrewd, smart, "cuts corners"
O	6	Self-assured, placid, secure, self-confident, complacent, serene		Apprehensive, self-reproaching, insecure, worrying, troubled, guilt-prone
Q_1	10	Conservative, respectful of established traditional ideas		Experimenting, liberal, free-thinking, non-moralistic, experiments with problem-solutions
Q_2	9	Group-dependent, depends on social approval, a "joiner" and sound follower		Self-sufficient, resourceful, prefers to make own decisions
Q_3	5	Undisciplined self-conflict, lax, follows own urges, careless of social rules		Controlled, exacting willpower, socially precise, compulsive, persistent, foresighted
Q_4	5	Relaxed, tranquil, torpid, unfrustrated, composed, low ergic tension		Tense, frustrated, driven, over-wrought, high ergic tension

The Sixteen PF verifies that John's problems are not due to a lack of intellectual endowment; he can take an analytic approach to a problem situation and identify whatever elements need to be changed to make an effective solution. The test also depicts John as an emotionally stable individual not bound up in excessive worry and ruminative concerns. It describes a man with a well-developed superego, one who has accepted societal values placed upon honesty, hard work, perseverance, and consideration of others.

The Sixteen PF captures two poles of a conflict in John's life, namely the conflict between dependent needs for affection, acceptance, and approval, on the one hand, and needs to go his own way and be independent, autonomous, self-assertive, and successful, on the other. One wonders if John is not still, at twenty-five, in the throes of late adolescence.

A second Sixteen PF was obtained from John three months after the first. In many respects this second Sixteen PF was consistent with the second MMPI. It depicts John as more extroverted and able to utilize his intellectual abilities (being more decisive and less bound up in ruminative worries), and less humble and self-effacing. However, at the same time this John shows less restraint; he is more impulsive than in the initial assessment, and ignores social rules and obligations to other people. The second testing portrays a more selfish and pleasure-oriented man than does the initial assessment. This John is less easily conned, gulled or exploited; he is more suspicious and distrustful, although less anxious and depressed, and more active in his life.

Other Dimensional Measures

The scores John obtained on the Sensation-Seeking Scales show that he has less need for sensation-seeking experiences than the normative comparison groups. His one elevation is on the Disinhibition Scale; this score suggests either that John is envious of individuals who act on their impulses regardless of societal prohibitions, or he is an unconventional individual who does so himself. Both these alternatives have typified his behavior at different points in his life.

John's scores on the Novelty Experiencing Scales indicate that he has little need for the kinds of experience measured by the External and Internal Sensation Scales and External Cognitive Scales. However, his mean score on the Internal Cognitive Scale is well above those for comparison groups. These findings suggest a person who is trying to understand himself, sort out the pieces, and determine who he is and what he wants from life.

Although he obtained a somewhat higher score on the Change Seeker Index than did college or army males, it is not markedly different from those reported for comparison groups; it suggests a conventional life orientation.

John obtained raw scores of 8, 13, and 1 on the Eysenck Extraversion, Neuroticism, and Lie Scales. These fall in the thirty-first, seventy-eighth, and twenty-third percentiles when compared with the industrial norms. These data depict John as a rather shy, unpresuming, and introverted man, and as one who suffers from more neurotic concerns than most male adults.

Integration

Any attempt to provide an integrative summary of the meanings of John's data encounters difficulties. The discrepancies among his test performances can be explained in several ways: Faulty administration of tests might be responsible; John might have been presenting a false picture of himself; his case might be a genuine one of dual personality or manic-depressive disorder, for he may be a person who goes into and out of states of withdrawal and excitement.

John's general willingness to cooperate in the investigation speaks against the idea that he was presenting himself falsely. He has nothing to gain by lying, particularly because he recognizes his own need for help. Clearly John knows, understands, and generally tries to live by accepted standards of behavior; he wants to be seen as hardworking and conscientious, as a gentle, introverted, and achievement-oriented person. Nevertheless, he shows signs of excessive self-criticism and depression, on the one hand, and an aggressive abandonment of social sanctions, on the other. John is aware of this and often feels uncertain and confused about exactly who he is.

Findings From Morphogenic Measures

Overview

John's morphogenic data describe what would have been only a minor personality maladjustment if it had appeared in an adolescent male or a young adult who had lived too long in an overprotected home. Appearing as it does in a twenty-five-year-old person, the problem must be taken more seriously.

John has romantic stereotypes about many people and situations in his life, and these do not serve him well in facing stern reality. Unfortunately, he does not know what to do or how to handle himself when his stereotypes fail. His self-concept is unintegrated, so he lives from one disappointment to the next. Cocaine serves to maintain the adolescent self-concept that John want so much to keep.

In his Q-Sorts John tried to present himself as self-satisfied, easygoing, independent, friendly, and adventurous. However, he showed a persistent tendency to produce deviant sortings at unpredictable times. It was as if another aspect of himself kept coming through despite his intention to appear in the best possible light. This other self is less self-confident, less happy, and more lonely than John's idealized stereotype; it is subject to feelings of shame and ridicule. At the same time it is attracted to feelings of tension, excitement, explosiveness, and nervous energy. Consciously, this energy appears to derive from sheer juvenile adventurousness; unconsciously, it stems from an undirected hostility which may be a reaction to rejection of his dependency needs.

The Rep Test confirmed that while John knows what he should and should not be he does not know who he is. He feels victimized by those who provide him with drugs, feels confused and uncertain, and occasionally doubtful of his own sanity and self-control. His conflicts were much more apparent on the Rep Test than in the Q-Sorts. On the Rep Test he seemed like a person who cyclically indulges his impulses and later feels sorry about having done so. At the same time he does not have the internal strength to prevent himself from going through this cycle again and again.

Surveys of his activities indicate that he is engaged in a program of self-improvement that is very demanding. One can only hope it will bring about essential internal changes as well as an external conformity to stereotypes of social expectations.

Q-Sorts

Standard Items

Although the general picture is of reliable and consistent use by John of the standard Q-Sort items, one of his descriptive sortings stood out from the rest. It was the first description of his usual self, provided at the first assessment session. Its reliability is low, both within that test session ($r = .149$) and in relation to other self-descriptions provided under the same instructional conditions at the first and second reassessment sessions ($r = .172$ and $.130$, respectively).

This finding could result from John's confusion about the requirements of the test, or it could represent a sudden shift in John's strategy of self-presentation. In the latter case, the sorting may reveal tendencies which John would rather not admit. In view of the fact that his other sortings, including descriptions of his usual self, were reliable, and in consideration of the actual content of this maverick self-description, the second hypothesis is more tenable. Factor analysis later disclosed that this atypical self-sorting turned up alone as an independent factor; it is described in greater detail later in this discussion.

The overall median of the reliabilities of John's other descriptions of his usual self was .708. The overall median of all other descriptive sortings was .656. Both values are satisfactory for psychometric purposes.

John reported being relatively self-satisfied (for usual self vs. ideal self, median $r = .629$). He also regarded himself as fairly typical of cocaine users as he saw them (median $r = .559$). Further, he said that this was a desirable state of affairs; the median correlation between his ideal self and his conception of the typical cocaine user was .513. The overall impression John conveyed, then, was of a self-satisfied cocaine user who feels little or no guilt about this activity.

Factor analysis. Three factors appeared, but the patterns of loadings on the first two were not sufficiently distinct to warrant analysis of each separately. Both depict John as being an independent, easygoing, friendly, and adventurous person who is not wishy-washy, self-effacing, or tied to anyone's apron strings. Since John identified himself as a typical cocaine user and said that his usual self is consistent with his self under the influence of cocaine, this self-presentation may be assumed to apply in those instances as well.

The highest loading on the third factor was the first (unreliable) description of his usual self which John provided in the first assessment session. In this atypical self-description John also described himself as independent, easygoing, and nonviolent. However, in this factor his independence was a function not so much of being free as of being lonely. John also said he was sad, depressed, and wishy-washy; that he does not impress others, is not responsive to them, and is neither adventurous nor wise. Though he described himself as sad, John gave the overall impression of being not so much depressed as disappointed, seeming like an adult who has found that adolescent dreams are not coming true but who is not yet ready to accept the implications of that discovery.

Individualized Items

In the context of a generally reliable set of sortings a few important exceptions provided revealing insights into John's personality. For one thing, the instability of his concept of his usual self again appeared with his production of an atypical sorting. This time the deviant sorting was the last one he provided. This sorting correlated at only .355 with the other self-description at the same session and at a level below .300 with self-descriptions from other assessment sessions. Once more John showed himself to be a person who cannot stave off breakthroughs of inconsistent thoughts.

John was also unsure about what he is like when wanting to get high on cocaine. The highest level of probability must go to the hypothesis that John simply did not know what he is like under these circumstances. He is inclined to mistake wishes for reality, a tendency that makes it difficult for him to interpret reality correctly under any but the most obvious circumstances. A similar difficulty in consistency was evident in John's conceptions of what non-users of drugs are like. The correlation pattern in his data indicated that a major shift in these sortings took place at the second reassessment session.

John's last description of his usual self correlated negatively with his description of his ideal self (−.347) and positively with that of his bad self (.511), reversing the trend in the rest of his data. Possibly some incident occurred that caused John to suddenly change his opinion about himself. But if that were the case one would expect to see the change in both of John's descriptions of his usual self at this session; such a change was not evident. Consequently the conclusion again seems warranted that John suffers periodic breakdowns of defenses. These breakdowns are temporary; they relieve strain but bring about no lasting development of personal strength or resilience.

TABLE 8.2. Individualized Q-Sort Items: John B.

Achievement
Positive
1. Obtaining a goal

*2. Accomplishing what you set out to do

Negative
*3. Winning is more important than how the game is played
4. Obtaining your success by someone else's loss

Affect
Positive
5. Feeling good
*6. Pleasant

Negative
7. Feeling lousy
*8. Depressed

Anxiety
Positive
*9. Mellow
*10. Has inner peace

Negative
*11. Nervous
12. Uptight

Dependence
Positive
17. Accepts friendship, can lean on others
*18. Accepts help gracefully

Negative
*19. Tied to someone's apron strings
20. Helpless without others

Dominance
Positive
21. Forceful
*22. Influential

Negative
*23. "Wishy-washy"
24. Indecisive

Excitement
Positive
25. Being ready
*26. Adventuresome

Negative
*27. Explosive
28. Full of nervous energy

Independence
Positive
33. Takes care of himself

34. Self-supporting

Negative
35. Does not accept help or friendship when it's offered
*36. Self-centered

Knowledge
Positive
37. Smart
38. Intelligent

Negative
39. Dumb
40. Stupid

Restraint
Positive
*41. Self-controlled
42. Self-restrained

Negative
43. Cannot get it together
*44. Dull and boring

Sexuality
Positive
*49. Physically sensuous
50. Doesn't care about any-thing

Negative
51. Runs around on his wife
52. Doesn't care who he's out with, as long as he is out

Interpersonal Relations
Positive
53. Helpful to anybody
*54. Friendly with both feelings and actions

Negative
55. Mean
*56. Cruel

Social Recognition
Positive
*57. Respected
58. Treated with honor

Negative
59. Butt of a joke
*60. Laughed at

Chastity

Positive

13. Not having sex as often as you could, because "who" is more important than "how often"

*14. Sexually faithful to one partner

Negative

*15. Afraid to have sex, but wants to

16. Cannot please a woman sexually

Humility

Positive

*29. Humble

*30. Modest

Negative

31. Left out

*32. Lonely

Self-satisfaction (Stasis)

Positive

*45. Self-satisfied

46. Has obtained what he wants and is hanging on to it

Negative

47. No ambition

48. Doesn't care about anything

Note: Items marked with an asterisk (*) are not significantly altered from their original (standard) wording.

Factor analysis. Four factors were extracted from John's data. On Factor I, several descriptions of John's usual self loaded fairly heavily, as did two descriptions of his ideal self and several descriptions of himself in various stages of cocaine use. The factor seems to correspond to the general self-presentation John produced with the standard items. It was called, somewhat hesitantly, a Good Drug-Self.

Factor II seemed like a Bad Drug-Self. All descriptions of John's ideal self loaded negatively on this factor, and all those of his bad self loaded positively — as did all descriptions of how he feels after a cocaine high.

Although the descriptive terms "good" and "bad" were used in naming these first two factors, they are not opposites but are independent. The two states are therefore not mutually exclusive; John is capable at times of feeling both at once. This undoubtedly contributes to his confusion about his identity.

Factor III was associated with amphetamine use. It also included a high loading on one of John's descriptions of what he is like during a cocaine high (.824 at the first assessment session). No descriptions of his usual self have high loadings on this factor. Consequently, Factor III describes a kind of drug response, but apparently not one that John cares to admit into his self-concept.

Factor IV contained the deviant self-description which John provided at the first reassessment session. Two of his conceptions of non-users were negatively loaded on this factor. Apparently, John was contrasting himself with most people and found himself to be deviant.

Factor I reveals how favorably John wishes to present himself. As with the standard items, he said he is: active and adventurous, sexually active and attractive, pleasant, feeling good, helpful, and friendly. Rejected from this picture of himself were suggestions of: dependence on others, being cruel or mean, being laughed at, or being wishy-washy.

Evidently John must see things as totally good or totally bad, with little allowance for shades of gray in between. His bad self (Factor II) is as stagnant as his good self is vibrant. He described this bad self: nervous, uptight, feeling lousy, depressed, left out, lonely, dull and boring. In this state he cannot get it together, good feelings are gone, and he does not feel smart or intelligent.

Factor III, John's other drug self, is similar to Factor I in many respects. This drug self is also excited, pleasant, helpful, and friendly. However, here John admits feeling nervous and uptight and being more explosive and full of nervous energy than his other drug self. Factor III, therefore, reveals a more tense and ambivalent personality than any which has appeared before.

In Factor IV — his deviant self — John described himself as dependent in both desirable and undesirable ways and as being laughable, fit to be the butt of jokes. This time he described himself not as exciting but as having no ambition and adventurousness. As has been shown, John possesses an idealized, adolescent conception of what he would like to be: lovable, adventurous, friendly, liked by others. Factor IV shows, first, that he does not always believe he is this way and, second, that when he is not this way he feels others will make fun of him and laugh at him. All in all, John is a person sensitive to the reactions of others who has an immature conception of his own desirability and suffers when he does not see evidence that other people love, accept, and admire him.

Rep Test

Role Groups

The instability of John's conception of himself showed again in the relatively low reliability of his description of his usual self (median $r = .417$). By contrast, his conceptions of his ideal and worst self were stable (median $r = .823$ and $.906$, respectively). Psychoanalytically, one might be tempted to say that John has a well-developed superego, a powerful id, and a weak ego caught between the two.

The interpersonal constructs invented by John were as follows:

Interpersonal Constructs

1. Insecure
2. Would sleep with me
3. Exercises good judgment
4. Lacks self-control
5. Unstable
6. Honest
7. Expensive life style
8. Thief
9. Loud, boisterous
10. Failed to take advantage of opportunities
11. Outgoing
12. Hard working
13. Spends a lot of money on fun
14. Enjoys social and legal pleasures
15. Involved only in self – not others

Factor analysis. Though revealing in many respects, the results of factor analysis of John's descriptions of others are not easily summarized. As usual he did well with stereotypes, but his thought-processes were not otherwise clear. For example, his first group factor contained what might be called Ideal People: mother, father, ideal self, liked employer, successful person, and interesting person. These people all exercise good judgment and are honest, hardworking, kind, helpful, strong, and wise; they enjoy social and legal pleasures.

His second factor was a combination of John's usual self, a person he feels sorry for, a person who drinks a lot of alcohol, and a person who behaves strangely. These people are honest, outgoing, hardworking, kind, and helpful, but they are also unstable, insecure, and lacking in self-control. This factor may provide an accurate description of what John himself is currently like – trying to live up to a socially acceptable image, but troubled by doubts that sap his self-confidence and impulses that make him worry, even about his own sanity.

John's third factor stressed sexuality: wife or girlfriend, cocaine-friend of the other sex, and person who needs you most. These people are sexy, and would sleep with John. This factor was bipolar, containing at its opposite extreme the person from whom John gets cocaine, clearly, the opposite of someone with whom he cares to be intimate, since this person is loud and boisterous, a thief interested only in self, not others, and who has an expensive life style, spending a lot of money on fun.

Finally, John described himself on cocaine in terms similar to those he used for someone who dislikes him. The inference is clear that John's socially acceptable self is something he rejects when taking drugs. In the latter state he spends a lot of money on fun and lives an expensive life style, but, in compensation for his backsliding, he is sexy and outgoing. Here too, one sees John's adolescent approach to pleasure and satisfaction. But in this factor he expresses conflicts for the first time between his desired self and this drug self.

Construct Groups

Factor analysis revealed four factors in John's interpersonal constructs; two of these were complicated by being bipolar. Thus, his interpersonal space showed up as rather complex in construction.

Construct Factor I extends from good to poor judgment. Poor judgment to John means lacking self-control, failing to take advantage of opportunities, and being insecure and unstable. Good judgment means being strong and wise. John described his usual self as being at the poor-judgment end of this factor.

Factor II is honesty versus dishonesty. To be honest — as John regards himself to be — is to be hardworking, kind, helpful, and able to enjoy legal pleasures. To be dishonest is to be selfish, involved only in oneself, and a thief.

Factor III is not bipolar and includes two main constructs: outgoing and spends a lot of money on fun. This is a "Good-Time Charley" construct, and most of the time John applies it to himself.

Finally, Factor IV is sexuality, pure and simple. It contains the constructs: sexy and would sleep with me. It applies primarily to: wife or girlfriend, person of the other sex with whom John takes cocaine, and person who needs John most.

In summary, John regards himself as a person who is basically honest but uses poor judgment, spending too much money on fun and good times. John seems to regard cocaine use as resulting from his own poor judgment; however, it also fits into his needs for excitement and sensory (as well as sensual) stimulation. To give those up means to give up components of the self which John is reluctant to leave behind. He looks in this respect like a case of adolescence that has been prolonged beyond its normal span of years.

Setting Survey

John's patterns of daily activity and satisfactions were stable. This observation merits comment only because it establishes that, whatever John's problems may be, they do not adversely affect his everyday life. John appears to be engaged in a vigorous and demanding schedule of activities. He works forty-eight hours per week and participates in educational activities almost nine hours per week. This is the schedule of a person trying hard to engage in a program of self-improvement. It is certainly not the pattern of the Good-Time Charley John sometimes wants to be.

John is now engaged in a deliberate program of rehabilitation; he is probably overdoing it, and may end up disappointed with the effort. His satisfaction ratings were interesting in this regard: At the first assessment he reported himself to be very satisfied with his educational activities and moderately satisfied with social-recreational activities. By the second reassessment, the first rating (education) dropped, but the second increased. John's ratings of work experiences have never been high, and John deserves credit for staying with this as long as he has, but one wonders how long he will be able to keep it up.

Integration

John's Q-Sort data showed several deviant responses and inconsistencies. While he generally tried to present himself in desirable terms, several sortings revealed aspects of his self-concept that he prefers not to think about. Apparently, he suffers periodic breakdowns of his defenses. When these occur he feels nervous, depressed, left out, and lonely. He is also subject to periodic bursts of excitement and tension from which he fears social shame and censure. He wants to be loved, respected, and admired, but often feels rejected and unworthy.

John's uncertainty was confirmed on the Rep Test. This also showed how strongly he relies on stereotypes for evaluating himself and others. Because of his devotion to stereotypes and his desire to please and do well, John works hard and tries to be good. However, he has been incapable of sustaining these well-intentioned efforts which raises doubts about the permanence of his current adjustment. John is married now and may have in his wife a strong ally who can help him through the episodic periods of confusion, turmoil, and disorientation in his life.

STYLE OF DRUG USE

General Pattern

The first drug John ever used was alcohol (table 8.3). "When I was about fourteen or fifteen, I would drink off and on with my friends. We couldn't buy beer ourselves, but one of the guys' older brothers would get it for us. By the time I was sixteen, I was drinking quite a bit — beer and hard stuff, too. I still drink quite a bit, mostly beer, but occasionally some bourbon and vodka."

TABLE 8.3. Genealogy and Pattern of Drug Use and Abuse: John B.

Drug Substances	13	14	15	16	17	18	19	20	21	22	23	24	25	Frequency of Drug Usage	Comments
1. Alcohol		↕	----	↕	←—————————————————————→								→	Regular	I like to drink.
2. Inhalants (glue)				↕ ---- ↕										Rare	A kid thing.
3. Amphetamine				↕ ←→ ↕										Rare	I did them for a while when doing over-the-road truck driving. I ate them.
4. Marijuana					↕ ←—————————————————→ ↕									Daily	It relaxes me.
5. Hash						↕ ---- ↕ ←————————→								Daily if available	Good hash is hard to come by on a regular basis
6. Barbiturates						↕ ←→ ↕								Rare	I did some phenobarbs but didn't like it.
7. Hallucinogens (Psychedelics) Peyote, Mushrooms, Cactus, LSD, DMT, STP						↕ ---- ↕								Rare	It was just part of growing up. I had to try it all.
8. Heroin						↕ ---- ↕ ←————————→								Daily	I would do it regular if available. It buffers coke well.

276

Drug		Frequency	Comment
9. Other opiates Dilaudid Opium		Regular	Used it when heroin not available with coke. I smoked and shot opium. It was a treat.
10. Cocaine		Daily	Coke makes you feel nine feet tall. I did some snorting earlier, but didn't like it till I scored some high-grade coke.
11. Psychotropics (Librium, Valium, etc.)		Intermittent	I used them to relax. I ate them.
12. Illegal methadone		Intermittent	I had to try it and see what it was like.
13. Polydrug (heroin/cocaine; Dilaudid)		Daily if available	Sometimes I mixed. You get the best of both.
14. Non-prescription, over-the-counter drugs		Only once	I tried Robitussin once. I didn't like it.

Legend
——— Denotes regular usage
- - - Denotes intermittent usage

During the period from sixteen to seventeen years of age, John tried glue-sniffing ("off and on") and took some amphetamine. "After I left home I did some truck driving for this guy. I ate amphetamines to keep awake; they kept me awake okay, but made me feel edgy all the time. I can't say that I liked them at all. I stopped using amphetamines when I went into the navy."

One of John's most regularly used drugs is marijuana. "I've smoked reefers since I was seventeen. I always look forward to going home after work and smoking a joint or two; they make me feel good. A little after I got into smoking reefers, I got into hash, too. I guess I was about eighteen years old then. I like hash better than reefer, but it is hard to come by. I would do it every day if I could."

At age eighteen, John experimented with barbiturates. "I shot barbs for a year or so. It was like getting drunk on alcohol, but I gave it up after a while. About the same time I did some LSD, some mushrooms, some DMT and STP. I also did some peyote. The trips weren't bad. I tripped on stuff like that for a couple of years while I was in the service and then after I got out.

"When I was about eighteen I did my first heroin; I shot heroin for a year or so. After my divorce I did a lot of heroin and Dilaudid. They make you nod off, and I was pretty down after the divorce — they helped at the time. I still use them with cocaine. You don't get so much of the adverse reactions with coke doing them together, and it makes the coke stay longer.

"I did my first cocaine when I was eighteen in the navy. I shot it, but it didn't do much for me. I snorted some, too, during that period, but I didn't get much of a high with it. I was twenty-two years old before I really got into coke. I lived with this gal I told you about, and had all the coke I wanted. That's when I really got turned on to coke, and I have done it every day I could since then. I used it alone, but I also mixed it with heroin and Dilaudid. Sometimes I mix and shoot the two but more often I use the heroin to come off a cocaine run.

"I also tried some illegal methadone; I had to try it and see what it was like. I did it off and on for a couple of years. It's not bad, but it's not as good as Dilaudid. When I was twenty-three I tried drinking some Robitussin, but I only did that once; I don't know why people drink that stuff regularly. I also tried tranquilizers about this time but never used them regularly."

At one time or another, John tried almost all the major drug substances available. However, the only drugs he has continued to use over any extended period of time are alcohol, marijuana, the opiates, and cocaine. John states that a daily cost of his drug use is difficult to calculate. "Good pharmaceutical cocaine is about seventy to ninety dollars a gram. On the market it would probably cost me one hundred and fifty to one hundred and seventy dollars a day, but for two years I lived with a chick who was a dealer, and she always had enough cocaine for us. A dealer takes his share off the top before he cuts it, so it wasn't costing me anything. Besides, there were several of us busting drug-stores. I guess you could say I was a pretty fair second-story man. I am not proud of it. Back to your question, though; I didn't spend much money for cocaine when I was living with that chick and I was doing one or two grams a day. After she left it probably cost me only fifty to sixty dollars a day for the next year because I cut down. I still had good contacts, though, and I could get drugstore cocaine almost whenever I had the money to buy it."

John stated that he only overdosed two times. "I was shooting 100 percent cocaine; all of a sudden I felt like I couldn't breathe. I fired up some Dilaudid and went outside and walked till I got to feeling better. I was alone both times. It's a scary feeling, that's for sure."

When asked the longest time he had stopped using drugs on his own, John stated from three to four weeks. "I have only been able to do that since I married Susan. I could never leave dope alone by myself. I fall off the wagon every three or four weeks now, but that's a hell of a lot better than every day."

Preference Rankings

The data in table 8.4 indicate that speedball mixtures of heroin and cocaine, cocaine alone, and heroin alone are John's preferred drugs. Marijuana, LSD, and beer occupy the intermediate preference range while hard liquor, amphetamine, and barbiturates are the least preferred. John seeks the lift which cocaine provides, but if he can he buffers its effects with heroin. He would rather use marijuana, beer, or LSD than hard liquor, amphetamine, or barbiturates.

TABLE 8.4. Drug Preference Rankings: John B.

Substance	First Assessment	First Reassessment	Second Reassessment	Mean	Composite Rank
Amphetamine	8	8	8	8.0	8
Barbiturates	9	9	9	9.0	9
Beer	6	5	5	5.7	5.5
Cocaine	2	2	2	2.0	2
Hard liquor	7	7	6	6.7	7
Heroin	3	3	3	3.0	3
LSD	5	5	7	5.7	5.5
Marijuana	4	4	4	4.0	4
Speedball	1	1	1	1.0	1

Ratings

In John's semantic differential data, only the first two factors were easily interpreted. Factor I includes cocaine and speedball as well as drugs-in-general. These substances are described as providing all the benefits John wants as part of his usual self. They are: active, strong, positive, beautiful, exciting, major, pleasant, mighty, hard, fast, and clean.

Factor II contains marijuana at one pole and amphetamine at the other. This means that the factor can be described in pairs of opposites. In the following list, the first term applies to marijuana, the second to amphetamine (largely unfavorable):

Passive — Active
Positive — Negative
Secure — Insecure
Minor — Major
Clean — Dirty
Good — Bad
Safe — Dangerous
Weak — Strong
Calm — Exciting
Healthy — Unhealthy

Factor III contrasts heroin with beer. The basis for some of the contrasts was not clear, but some of the more comprehensible comparisons are:

Hard — Soft
Strong — Weak
Negative — Positive
Hazardous — Sheltered
Valuable — Worthless

The last factor contrasted LSD and hard liquor. The contrast was similar to that between heroin and beer, but LSD was described as more exciting and beautiful than heroin.

Pattern of Use

John first used cocaine at age eighteen when in the navy. "Some other guys and I were shooting some Dilaudid. This striper came by and said he had some cocaine. It was the first time I had ever seen coke. He wanted seventy dollars a gram; we bought two grams and tried it. I really didn't feel anything much. It was disappointing, because I had heard so much about how good it was. It had no real effect, and it was too short a high. Also, I guess maybe I had expected too much, I don't know. I did some snorting of coke later, but it was never much, either.

"I never got turned on to cocaine till I was older. Then when I was living with this girl who was dealing it, I got some good drugstore cocaine. That was different! Then I really got turned on. Even snorting pharmaceutical cocaine was better; I snorted coke every day for nine or ten months, but when I 'pulled up' on it I felt the need for that 'zing' it gives you."

"While I was living with that chick, I started shooting coke every day. There is a helluva difference between snorting and shooting drugstore cocaine. I did a lot of snorting in bed with gals and you can stay up a pretty long time; you can keep a helluva erection if you put the coke right on the head of your dick. In my opinion, coke is not the aphrodisiac everyone says it is, though. When I was shooting I was after the flash and you are not interested in sex, just the flash. It only lasts a few minutes, so you have to keep shooting up every ten or fifteen minutes. You get a longer high snorting coke, but it is a helluva lot less intense.

"Coke generally doesn't make me suspicious or paranoid. Sometimes, I did get a funny feeling that people might be talking. I never really heard voices, where I could understand what was being said, it was just a feeling. I would get suspicious and paranoid on a long run though; sometimes I was afraid the cops might break in at any minute.

"Coke never made me violent. I would score a gram an evening and it wouldn't make me violent. The only drug that ever made me violent was alcohol. I have done a lot of cocaine with a lot of people, and no one ever acted violent, that I recall. Maybe it depends on the circumstances, the surroundings. Maybe if you get violent it's because violent dudes are taking it. That doesn't make too much sense, though. For two years, when I was living with the chick, I carried a gun. I was living with thieves, murderers, and robbers. Everyone carried guns, it was part of the whole scene. I was paranoid, but I couldn't tell you whether it was because of the coke or the company I was keeping. Everyone was suspicious; you were always watching out for John Law or the Narcs. You had to be paranoid with those dudes — the guys I lived with — though. It could have been either the people around me or the coke that made me so suspicious. Everybody was paranoid."

Social Context

"I use cocaine because it gives me an instant lift out of depression. It is not like heroin, which makes you nod off and not think about anything. It lifts you right up and makes you feel nine feet high. I like to feel like that; I sure as hell don't when I am not using drugs. I guess maybe I am a guy who walks around setting up rejection situations. Sometimes I'll do dope, mostly cocaine when I am down. It's funny — no, not so funny — but sometimes I'll lose my self-respect in order to get that high feeling again."

John estimates that 85 percent of the cocaine he has taken was with one other person — "It was usually this gal I was living with or with one other friend of mine". Approximately 10 percent of his total usage was when alone and 5 percent was with from two to four friends, mostly male.

John consumed an average of a gram of pharmaceutical cocaine per day for more than two years. "I would do about a gram of coke a day, sometimes two when it was available. To do that much I would be shooting, off and on, all day. I wasn't working at the time, so there wasn't much else to do. The largest amount of cocaine I ever used in a single day was two-and-one-half grams on a run from noon till noon without any real bad effects. I came down on Dilau-did."

John preferred cocaine runs when possible. "I must have done about fifty runs over a four-year period. I would do short or long runs: A short run might be doing coke every day for a week to ten days, come off of it with heroin or Dilaudid at night so I could sleep, then get up and start all over again. A long run was doing coke every day for a month or more. I wouldn't be doing coke constantly for a month or anything like that; we would lay off a day or so, then come back for three or four days, then off for a day or so, then back on again. That chick and I shot up two-and-seven-eighths ounces of pharmaceutical co-caine doing runs like that. I couldn't afford anything like that after she left; at that time an ounce of sealed pharmaceutical cocaine would cost anywhere from $1,800 to $2,300. I didn't have that kind of money."

John reported only two circumstances that would trigger a cocaine run. "The money and availability of the coke were what would set off a run. Usually, this chick would start the run when a batch of coke came in. We'd have at it whenever it arrived; we'd shoot, and I'd help her cut it and get it ready to sell. It usually didn't last long; she had a good reputation as a dealer and it would move fast." Certain life events would also trigger use of cocaine. "Being de-pressed would make me want to do cocaine. Sometimes a little or insignificant thing might set me off. If I got my feelings hurt I would want to do cocaine. Sometimes a disappointment would do it. My girl — that dealer — wanted to go to Texas. I didn't go, but she went ahead anyway; that triggered a big run."

John's daily pattern was distinctive. "Usually I would start doing coke in the late morning, say ten or eleven o'clock. I always tried to eat a good breakfast and then wait an hour or so before I would start to fire up. Sometimes coke makes me gag or vomit, and that didn't happen if I had something on my stom-ach. However, I would be less than honest if I told you I always did it that way. A lot of times I would just do it whenever it came."

When asked how he distinguishes grades of cocaine John stated, "The only two ways I know is by the source and firing it up. I've heard guys talk about different techniques to determine the grade of coke, like burning it, the smell, watching it dissolve in water, pouring it in Clorox, but I think it's a lot of shit. Street coke is cut with a lot of garbage; you don't know what you're buying. Street coke was probably what the striper sold us the first time I tried coke. However, I have been lucky because I have always — almost always — had access to pharmaceutical flake cocaine that is 100 percent pure."

John felt that during a run his body did develop tolerance. "All I know is that initially I would fire up only this much [he demonstrated on the tip of a pocket knife]. After a while I would have to start increasing each hit every twenty to thirty minutes to get the flash. I might be shooting a quarter of a gram by the end of the day. After I slept and we started again, it would require half as much again to get the flash as it did the first day. However, if I were to lay off coke for two or three days I could start at the bottom again and get a good flash; I think it must take two to three days to get all the cocaine out of my system.

"Withdrawal from coke was not too bad for me. But I would really be tired and depressed as hell that the coke was all gone. I felt worn out, exhausted, kind of empty and washed out. If you used heroin or Dilaudid after a run you could sleep it off. However, the longer you run, the lousier you feel when you come off of it. I never did have hallucinations, feel like bugs were crawling on me, or stuff like that. I would begin vomiting it up if I had done too much."

Reactions to Cocaine

Physiological Reactions

The physiological reactions reported regularly by John (table 8.5) are those associated with stimulation of the CNS and sensitization of the autonomic nervous system. The sympathomimetic signs include: dizziness or a feeling of light-headedness, palmar sweating, light sensitivity, increases in heart, pulse, and respiration rates, dryness of the mouth and throat, loss of appetite, flatulence and bowel evacuation, eradication of sensations of fatigue, local anesthesia, and accelerated mental activity. Collectively such physiological reactions would be clear signals to John that he had been turned to an "on" position.

A second cluster of regular but less frequent reactions which John estimates occurred during 50-75 percent of his cocaine usage, includes a ringing sensation in the ears accompanying the flash or rush, vomiting or a gag response, and gooseflesh. In addition, John reports that he felt headaches and tightness or pains in his chest approximately 20 percent of the time with cocaine. For John headaches were usually associated with a big hit and were regular occurrences with cocaine withdrawal.

John never experienced reactions associated with snorting: increased sensitivity to allergies, infections or hepatitis, yawning, muscle spasms, deep tendon reflexes, fainting, or convulsions.

Psychological Reactions

The psychological reactions that John reported as always being associated with his intravenous use of cocaine (table 8.6) include: increased restlessness and excitement, feelings of increased assertiveness and self-confidence, euphoria and exhilaration, the feeling that his mind was quicker, accelerated imaginal activity, garrulousness, indifference to pain, insomnia, depression, and anxiety. A considerably less frequent reaction which occurred to John on cocaine runs was one of suspiciousness, paranoia, and an irrational fear that the police might break in at any moment.

John reports that his experience with pharmaceutical cocaine was never associated with feelings of greater self-control — he thought, on the contrary, that he was losing control — increased physical strength, failure of ambition, the feeling that everything was perfect, terror or panic reactions, visual,

TABLE 8.5. Physiological Reactions to Cocaine Use and Abuse: John B.

Commonly Reported Reaction to Cocaine Use/Abuse	Reaction Observed Yes	Reaction Observed No	Percent/ Time Observed	Qualifying Comments and Observations
Dizziness – feeling of light-headedness	Yes		90	There have been times with pharmaceutical coke that I felt like my head was about two feet above my shoulders.
Sweating – perspiration or increases in temperature	Yes		100	My palms were always sweaty and sticky.
Rhinorrhea – running nose		No		You get that snorting.
Tremors – muscle spasms		No		I didn't tremble, but I always had a strange feeling in the pit of my stomach.
Lacrimation – tears to eyes		No		You do snorting, sometimes.
Mydriasis – dilation of pupils, light sensitivity	Yes		100	Bright lights hurt your eyes on cocaine.
Gooseflesh	Yes		50	I'd get goosebumps about half of the time. I don't know why, though.
Emesis – vomiting	Yes		5	You feel you're going to vomit almost all the time.
Reactive hyperemia – clogging of nasal air passages		No		You do snorting.
Anorexia – loss of appetite, sensation of hunger	Yes		100	You're just not hungry.
Dryness of mouth and throat, lack of salivation	Yes		100	They are dry as hell.
Increased heart rate	Yes		100	Your heart rate increases. You can feel it.
Tightness in chest or chest pains	Yes		20	I don't get chest pains but you do feel tight.
Local anesthesia, numbness	Yes		100	If I shoot over a gram my whole head is a little numb, but it is a little spot under my nose that I notice most.
Nosebleed		No		I never had that happen snorting or shooting.
Elevation of pulse rate	Yes		100	It's more pronounced shooting than snorting.
Increased respiration rate	Yes		100	I start breathing harder when I am shooting.
Cellulitis – inflammation following administration		No		You can get that snorting if you don't rinse.
Infection of nasal mucous membrane		No		Never.
Yawning		No		I never noticed it.

284

Hyperphrenia — excessive mental activity	Yes		Your mind goes like hell. It is more pronounced shooting.
Weight loss	Yes		It's simple, when you shoot you don't eat.
Fainting	No		I never fainted on coke.
Increased sensitivity to allergies	No		I don't have any allergies.
Diarrhea or explosive bowel movements	Yes	100	I didn't have diarrhea. I just had to go to the john 20–30 minutes after I got off. It happened every damned time.
Hepatitis or liver infections	No		You don't have that problem with new needles.
Headaches	Yes	20	I would only get headaches with a big "fix." Then, sometimes I would have a ripping headache with the rush, but it wouldn't last too long.
Loss of fatigue	Yes	100	You have no sensation of being tired. You can go on and on.
Ringing in the ears	Yes	75	Your ears will ring with high quality coke most of the time.
Convulsions	No		I never had anything like that. I will start vomiting if I do too much.

285

TABLE 8.6. Psychological Reactions to Cocaine Use and Abuse: John B.

Commonly Reported Reactions to Cocaine Use/Abuse	Reactions Observed Yes	Reactions Observed No	Percent/ Time Observed	Qualifying Comments and Observations
Increased feeling of self-control		No		No, instead I always felt like I was losing control because I had to do more.
Increased optimism, courage	Yes		100	I felt more self-confident and more aggressive.
Increased activity, restlessness, excitement	Yes		100	I just felt more restless and excited.
Feeling of increased physical strength or ability to do physical work		No		I was *never* thinking about working when I was shooting coke, just the next "fix."
Intensified feelings of well-being, euphoria, "floating," etc.	Yes		100	Yes, I felt great!
Feeling that everything is perfect		No		Hell no, I was just getting high!
An exquisite "don't care about the world" attitude		No		You get that sometimes with high grade heroin though.
A physical orgasm in the "rush"		No		Never.
Increased thinking power and imagination	Yes		100	Your mind and your imagination are both going crazy.
Feeling that the mind is quicker than normal, the feeling that one is smarter than everyone else	Yes		100	I felt my mind was quicker than normal.
More talkative than usual, a stream of talk	Yes		100	If there is someone with you, you just rattle on.
Indifferent to pain	Yes		100	You don't feel any pain. You don't notice it at all.
Decreased interest in work, failure of ambition, loss of ambition for useful work		No		There was no work involved. I wasn't working when I was doing coke every day. I was just doing coke. I didn't have a job to worry about.
Insomnia	Yes		100	You can't relax. You can't sleep unless you take something to come off coke.
Depression, anxiety	Yes		100	Shooting cocaine makes me more anxious. Sometimes, I would get depressed afterwards. I was always depressed when I come off cocaine.
Prolonged sexual intercourse		No		Only if you applied it directly to the penis or clitoris.

An aphrodisiac or sexual stimulant	No		Not for me.
Better orgasm on coke	No		Hell, I have never had a bad one. The worst I ever had was exquisite.
Irrational fears	Yes	10	Particularly on a run. I would get paranoid.
Terror or panic	No		I've been scared at times, but never felt terror or panic.
Tactile hallucinations — the feeling that insects are crawling on or under the skin (particularly fingertips, palms of hands, etc.)	No		I never felt anything like that. You get more of that with amphetamines.
Changes in reality or the way a room or objects look — the wall waving or in motion, etc.	No		Nope.
Paranoid ideas — the feeling that people are after you. You believe you are being watched, talked about or threatened, a wife or girlfriend is unfaithful, untrustworthy, etc.	Yes	10	I was afraid the cops would break in several times. You shut the doors and windows and lock the place up, but you're still scared they are coming.
Causes one to carry a gun or run from imaginary enemies	No		I carried a gun for two years. Hell, I was living with thieves, murderers and robbers. Everyone carried a gun. I don't know if I was paranoid because of the coke or the company. You had to be paranoid around those dudes.
Visual hallucinations	No		No, I never saw anything that wasn't there. It's all in your head.
Auditory hallucinations — hearing voices talking about you, threatening, etc.	No		I never heard it, but just had a funny feeling that people might be talking. I could never understand what was being said. It was just a feeling.
Olfactory hallucinations — new odors, smells, etc.	No		Just the smell of drugs and blood.
A trigger for violence	No		Cocaine will not make you violent. It never made me that way. If you get violent it is because violent dudes are taking it.

auditory, tactile or olfactory hallucinations, or changes in perceived reality. Although John is sexually active, he reports that he never experienced an orgasm with the flash; he does not feel cocaine is an aphrodisiac or produces a more spectacular sexual orgasm. However, he did assert that cocaine applied directly to the penis or clitoris would prolong sexual intercourse. John does not feel cocaine is a trigger for violence, although he feels that a violent man taking it might have some tendency to become more so.

Integration

John has tried most if not all of the major drug substances. However, he is not a polydrug user in any strict definition of that term. His adult use of drugs has stabilized with alcohol, marijuana, hashish, opiates, and cocaine. As he describes it, his opiate use is simply an adjunct to cocaine; it prolongs the cocaine high and curbs adverse cocaine reactions.

Regular use of cocaine has served several important purposes in John's life. It (1) gives him an instant lift out of depression, (2) buoys him up and obliterates his uncertainty and self-doubts, (3) helps him shake off slights and disappointments, and (4) with its exhilarating euphoria makes him feel more aggressive and confident. Using cocaine he becomes the shadowside of his personality, the bold and decisive man who takes what he wants from life. These reactions are in such contrast to John's typical state that he has been drawn repeatedly back to the drug in efforts to recapture these powerful but fleeting experiences of well-being.

Apparently, John is not taking cocaine as heavily as before. He still suffers intermittent and at times almost disabling bouts of depression. However, they are not daily occurrences. It may be that in his second marriage he has finally found the affection, emotional support, and encouragement he needs.

LIFE ACTIVITIES AND EXPERIENCES: IN JOHN'S OWN WORDS

Overview

The following sections are accounts of two days of John's life. They cover a period in 1975 from April through May.

John works the day shift in a service station that services from 300 to 400 cars daily. Gene, the station owner, is in and out during the day. He watches his employees closely because he thinks they are stealing money from him; if the daily cash report doesn't balance closely, he accuses everyone of theft. John resents this. This service station only pumps gasoline; it is against the owner's policy to provide ancillary services for customers — washing windows, checking the oil, tires, and so on. However, John sometimes provides these extras for customers; they then learn to expect the extras and are irritated when he fails to provide them. Sometimes John is not sure he likes people.

On the first day, John and his wife leap out of bed, dress and race to work. John wants to be on time today; the station owner has asked John to become the day manager with a large raise. John is also looking forward to getting off work early and riding in a friend's hotrod.

John is irritated that the night shift did not do their work. He and his assistant are busy all morning. At mid-day John goes home to meet his friend. His friend takes John's car and John has the afternoon to drive his friend's hotrod with "600 h.p. under the hood." He shares how he feels driving this superb machine, and provides an apt description of how he must feel when he takes cocaine: fast, powerful, and unbeatable.

John has to work at the station that evening to "pay for" his afternoon off. John shares how he feels about his boss. When the station closes that night a friend, Fred, and his girlfriend bring John's wife to the station to go out and have a pizza. John does not respect Fred because he had impregnated his wife and then left her. Although it upsets Susan, John tells Fred in no uncertain terms that he is tired and is going home to bed, and then does just that. As he says, "I have to get up and go to work tomorrow!"

The second day occurs a month later. John had accepted the promotion to station manager; during the last month he has worked from twelve to fourteen hours a day, has turned the station around, reduced cash losses to almost nothing, and established tight supervisory control over other employees. However, the owner has never given him the promised raise. John feels he has been taken for a sucker.

Throughout this day John broods about this dilemma. He fears that the only recourse left to him is to leave the job. Though he has done all that anyone could expect of him, he sees no reward for his efforts. By withholding the promised raise the station owner has thrust John into the emotional state he has so painstakingly attempted to avoid in his life, namely, anger. He fears he might lose control, explode in a rage, and hurt someone; he has the physical capability to do that. Now he is a prisoner of his anger; it permeates everything. It is only late in the day when working in his garden that John is able to obtain some feeling of relief.

A day later the anger had dissipated somewhat, but had been replaced by a pervasive sense of depression and dejection.

Activity and Experience Audits

First Day: A Wednesday in April

6:30 a.m.–12:00 n.

I woke up late, jumped out of bed, cleaned up quick, and woke Susan. She got dressed quick. We were racing. She drove me to work. Gene, the owner, wants me to run the day shift now, so I didn't want to be late. I'm usually there by 6:45 to open up. Really though, I was already waiting for the day to pass. I had a friend of mine with the damndest hotrod you've ever seen coming into town today. He was gonna let me drive his hotrod while he tried to score some coke. I was feeling okay.

I opened up with John — Brad had quit and taken another job. As I told you, John's my age, kinda slow mentally; he's not real sharp but he's a hard worker. He doesn't talk too much, which is okay with me. People were sitting on the drive to buy gas when we got there, and business was steady till noon.

As John and I got time, in between cars, we took the stuff out and opened the outside. The night before, I had told one of the guys to get the salt off the drive; this morning it was still there. It pissed me off! It's a small thing to ask of a guy, but the guys who work the night shift do nothing. They leave everything for the guys who work days. It's not fair.

The repairmen came, five of them. They were there most of the day, and two were in and out most of the day. They were fixing the exterior and hanging new lights. About 8:30 the owner, Gene, arrived to watch them. He also was hiring some new guys and had a bunch of applications in the office; I bet he asked me ten times if I remembered the guys who had applied and ten times I told him no, that Brad had interviewed them and I had been working the drive. Then he would start telling me about them. Damn!

We worked steady all morning. In between cars I helped two of the electricians hang some lights; when they found out I knew how to do the wiring, they seemed glad for my help.

12:00 n. –1:30 p.m.

John left at noon and David came on. I like John better; all David wants to do is talk hotrods. He always wants to help. I appreciate his offer, but I would rather do my work myself.

At noon I started to do my reports for the day. It takes about an hour and a half to do all the bookwork when you can devote full time to it. You have to count the money; you count the gas you've pumped, the products sold, products left, add up the credit-card purchases, and try to balance the books. I came up nineteen dollars over. I tried to find the error, but couldn't.

I told Gene about it. He said not to worry if it was that close. We would probably be twenty dollars short the next day. You're just as much in trouble if you're long as if you're short.

1:30–6:30 p.m.

The other guy, Mike, came in. He's tall, thin, and lazy as hell. I don't know why Gene hired him. I split out, drove home hoping my friend would be there. As I rounded the corner, I saw his car at the house.

Clarence, the guy, was having some trouble with his car, so I helped with it. We opened the hood, and Jesus Christ, there were 600 'horses' in there. It had a short in the wiring. We found it and fixed it.

We opened some vodka and stuff in the house and proceeded to get high on booze. I don't keep any rigs anymore. We are starting to get some new friends. A doctor and his wife and kids were over recently; Susan and I like them, and I'm not gonna take any chances of fucking it up. Man, it's hard to break out of the drug culture. It is hard as hell to make friends who are straight but someone you would like to know. Clarence and I visited awhile.

He took my car to get what he wanted; he wanted to score some dope. I took his hotrod. He said he would pick up Susan at work, so I went driving in that hotrod! Shit, man, it was exquisite! He has about ten thousand in it. He can't keep a transmission in it to go with a motor like that, though. I cruised up and down the streets and highways. I got in some races. Shit, you step down on it and she moves! It has so much torque, you crowd it into third and she'll turn completely around. You'll be going the other way! You're riding only about a foot and a half off the ground!

It was a nice day, and when I got out on the highway there were a lot of kids tooling around. They saw that car and they wanted to go! Even though it is highly muffled, that s.o.b. would just sit and shake at the stop signs. I literally walked away from those 240Zs, big Mustangs, and Corvettes. I ate them up, just disappeared! Shit, the police couldn't catch you with a car like that; they'd have to have a helicopter to keep track of you. You turn a corner, step on it, and you're three blocks away! It was wild! It made me feel high as hell!

I used to have a hotrod in high school but nothing like that damn thing! Guys would just look at you when you pulled off and left them. They couldn't believe their eyes! They might catch up with you later at a stop sign and say, "What the hell you got in there?" I told them just a stock motor. The damn thing was so powerful, by the time you're in second gear you're doing 80 m.p.h.! By the time you got to third, you were doing over a hundred!

I got back about 6:00. Clarence and my wife were home. He asked how I liked it. I said that was one fine car! He smiled.

Susan told me Mike had called from work, so I called him back. Mike laid some shit on me about relatives coming in that evening and asked if I would work for him. I didn't want to, but he agreed to work for me Saturday night, so I said okay.

I told Susan I was going back to work. I didn't eat; we were going out with some friends after work.

I smoked some reefer and split for work. I drove back to work feeling very good; I was thinking how I wanted Mike to work the next day. He didn't.

6:30–10:00 p.m.
I worked the place till 10 p.m. Business was pretty slow that night. I scrubbed down the driveway keeping busy.

Gene came in and out all night. He told me he appreciated me cleaning the drive. I thought, "If you weren't so damn cheap and would buy some cleaner, we could get the grease off the drive, too!" There was only one guy, David, there. I let him work customers on the drive while I scrubbed it down.

The guy who I told to scrub the drive down the night before was there; he came over and apologized and started helping me. The s.o.b. figured I would do it and not say anything. I guess he was right. Gene knew about it and was not on his ass. All the kids he hired were friends of customers, and Gene doesn't want to antagonize anyone. He tells me to handle it in any way I choose. He puts the shit on me, and I resent it, I guess.

10:00–11:30 p.m.

Susan and two others — the crazy guy, Fred, and his new chick — pulled in. Fred had split with his wife and was living with this chick on the Plaza. He's knocked his wife up and then left her.

I closed the place and locked the door. Gene asked how much gas we had sold, and I told him. He said not to stay, 'cause it would increase the risk of getting robbed. Hell, I was leaving!

Susan and I got in our car. The guy and his gal were going to follow us. I found out they wanted to go to another town for a pizza! I told Susan to hell with that shit, I didn't want to go that far. I told them I was tired and didn't want to go that far; I wanted to go home to bed! They said okay.

Susan and I drove home. She was wondering if they were pissed that we didn't go. I told her they were not disappointed, they knew I had worked a long day. I told her the guy understood. Frankly, I didn't give a shit whether he understood or not! He's a nice guy, but he's a fuckup, anyone who would treat his wife that way. I told Susan, hell, I have to get up and go to work the next day.

At home, Susan fixed a light dinner while I cleaned up. She and I ate and went to bed.

I went straight to sleep. My wife was tired too; she had had a hard week at work.

The Day: It was a pretty good day; I drove the car and got high.

Second Day: A Monday in May

(John was "down" and depressed. His body sagged in the chair and he stared vacantly at the floor. His eyes were red; he was unkempt and spoke in a low, halting, almost inaudible tone. It was difficult to hear him.)

6:30–7:00 a.m.

I woke up, cleaned up, and got dressed. My wife Susan was feeling bad; she had come down with the flu. No sex today; I am too depressed and Susan is sick. I am too down to do sex.

She got up, though, and took me to work. I was thinking about a lot of things at work — and that idiot boss of mine. I was feeling angry about the whole fucking thing! I had done what I said I would. I thought it was only fair he did his side of the bargain, but he hadn't!

7:00 a.m.–2:00 p.m.

I opened that fucking place up! You know that damn routine almost as well as I do now: We put out the barrels, opened the oil display, counted the gas sales from the night before and all of that shit! There was another kid, Paul, there helping me. I sent him over to get us some coffee and rolls while I opened the fucking place. He's only been working two or three weeks. Paul is a kid, eighteen or nineteen years old; he's a hustler when I tell him to, but he sits on his ass otherwise. He's okay, I guess.

Business was real slow. People are pissed off about the price of gas going up. It was a slow day; we probably only serviced seventy cars from 7:00 a.m. to 2:00 p.m. I am thinking about going back to work on the railroad; I would be working mostly out in the country. I would rather be doing that than sitting at that damn station! I am kind of trapped there till I settle the shit with Gene, the owner. I was figuring that if I am going to have to work my ass off, I might as well be getting some bread for it. My wife, Susan, feels the same way! It would have been different if Gene had given me the raise he had promised, but he has not done it, the idiot! I am fussing with all of this shit!

I am trying to put my cycle back together. My dumb brother ran it into a tree and wrecked it. I am thinking about this, too; I'm thinking it will take about $400 to get the cycle fixed. I am feeling kinda low down with the whole fucking deal! The whole thing of my life right now is kind of screwy. I am pissed about it all!

At the station about all of the customers know me. I've got our day customers to a really good point now. If I could only make the money Gene promised me, it would be okay there, but shit, it looks like that's all been for naught!

Brad came by and brought me something to eat! He didn't bring much, but it was something. He stops in every once in a while and visits with me — I was glad to see him. He's doing real well on his new job. He drives six to eight different cars for this rich dude. He said the old fellow bought him $400 worth of clothes to work in. I was telling Brad about Gene; he said that Gene had taken advantage of me as long as he could. He told me I should find out where Gene was at and see if he was going to honor his promise to me.

I simply couldn't believe Gene would pull all of this shit on me after all I had done to help him! I was thinking I will end up quitting, and it will cost the idiot a third of his business!

Brad left.

I did the fucking report; it took an hour and a half. I was less than two dollars short. That's the way it has been coming out since I became the day manager. I have come as close as thirty-five cents of being even, and shit, that's almost impossible in an operation like ours.

Gene comes in or calls every day. He says he's real busy doing some other stuff. He will be in tomorrow to pick up the time cards, and I intend to corner him and find out where the fuck we are with the raise he promised. I am angry, hurt, and disappointed with the s.o.b.! I guess I am just seeing him for what he really is, a fool!

2:00–4:30 p.m.

Susan came back, and we left the fucking station! I was supposed to pick up some air conditioners and help my brother put them in. I was still thinking about the idiot, Gene. You know, I pretty well gave up trying to make it at school when Gene offered me the raise; I put all my effort into getting that damn station turned around. It looks like I'll be going back to the railroad and all of that work will have been for nothing!

We drove over to my mother's place. I am really pissed at Susan! There wouldn't be any sense in going over there if she had called my brother before-hand like I asked her to! It was her damn stupidity. When we got to my mother's place I called my brother. He was leaving and said he didn't have time to do the job that day. I told Susan she should be very fucking glad I had not gone down there with those damn air conditioners and found him gone! Yesterday I laughed with her about it, but I guess I am angrier today talking about it than I was then.

We visited with my mother a few minutes. I ate some pie and a couple of apples. We just bullshitted around with my mother a while.

That fuckup, idiot s.o.b. Gene makes me mean! He's made me an angry man!

Recently I ran into another dude, a strong-arm robber who had owed me $1,000 for two years. I have been upset over that, too! I saw him drive by in a new car. I am going out one of these days to collect my money. If he doesn't pay, I'll just have to beat the shit out of him!

4:30–6:30 p.m.

Susan and I drove on home. She's not feeling very good. The flu has worn her out. I was kinda pissed at her, but I also wanted to get her back home where she could rest.

When we got home I laid down a few minutes and smoked a reefer. Susan went out to do some shopping instead of going to bed!

I got up, ate a sandwich, and walked out to the garage and worked on my cycle for a while. My brother tore the shit out of it! I was trying to keep the anger out of my mind. I go through periods where I very deliberately don't think of anything at all, because I am afraid if I think about it all of the time I might do something rash.

I have put in a big garden out in back of our house and I work in it every night after work; it kind of takes out my frustration. I left the tore-up cycle and worked in the garden. It's a nice one. I was having a good time working there; I got off into thinking about everything I had been growing there. I have found that the garden is really self-satisfying. I puttered out there.

I was thinking I am not going to blow up and bust Gene for fucking me around. I'd get put in jail for hitting him, and I don't intend to go to jail for hitting his fat ass!

6:30–9:00 p.m.

I went in the house, cleaned up a bit, and took a nap.

At about 8:15, Susan woke me. She was home, she had bought a bunch of garden stuff for me, to help me feel better, I think. She bought me a new garden hose, a cooler, and stuff. She was trying to get me in a better mood.

It took me about thirty minutes to wake up; I had been sleeping hard. I took the new hose out and watered the garden down good while she started on supper.

9:00–11:30 p.m.

I came in and helped Susan get the stuff together for dinner. I was feeling okay, but was still griping and complaining about that damn Gene. He screwed me, and I didn't think he would.

We ate dinner. I was pretty hungry. I didn't have much to say; there were long periods of silence.

I picked up the dishes. Susan went on up to bed. She was wiped out.

I took the dog outside, and then about 11:30, I went to bed.

The Day: It was an okay day, I guess. I did everything I had set out to do. I was pissed at myself, though, because I was letting people run over me, and I don't like that!

9

Willie M.

LIFE THEMES

Willie M. is a proud and stoic black man who has suffered much; he is 44 years old and has "seen it all and done it all" in a violent, drug-ridden, ghetto community. For several years Willie was a highly successful cocaine dealer. The major themes in this man's life are the following:

- I was exceptionally talented and should have made it to the top, but because I am black I never had a chance. Nevertheless, I kept trying, only to be excluded again and again.
- I turned to drugs to escape the hatred these frustrations built up in me.
- Selling drugs also gave me some of the success I deserve.
- Now, though I am important in the drug community, I am bitter and I grieve over the hopes and dreams that were denied me.

Cocaine Use in Relation to Life Themes

Willie is a daily, high-dosage (four grams per day), intravenous cocaine user. Willie uses cocaine because it

- helps him tolerate a life of isolated self-sufficiency,
- helps him tolerate the failures, missed opportunities, and crushed hopes of his life,

• helps him shake off his heavy protective armor and occasionally enjoy a good time with a few close friends,
• makes him feel briefly vibrant and alive, and
• obliterates temporarily the anger and despair that dominate his life.

For these palliatives Willie pays a high price in terms of the adverse reactions the drug produces.

EVOLUTION OF LIFE STYLE

Introduction

Willie is a tall man, not muscular like Muhammad Ali but broad-shouldered, angular, and lean like Bill Russell, the basketball star. He displays little motor tension and moves with the loose, relaxed grace of a well-trained athlete. Typically, he wears tasteful dark-colored slacks, a quiet sportshirt, dark shoes or loafers, a leather jacket, and a snap-fastened "Big Apple" billed cap. If one saw him on the street, one would probably notice him briefly, but then pass on to look at others, for Willie prides himself on his anonymity; he deliberately dresses "down" to enable him to move unobtrusively in and out of the ghetto scene. His demeanor is consistent with his dress: Willie is always poised, relaxed, and at ease. At no time at interview sessions did he exhibit the slightest flicker of tension, anxiety, or breaks in what was obviously a well-learned stance of poise and composure. At no time did his cool, calm self-assurance break, falter, or fail him; he always seemed to know exactly what he was doing. Though he has an engaging boyish grin, Willie rarely smiled; his face was so impassive that it soon became clear that to understand him one must listen closely and watch his eyes — which, unlike his face, are highly expressive. Willie communicates the aura of an alert diplomat or prince from another country, another world, another era. It seems clear that whatever country, world, or era he represents, it is not necessarily a friendly power.

Always alert, formal, and reserved, Willie is an articulate man whose responses flow smoothly; however, he carefully weighs his words. He is complex and subtle, adept at innuendo and indirection. Despite Willie's distance and caution, he worked diligently. He was honest and direct — though careful about how he expressed his feelings and ideas — and reliable; his word is his bond. Yet he never relaxes completely. Perhaps he cannot do so.

Developmental Experiences

Willie was born in Kansas City, Missouri, the second of four children in a black family. He has one older sister, age forty-six, one younger brother, age forty, and a younger sister, age thirty-eight. Although his father was the basic family provider, his mother also worked during Willie's developmental years.

Willie's father is now in retirement. However, during Willie's early years his father had a successful business providing janitorial and cleaning services on a contract basis for several large office buildings in the city. "My father worked almost his whole life to take care of his family. It seemed like he had to work all the time to do it. He was a farm boy with only a fourth-grade education. He started off doing menial labor; then, during the war, he worked in several war plants. After the war, he set up his own business and was very successful with it. He retired six or seven years ago. He has aged tremendously since then; I am afraid he's getting senile. I wish there was something I could do to help him, but there isn't. He is a good man, a hard worker who never harmed anyone."

When Willie was asked what his father was like during his developmental years, he stated, "He was kind and considerate, a good provider. He'd take me to basketball and baseball games and sometimes to the movies. Sometimes we would go squirrel or rabbit hunting together, too. He was never involved in much, outside of work and his family. He was very affectionate, but not as disciplined as my mother. He was very proud when I was selected for the city all-star basketball team. I guess you could say maybe that he guided me in the direction of basketball. He would take our whole basketball team on trips when we played out of town."

When asked how he would change his father if he had his life to live again, Willie stated, "I'd change his way of doing things quite a bit. I wish he had disciplined me more and given me more attention and guidance. I needed help. I was stubborn and hard-headed. I needed some guidance when I was growing up. He could have taught me to fight to get the breaks I needed; he didn't do that. A man has responsibilities to his children, his sons. He should guide them and show them the right way."

Willie said his mother was "a lot of woman," adding, "She was very personable. She worked some when I was a kid, but she was more or less just a housewife. My mother is always willing to help someone. However, she could be stern and would discipline us kids when we needed it. She showed the leadership and direction in our family. She had more education than my father; she had a year of college. She paid all the bills and handled all the finances for the family and my father's business too. When problems arose I would always discuss them with my mother, not my father. My mother was involved in church, school, community groups, a lot of things. She is still very alert and active, even though she is almost seventy.

"I would always rather my father spanked me than my mother. She would get mad as hell and would prove to you in no uncertain terms that she meant what she said! You couldn't con or manipulate her, she would see through you in a minute. I think she probably over-disciplined us. I remember she wouldn't let me out of our front yard until I was twelve years old. That's a bit much, I think, but she is still a good woman."

When asked how he might change his mother if he had his life to live over, Willie stated that he would not change her at all. "I love her the way she is. I only wish my father had had some of her strength."

Willie was not close to his brother and sisters. "There is one exception, my older sister Joyce. I was quite close with her; I still am. My brother Tom and I were never really close, but we got along OK. He's pretty square, works regular, has a family; he hasn't been through the hurts and disappointments I have, maybe because he didn't dream as big as I did. My younger sister and I never had much in common. I guess I am distant to an extent with my brother and my sisters, but I still am close with my parents. I go by to see them once or twice a week to see how things are going."

Willie's family was stable. "We were probably better off financially than our neighbors. My parents didn't fight a lot; my father would do what my mother said. That bothered me some. I wish he had stood up more for himself, but he didn't. The biggest single problem I faced was trying to get out of our front yard. Maybe that is why I like to travel so much now, go to new places, meet new people, see new things."

When asked what he was like as a child, Willie stated, "I was mischievous; I instigated a lot of things. I used to set up pranks, but I was a kind of loner even then. I had to find out all of the things I needed to know by myself. I really didn't confide much in people – anyone."

"I did OK in grade school and junior high school. I was a good athlete, but only an average student. The fact is, I was an exceptional athlete; I was captain of our high school basketball team and was on the all-city all-star Team for two years. I always had a dream of going to this large university on the West Coast and playing basketball. I followed their team in the papers and sports magazines all those years; they were the only team I was interested in. It was my dream to have a family by the time I was twenty-one and be in California going to school and playing basketball there. I was good enough, but I didn't know how to get a chance. I wrote the coach a letter – he was a white guy – and told him about myself and how I would like to have a chance for a tryout. I even sent my clippings from the *Star*. The coach never even answered the letter.

"I was crushed. I thought about going out and seeing the coach myself, but somehow I was so hurt, I didn't. Later, I always wished I had done it anyway. It didn't make me feel any great love for whites, though; it took something out of me and left a kind of bitterness towards whites and the world. It also left me with another problem: What was I going to do with myself after I got out of high school?

"I only wanted to be a basketball star. My coach sent letters to a lot of black schools and by spring I had a number of offers and accepted one from one of the biggest black universities in the South. My folks were very proud, but it wasn't where I wanted to go — that was out west. I played on the freshman team and was the star; I'd make anywhere from twenty to thirty points a game. I stayed there for a year and a half. The coach said I was one of the best young players he had ever coached. But something was wrong; I couldn't discipline myself to study, I wasn't happy. I don't know why to this day, but in my second year I just quit school and came on back to Kansas City. The coach wrote me a letter asking me to come back, but I was too proud. I needed help, but I didn't know where to find it.

"The upshot of it all was that I enlisted in the army. The Korean War had started and I wasn't in school, so it was either enlist or be drafted. I made sure the officer who enlisted me put my basketball experience in my record, and, sure enough, as soon as I was out of basic I was picked for a post basketball team.

"I was making my twenty to thirty points a game, and began to make a name for myself. But I had trouble living with the rules and regulations, saluting officers, and taking orders from dumb-asses. Well, I got into heroin; it took anger and everything else away and made me feel relaxed and mellow, but two or three of us were caught shooting it. I received an undesirable discharge. I didn't mind getting out of the service, but the undesirable discharge hurt.

"I came on back to Kansas City, and had an offer to play on a well-known black professional basketball team. I took it. The money wasn't great, but enough to get by on OK. I traveled a lot; I enjoyed that. I played with the team three or four years. In those days there was no place for a black athlete to go. Young black athletes now don't know what it was like twenty to twenty-five years ago. I get to thinking if I had been born ten years later I could have made it. It all makes me feel very bitter at times.

"I married a beautiful woman while I was playing ball. I have a way with women; I always treat them with courtesy, respect, and dignity until they show me they don't deserve it. Anyway, I married Agatha. She was like my mother in a lot of ways. She was nice, outgoing, gregarious and affectionate, outspoken and direct; she had a lot of drive too. She was good to me and good for me. We had two children, two boys. I loved them very much.

"I had a number of jobs after we moved back to Kansas City. I worked making cinder blocks, as a porter, a stack man in a factory, a delivery man — but I always thought I was capable of doing better. I had trouble working for the other guy; I liked my independence too much.

"After a couple of years my marriage began to come apart; it was the drugs. I was addicted to heroin the first time when I was twenty-one. I broke that one cold-turkey, but after I came back to Kansas City I got more into heroin, till I was spending almost everything I made on it. Agatha was working, too, but she couldn't support a family all by herself. She begged me to stop, but I couldn't. I was using up all our money supporting my habit. Finally, Agatha told me she loved me, but she couldn't live that way. She divorced me, took our sons, and moved to California.

"I was twenty-seven then. I had lost the best thing that had ever happened to me. Agatha later remarried and some other man raised my sons; they're almost grown now. I got involved in drugs more heavily after that; I did a lot of heroin, morphine, even barbiturates. Drugs took me to rock bottom. I was arrested for vagrancy and spent several months in jail for writing bad checks and script. I was what everyone thinks of when they think of a heroin addict.

"I have been addicted four or five times in all. I guess I naturally drifted into dealing. It was hard to get a job, no one wants to hire an addict. Anyone who does drugs deals some. At first you deal to cut your own drug costs. Gradually, I began dealing more and more. It's hard business; you can get rich quick and you can be killed quick. Addicts are vulnerable people; they are vulnerable to their dealer and they are vulnerable to the law. The dealer has to be prepared to strike fast when addicts try to take advantage of you — and they will. You can't even trust your best friend. I have a friend, Terry. He's a jewel, a charmer, he's my number one man, but he's an addict, and I know he wouldn't hesitate to take advantage of me if any real amounts of heroin were involved.

"The dealer builds a reputation as a man not to be messed with by examples. It's brutal but necessary. People do not mess with me. A smart dealer doesn't get too high in the business or too low: If you are too high, you're too visible; if you're too low, the police are always pulling you in. You're alone and always in danger — it's a jungle. I made it a point to be Mr. Anonymous and I established a number of very complex ways to protect myself — which, by the way, are none of your business. Also, during the five years I dealt cocaine I surrounded myself with violent men, men who wouldn't hesitate to hurt people if necessary. Finally, I tried to keep a legal job to cover me; police won't bother you too much if you mind your business and have regular employment.

"You have to be cautious, careful, and bold at the same time, if you know what I mean. Sometimes boldness will carry you through where nothing else will. The drug world is a violent world. You have to be prepared to be murdered or murder someone else. It's that simple; kill or be killed.

"I did well as a cocaine dealer. The cocaine I sold was Bolivian rock crystal. It was brought into the country in diplomatic pouches. It came every month. I would purchase a half kilo or a kilo at a time. My man was a nephew of the embassy contact, so there was a regular monthly supply. I would cut it and sell it, to blacks and to whites, too. The drug world is integrated; people who paid the price got a good grade of cocaine.

"I lived well, but never was involved in much public display here in town. If I wanted to have a good time I would catch a plane to some place like Los Angeles or New York, vanish in the city, and have a good time. Here I tried to be quiet and unobtrusive.

"When I was thirty-eight, I got a job helping out in the kitchen of this big restaurant. I felt humiliated, but I needed a job. Surprisingly, they didn't check references, they just hired me. I learned a lot about food preparation, it's an art. The restaurant manager took a liking to me. Several times he asked why a man would take that kind of job. I finally told him I had been an addict, but was trying to put my life back together (which was true). Funny, he accepted that. After that, whenever a waiter would be sick or on vacation, he would call me to cover. I learned how to be a waiter and a damn good one. I learned that you can serve other people and still be a proud man. Later, I became a waiter full-time, and now I have worked myself to head waiter behind the maitre d'. I intend to go to maitre d' school back East next year; a good maitre d' can always find employment. There is a lot of grace and art and even a little showmanship, muted of course, in being a good maitre d' — I like that part of it. Life can be paradoxical; I never set out to be a maitre d', I wanted to be a professional athlete, but here I am.

"At about the same time that I went to work in the restaurant I remarried. She was an addict, too. She had a son and a daughter. I married Betty because she was amorous, and because I was tired of the loneliness. Even though we should've never married, it gave me stability when I needed it. I love the children, particularly my stepson; he is about ten or eleven, a beautiful boy. Having children around gives me responsibility — I need that.

"As it ultimately turned out, the children were the only thing Betty and I had in common. I am divorcing her. It would be easy if it were just Betty and I, but I love my stepchildren and that tears at me. Betty will get the children; but she won't know how to support them, how to love them. The boy, Randy, wants to come and live with me, but I work nights at the restaurant. Who would look after him?

"As I have gotten older I have gotten away from heavy use of drugs. I am not an addict anymore; I haven't been for a couple of years. I am very much against doing cocaine anymore. It gives me an exceptional high, but it tightens me up, turns me against people, and makes me intensely paranoid. I don't want any more of that. Betty is still into heroin and keeps trying to pull me back into it. An addict can't tolerate an ex-addict, they will go to extremes to try to bring them back into it. When I was dealing, it was common practice to give an addict coming out of the penitentiary free heroin for a while. It was designed to draw him back into it, and it works most of the time.

"I moved out for a couple of months. I went back because of the kids and because Betty said she would try to do better, but she hasn't, so we're separated again. I will divorce her this time, but it makes me sick to think about what will become of my stepchildren.

"I am not heavy into dealing drugs now. I kind of edged out of it over the last four to five years. The players in the drug world change so fast that one can do that if he is careful. The drug world is a young man's world. I have done many things that my parents would consider brutal, evil, or abhorrent, but when you are dealing they are simply necessary to survive. At times one is tempted to get back into it, because you can get rich overnight if things break right, but I am tired of looking over my shoulder all the time. I have seen enough of deceit, violence, and killing. When I look back at the opportunities that I missed, the things I might have done, I become very depressed.

"I would like to go into some type of business of my own. I would like to be able to travel, go to superbowls, the fights, and things like that, but if I had a business of my own I would probably goof off a lot. Realistically, I'd like to become a good maitre d' in a big restaurant or a big hotel, something like that.

"I am forty-four years old now; much of my adult life has been a shambles. I am still alone. Maybe I will never be able to trust anyone; I can live with that, I suppose, I always have. Maybe I can find some peace in my life, I don't know."

Interpretive Integration

At least seven modal factors in Willie's early life provided the framework for the evolution of his life style:

- A childhood spent in a relatively secure, black middle-class family
- A work-oriented but gentle father who permitted his wife to assume major responsibilities for management of the family
- A resourceful and dominant mother — an affectionate woman but a disciplinarian who filled the void left by the father
- A reasonably secure but somewhat overprotected childhood
- A developing awareness that he was an exceptional athlete
- The crushing defeat of his childhood dream to play basketball at a large, well-known university
- Subsequent bitterness toward whites and the world for his inability to capitalize on his exceptional talent — a rationalization he could fall back upon in succeeding years to account for his failure to achieve things he desired.

As a result of these experiences, Willie developed a pattern of adjustment characterized by the following:

- Difficulties in developing a stable and secure identity
- Chronic feelings of resentment toward persons in positions of authority
- Difficulties in pursuing long-range goals in the face of adversity
- A tendency to become discouraged, give up, and withdraw
- The use of drugs — primarily heroin — to obtain relief from the rage he felt toward an uncaring world
- Development of a cynical view of the world in which people are seen to be dishonest, hypocritical, and motivated by selfish interests

· Efforts to build an invulnerable existence characterized by (1) complete self-sufficiency, (2) pervasive distrust of other people, (3) superficial warmth and charm without any willingness to permit intimacy, (4) willingness to take violent action against anyone who poses a threat, (5) denial of dependency needs as making him vulnerable to exploitation or attack by others, and (6) depression and malaise as a consequence of his efforts to maintain an impossible existence.

Willie is a strong, disciplined, and self-sufficient man. As a youth he desperately needed fatherly guidance; had this been available, his life might have gone in a much more rewarding direction. At age forty-four, Willie has finally found employment which, though far below his youthful aspirations, provides financial stability, a challenge, and some future. It has been a hard struggle and he has paid a high price to regain control of his life. He has fought his way out of the ghetto drug community. Apparently he functioned very effectively in this dangerous and violent world; he is still known, feared, and respected there. Obviously, he obtained gratifications from being a dealer that went beyond the financial rewards. Perhaps it was the sense of having power over people's lives. More likely, however, Willie (like some gamblers) took pleasure in the excitement, danger, and competition, and from operating an illegal and clandestine business without being caught.

Willie may never be able to shake off the cynicism, depression, and malaise that is always with him. And of course there is no way he can recapture the years of his life that are lost. Willie knows this, and that may account in part for the sense of meaninglessness in his existence. Perhaps he can come to terms with it. Perhaps this is why he talks about needing peace and tranquility.

Willie's responses on the Metaphors Test tell of his stance in life. When asked what kind of animal he would be if he had the choice, Willie stated, "I would be a tiger, a big cat. They are strong and independent. Others fear them. They provide for themselves. They don't run in packs, they are loners like me." When asked what kind of car he might be, he stated, "I would be a luxurious car, a Cadillac or a Lincoln Mark IV." Finally, when asked what flag he would fly from his car antenna to convey his uniqueness to the world, Willie stated, "I don't know. Well, no, I would have a flag with three stripes across it: bright blue, white, and blue. It tells everyone that I am distinctive, but they won't know what the symbolism means. I have always tried to be anonymous; the flag I described would be distinctive, yet still would be anonymous."

FORMAL PSYCHOLOGICAL ASSESSMENT

Dimensional Test Findings

Intelligence Tests

Willie performs in the Bright Normal range of intelligence. Thus, he has somewhat more ability than does the average man in understanding problems, engaging in planned behavior, and acquiring new learning.

MMPI

MMPI results (figure 9.1) present the picture of an adjustment characterized by well-developed self-controls, resentment of authority, depression, and tendencies to bind tension in vague psychophysiological complaints (headaches, gastrointestinal symptoms) and in ruminative concerns. It is a picture of a chronically unhappy man. There is no evidence of a serious mental disorder, although there are some suggestions of neurotic difficulties. The relatively low Validity scores indicate that Willie attempted to answer questions honestly.

Willie appears to be, first and foremost, a controlled individual. There are often marked differences between what he feels and what he does. Although he can make appropriate decisions easily, he carefully considers consequences before he acts, and worries about them. Given the stakes involved in his decisions, that he would worry on occasion is hardly surprising. Willie is an introspective man who values self-understanding and understanding others.

Willie tends to dominate and control others. Though he may be somewhat sentimental, he does not allow such feelings to interfere with his actions, nor does he express them to others. He is probably seen by others as strong, personable, smooth, and socially sophisticated. He strives to be sufficient unto himself, impervious to censure, and to live by his own personal code. Though not paranoid, Willie is distrustful, and allows himself intimacy with only a few carefully selected friends. He is not a man who allows himself the luxury of anger; rather, he gets even quickly, settling accounts in a cold, businesslike way.

Internally, however, Willie is anything but "smooth and calculating." He is an emotional person. He tends to experience feelings strongly, often overreacting internally. He uses his intellect to monitor his expression of these feelings, and for this he pays a price.

Willie is a pessimistic and unhappy man, dissatisfied with life and cynical regarding interpersonal relationships. This cynicism is fed by his intense, unmet dependency needs; he would like to let down and be taken care of but knows he cannot do so. He also internalizes his anger, resentment, and frustrations. Though he looks unruffled on the surface, he is prone to depression and somatic complaints. Willie tries to see himself as basically healthy and problem-free while the world in general is wrong and unhealthy. Willie knows he cannot change it, so he sets about to control it.

Sixteen PF

On the Sixteen PF Test (table 9.1), Willie describes himself as an assertive, dominant man who can be solemn, stern, and hostile. He is headstrong and competitive — he expects to win. Unconventional in his values, he none-

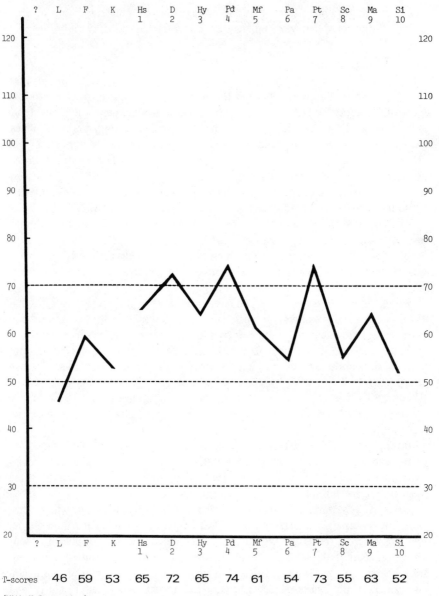

T-scores   46 59 53   65 72 65 74 61   54 73 55 63 52

(With K Correction)

FIGURE 9.1.   MMPI Profile: Willie M. *Reproduced from the Minnesota Multiphasic Personality Inventory Profile and Case Summary form, by permission. Copyright 1948 by the Psychological Corporation, New York, N.Y. All rights reserved.*

theless expects respect and deference from others. Willie tends to operate behind the scenes; he is not flamboyant or flashy. Yet though he tends to be understated and cautious, he can be bold and daring when a situation demands it. In periods of stress he tends to isolate himself and be self-sufficient; he evidences high autonomic stress.

These data also suggest that Willie is an emotional, changeable person who is easily upset and is generally annoyed and dissatisfied with the world. He experiences some psychophysiological complaints (headaches, insomnia, digestive distress); many of these are directly related to the way in which he deals with stress, for he is internally a volcano while externally cool, aloof, and detached.

Other Dimensional Measures

Willie's scores on the Sensation-Seeking and Novelty Experiencing Scales indicate that he is not a thrill-seeking adventurer. He does seek novel experiences, but these are usually quietly internal and cognitive in nature. He enjoys outfoxing his adversaries, and is challenged more by mental problems than by physical feats. He tends to eschew thrills and danger, getting his thrills from more sophisticated experiences such as travel, sporting events, music, art — or cocaine.

The Change Seeker Index reveals him to have a higher need for variety than the average person.

Willie obtained scores of 10, 10, and 2 on the Eysenck Extraversion, Neuroticism, and Lie Scales. These scores compare with normative scores at the forty-seventh, sixty-first, and forty-fifth percentiles among adult industrial workers. They suggest that Willie is a mildly neurotic man who is about as outgoing and gregarious as his peers. The moderate Lie score suggests that Willie was reasonably honest in his responses.

Integration

Findings from the formal dimensional measures are consistent with those reported in Willie's developmental history. Viewed from without, Willie seems cool, distant, self-sufficient, well-defended, intact, and in full control of his life. Viewed from within, however, he is seen to be a brooding, depressed, bitter, and lonely man. Willie has gained what success he possesses only because he has forged and tempered a will of iron. Though this protects him from the dangers of the world in which he lives, it has squeezed much of the meaning and joy out of his existence.

TABLE 9.1. Cattell 16PF Profile: Willie M.

Standard Score	Low Score Description	Standard Ten Score (Sten)	High Score Description
4	Reserved, detached, critical, cool, aloof, stiff, precise, objective	A	Outgoing, warm-hearted, easygoing, trustful, good-natured, participating
5	Less intelligent, concretistic thinking, less well-organized, poor judgment	B	More intelligent, abstract thinking, bright, insightful, fast-learning, better judgment
2	Affected by feelings, emotionally less stable, worrying, easily upset, changeable	C	Emotionally stable, mature, unruffled, faces reality, calm (higher ego strength)
10	Humble, mild, easily led, docile, accommodating, submissive, conforming	E	Assertive, aggressive, stubborn, headstrong, competitive, dominant, rebellious
6	Sober, taciturn, serious, introspective, reflective, slow, cautious	F	Happy-go-lucky, enthusiastic, talkative, cheerful, frank, quick, alert
4	Expedient, disregards rules, social conventions and obligations to people (weaker superego strength)	G	Conscientious, persistent, moralistic, persevering, well-disciplined (stronger superego strength)
2	Shy, timid, withdrawn, threat-sensitive	H	Venturesome, uninhibited, socially bold, active, impulsive
7	Tough-minded, self-reliant, cynical, realistic	I	Tender-minded, sensitive, dependent, seeking help and sympathy
5	Trusting, accepting conditions, understanding, tolerant, permissive	L	Suspicious, hard to fool, dogmatic

(Standard Ten Score (Sten) scale: 1 2 3 4 5 6 7 8 9 10)

Low Score Description	Factor	Score	High Score Description
Practical, "down-to-earth" concerns, guided by objective reality	L	7	Imaginative, bohemian, absent-minded, unconventional, easily seduced from practical judgment
Forthright, unpretentious, genuine, spontaneous, natural, artless, socially clumsy	M	5	Astute, polished, socially aware, shrewd, smart, "cuts corners"
Self-assured, placid, secure, self-confident, complacent, serene	N	5	Apprehensive, self-reproaching, insecure, worrying, troubled, guilt-prone
Conservative, respectful of established, traditional ideas	O	7	Experimenting, liberal, free-thinking, non-moralistic, experiments with problem-solutions
Group-dependent, depends on social approval, a "joiner" and sound follower	Q1	6	Self-sufficient, resourceful, prefers to make own decisions
Undisciplined self-conflict, lax, follows own urges, careless of social rules	Q2	6	Controlled, exacting willpower, socially precise, compulsive, persistent, foresighted
Relaxed, tranquil, torpid, unfrustrated, composed, low ergic tension	Q3	6	Tense, frustrated, driven, over-wrought, high ergic tension

Average

Findings From Morphogenic Measures

Overview

The pattern of Willie's morphogenic data seems at first to reflect vagueness and inconsistency in his thinking. However, close examination reveals that while Willie may suffer ambivalence and conflict his thinking is by no means confused. Rather, it is complex, like the thought-processes of a sensitive person aware of all possibilities and unable to avoid problems by self-deception.

The Q-Sort descriptions he provided made it clear that Willie is not happy or self-satisfied. He dislikes being hostile, cruel, violent, or sad, yet he admits that sometimes he is all of these things, especially when involved with drugs. Characteristic of Willie's Q-Sorts was his tendency to discriminate among people and psychological states by what they are not rather than by what they are. For example, he would describe someone as being "not foolish," but he would not describe that person as "intelligent." He often does not like what he does, but he seems to feel that hostility, cruelty, and dishonesty are sometimes essential. He resents having to be that way, and his resentment is aggravated by his feeling that he has not really achieved his goals.

Willie's interpersonal relations as described on the Rep Test reveal as much about his attitudes toward drugs as about his relations with people. Apparently, the two are closely related: On the one hand, he seems to use cocaine to facilitate social communication and enjoy a good time with friends; on the other, he can use it to escape from others. It is likely that Willie vacillates between times when he is sociable, easygoing, warm, and friendly, and times when he is aloof, bitter, and hard as nails. He knows this and does not like it, but feels unable to live any other way.

As regards environmental settings, his contacts with them are both varied and reasonably satisfying. Willie is able to continue behaving effectively and drawing sustenance from a world he does not like.

Q-Sorts

Standard Items

The most impressive characteristic of Willie's Q-Sorts is their apparent inconsistency. For example, at the first assessment session his two descriptions of his usual self correlate at a chance level (median $r = .095$). The median value of the between-session reliability of his usual-self descriptions was only .282. One cannot conclude that Willie is incapable of producing reliable descriptions, because the median value of the reliability coefficients for his ideal-self descriptions is .653, a satisfactory figure.

The most likely explanation for the apparent unreliability in Willie's usual-self descriptions is that he is so complex that he can provide several different descriptive sortings under the same set of instructions, and they are all valid.

The stability of Willie's description of his ideal self can be explained on the grounds that he has a strong moral sense which provides, perhaps, the only constant and dependable thing in his life.

Despite their apparent unreliability, some trends can be discerned in correlations among specific sortings; that such trends exist speaks against the hypothesis that Willie was providing meaningless data. For example, the correlations between his descriptions of his usual self and those of his ideal self became more negative as time went by, dropping from a median of -.152 to a median of -.414. It seems that Willie was undergoing an increase in dissatisfaction with himself. Associated with this increase in self-dissatisfaction was a slight but noticeable increase in self-identification as one similar to the typical cocaine user. There was also a marked increase in the negative correlation between Willie's description of his ideal self and his description of the typical cocaine user. These findings suggest that Willie's opinions of cocaine users and himself were changing in an unfavorable direction.

Factor analysis. Willie's data yielded four factors with a complicated table of factor loadings. Most characteristic of the first factor were the strong loadings of all three descriptions of Willie's ideal self. Although some other descriptive sortings had moderate loadings on this factor, these three were definitive, and the factor was therefore called the Ideal Self.

The heaviest loadings on the second factor were two descriptions of the usual self (at the first and second reassessment sessions) and one of the self during a cocaine high (at the first reassessment session). Two more descriptions of the usual self (at the first and second reassessment session) have moderate loadings. This factor was therefore identified as that of a Drug Self.

Each of the next two factors contained one high loading, each being a description of a typical cocaine user. No descriptions of the usual self or the ideal self loaded on either factor.

What Willie wants most in his Ideal Self (Factor I) is to be wise and logical, happy and pleasant, and to strive and accomplish. He dislikes most being hostile or cruel, violent or impulsive, feeling sad or depressed, and the possibility of being foolish or unintelligent.

Factor II (Drug Self) is possibly also a description of Willie's actual self. The person described in this factor is sad and depressed, but kind and friendly, respected, and well-known. He is not at peace with himself, sacrifices happiness and pleasantness, and gives up striving and accomplishing as well as wisdom and intelligence. If this is a self-portrait, it is not a happy one.

The first typical cocaine user (Factor III) is anxious, nervous, violent, explosive and impulsive, and stubborn and self-centered as well as a great many other undesirable things. This person is not happy or pleasant, controlled or restrained, or kind or friendly. The second typical cocaine user (Factor IV) is also anxious, nervous, and prone to violence or impulsiveness; but this person tends to become sad and depressed rather than stubborn or self-centered. Willie further characterizes him as not being foolish or unintelligent, as not being shamed or laughed at, and as not being sexually impotent or afraid. Willie typically makes discriminations more clearly in negative than in positive terms; the differences between the two cocaine styles are much more pronounced at the negative than at the positive end of the scale. Willie grants that the second cocaine user may be socially prominent; but he does not say that because he is not foolish he is therefore wise.

Individualized Items

As was the case with the standard items, the evidence on the consistency of Willie's sortings of individualized Q-Sort items (table 9.2) is mixed. Again, he provided consistent descriptions of his ideal self (median $r = .737$). His descriptions of himself as he is after cocaine wears off were also reliable (median $r = .725$), as were those of himself during an amphetamine high (median $r = .523$) and of his own bad self (median $r = .500$). Time trends were not marked in these data.

The negative correlation between usual self and ideal self was stronger and more consistent in these data (median $r = -.542$) than in the data from the standard-item Q-Sorts. As if to complement this finding, correlations between Willie's descriptions of his usual self and bad self were positive (median $r = .489$). Furthermore, correlations between Willie's descriptions of his usual self and those of most nonusers of drugs hovered around the chance level (median $r = .004$).

Factor analysis. Six factors were extracted from the data. As might be expected, the factor structure was complex and difficult to interpret. Only four of the factors were subjected to detailed analyses. The first factor we have called Drug Self 1. Its most consistent pattern of loadings occurs at the first reassessment session, where high positive loadings occur for Willie's descriptions of his usual self and of himself during a cocaine high, after a cocaine high, and during an amphetamine high. A strong negative loading appears for his description of what he is like when wanting cocaine. Descriptions of the ideal self tend to have negative loadings on this factor while descriptions of the bad self are positively loaded.

Factor II has high loadings only on Willie's descriptions of what most nonusers of drugs are like. Consequently, this factor was called Other People.

Factor III, called Drug Self 2, is closely identified with amphetamine use. (Although Drug Self 1 contains one description of the self while on an amphetamine high, it seems to be mainly concerned with cocaine effects.)

Only two sortings have high loadings on Factor IV; both are descriptions of Willie's bad self. This factor was therefore named accordingly.

Drug Self 1 (Factor I) is in a most undesirable state. Willie says he is tense, nervous, foolish, dumb, stuck on himself, and vain. He lacks self-satisfaction and wisdom; he is not happy, laughing, relaxed, or peaceful. Drug Self 2 (Factor III) is similar in some ways to Drug Self 1, but in Drug Self 2, Willie feels vibrant and thrilling and tends to lose self-control and patience. He feels less vain and

TABLE 9.2. Individualized Q-Sort Items: Willie M.

Achievement
Positive
1. Succeeding
2. Making progress
Negative
3. Successful by stealing
4. Using others to pull yourself up

Affect
Positive
*5. Laughter
*6. Happiness
Negative
7. Hurt
8. Crying

Anxiety
Positive
9. Relaxed
*10. Peaceful
Negative
11. Tense
*12. Nervous

Chastity
Positive
13. Pure, like a monk or nun
14. Disciplining yourself when no women around
Negative
15. Sexually incompetent
16. Cannot please a woman

Dependence
Positive
17. Not grown up
*18. Accept help gracefully
Negative
19. Helplessness
*20. Clinging

Dominance
Positive
*21. Strong
22. Aggressive
Negative
23. Passive
24. Weak

Excitement
Positive
25. Feel vibrant
26. Thrilling
Negative
27. Thirsty for violence
*28. Impulsive

Humility
Positive
29. Mellow
30. Cool
Negative
31. Overlooked
32. Pushed aside

Independence
Positive
33. Free
34. Self-sufficient
Negative
35. Stuck on himself
36. Vain

Knowledge
Positive
37. Smart
38. Ready
Negative
*39. Foolish
40. Dumb

Restraint
Positive
41. Self-control
42. Patience
Negative
43. Haven't bought a ticket
44. Boring

Self-satisfaction (Stasis)
Positive
45. At peace with himself
46. Has peace of mind
Negative
*47. Lazy
48. Stumbling along

Sexuality
Positive
*49. Romantic
*50. Sexually stimulating
Negative
51. Do sex forcibly
52. Adultery

Interpersonal Relations
Positive
*53. Kind
*54. Friendly
Negative
*55. Hostile
56. Cruel

Social Recognition
57. Someone like Mayor Wheeler
*58. Famous
Negative
59. Clown
*60. Laughed at

Note: Items marked with an asterisk (*) are not significantly altered from their original (standard) wording.

313

stuck on himself than when in Drug Self 1, but he is more inclined toward hostility and cruelty.

Willie's conception of other people (Factor II) is not flattering. They are vain and stuck on themselves, boring, and haven't "bought a ticket" (i.e., they "missed the train," are missing out on life). In compensation, they are succeeding or making progress and feel relaxed and peaceful. But they are not famous, violent, and smart.

The contents of Factor IV (Bad Self) should dispel any beliefs that Willie was using the Q-Sort items to present himself in a favorable light. It has already been shown that Willie identifies to some extent with his own bad self. That self is hostile, cruel, foolish, dumb, and will steal or use others to gain success. It is not at peace, it is not free or independent, and it is not succeeding, despite its dishonesty. The appearance of the bad self as a separate factor suggests that Willie is sensitive to this aspect of his character. Willie is not a self-deceiver; his life would be less unpleasant if he were. As it is, he is painfully aware of everything and is therefore condemned to try to make sense out of a conflicted world.

Rep Test

Role Groups

If a liberal criterion of .500 was set for acceptable reliability, eleven of the twenty roles Willie described here would be discarded from the data. Among his most reliable descriptions were: ideal self, mother, father, liked employer (described in exactly the same way every time), successful person, and person you would most like to help. These are all "safe" role-descriptions in that honesty here is not likely to reveal much of importance about Willie himself.

Among his least reliable descriptions were: usual self, worst self, wife or girlfriend, interesting person, person who dislikes you, person who behaves strangely, and self on cocaine. Possibly Willie had more than one candidate for these roles and shifted referents from test to test. Possibly he is truly uncertain about some.

The interpersonal constructs invented by Willie were as follows:

Interpersonal Constructs

1. Independent
2. Aggressive (pushy, forward)
3. Loner
4. Responsible
5. Stubborn, dogmatic
6. Respects feelings of others
7. Patient
8. Lovable
9. Considerate
10. Braggart

11. Talks too much about other people's business
12. Aspired to be a businessman, but no respect for the law
13. Can communicate with others
14. Rational
15. Hostile toward authority

Factor analysis. Willie's data yielded five factors, of which two are strong and three are weak. Only the first three have been subjected to closer analysis.

Factor I is a stereotype of the nice people in Willie's life. He includes both his usual self and his ideal self in this factor, which is quite a change from his behavior on the Q-Sorts. (There, his usual and ideal selves correlated negatively while his usual and bad selves correlated positively.) Other members of this group are: mother, father, liked employer, successful person, and interesting person. These people are lovable, considerate, wise, responsible, rational, and can communicate with others. They are not aggressive, mean, selfish, hostile toward authority, and are not braggarts.

Factor II is related to drugs: friends with whom Willie takes drugs, someone who drinks a lot of alcohol, person you feel sorry for, and wife or girlfriend. These people are like those in Factor I, but they are not responsible, rational, or wise. However, unlike people in Factor I they are sexy. This factor suggests that for Willie drug-taking is a way of getting together with friends and perhaps of abandoning temporarily consideration of the harsh realities of everyday affairs.

Factor III may be idiosyncratic. It is bipolar, containing at one end a person who dislikes Willie: This person is independent and responsible, but is also a braggart. The other end of the factor contains Willie's self while on cocaine. Despite the suggestion in Factor II — that he uses drugs to promote socialization — he describes himself on this factor as selfish and a loner. A reasonable guess is that Willie uses cocaine for both purposes: sometimes to facilitate socialization, at other times to get as far away from everything as possible.

Construct groups

Like everything else about him, Willie's interpersonal construct space is complex. Six factors were produced by the data.

Factor I has something to do with character strength, containing as it does the constructs: independent, responsible, rational, strong, and wise.

Factor II refers to potentiality for positive, affectionate interpersonal relations. It contains the constructs: respects the feelings of others, lovable, can communicate with others, kind, helpful, and sexy. Worthy of note is the fact that Willie places sexuality in the context of love, respect, and communication. His approach to sexuality seems, therefore, to be a mature one not complicated by problems of feared impotence or the need to prove his own masculinity.

Factor III contains undesirable constructs and seems to refer to others' aggression and lack of consideration. The traits it contains are: aggressive (pushy, forward), braggarts, mean. A negatively loaded trait here: considerate.

Factor IV refers to opposition to legal authority, mentioned in both of its constructs: aspires to be a businessman but has no respect for the law, hostile toward authority. Factor V calls to mind Willie's description of himself on cocaine as a selfish loner. Both Factors IV and V are important characterizations to Willie; they are highly specific in their referents.

Factor VI contains one heavily loaded construct: talks too much about other peoples' business. Aggressive (pushy, forward) also has a moderate loading on this factor. The factor applies to Willie's own worst self and to several people of whom he seems to be otherwise fond: wife or girlfriend, cocaine friends, and an interesting person. Apparently, this is a trait he dislikes but is willing to tolerate in others if they are sufficiently appealing on other grounds.

Setting Survey

In contrast to most of the other data, Willie's record of daily activities is reliable overall. He has a stable pattern of activities and satisfactions that repeats itself regularly. His life seems to be well-organized. Willie enters a wide variety of settings, leading what appears to be a well-balanced life. He works steadily but is also engaged in job-training and commercial and financial enterprises (about the nature of which the reader is left to speculate).

Apparently, too, Willie leads a satisfying existence. His satisfaction scores do not indicate any serious or permanent sources of difficulty. His least satisfying activities had to do with physical health rather than work or social relations. He is very satisfied with his mental health contacts, so it may be that he is currently attempting to work through some of his problems.

Integration

Willie's morphogenic data seem unreliable if examined superficially. However, he is a complex individual so sensitive to all possibilities that he can provide multiple responses to the same stimulus, and all of them are valid. He tends to see the negative sides of things, to be cynical, and to experience despair. He is not satisfied with himself, the world in which he lives, or the people in it. He admires and respects independence, rationality, strength, and wisdom, and is capable of love and affection. Yet he is unhappy and critical of himself and his environment. He feels that aggression and selfishness are necessary for survival, so he becomes aggressive and selfish almost against his own will; as a result he sees himself as a bad person. Probably this only makes him angrier at the world, for he believes that he is not bad by choice but by necessity, and he resents that necessity.

STYLE OF DRUG USE

General Pattern

Willie began drug use with marijuana at age thirteen (table 9.3). He used it off and on for two or three years, then began daily use that has lasted throughout his adult years. Apparently, he uses marijuana as a tranquilizer; he feels it is a relaxant. At age fourteen Willie drank alcohol for the first time, beginning regular use at about twenty-one and continuing throughout his adult life.

He experimented with heroin while he was in the service and was first addicted at age twenty-one. He continued to take heroin on a nearly daily basis for almost twenty years. Although he suffered addiction at least five times, he stated he has taken heroin only intermittently during the last two years. Shortly after Willie's first addiction to heroin he experimented with a variety of other opiates (morphine, Dilaudid, opium), and apparently has used them off and on for much of his adult life. Willie reported no use of illegal methadone.

Willie tried cocaine first when he was about twenty-four. He used this drug off and on until the age of thirty-six or thirty-seven; then he began relatively heavy use of cocaine — this was during approximately the same period he was a cocaine dealer. He gave up cocaine about two years ago; he wants nothing more to do with the drug because it made him exceedingly paranoid.

For a brief period following his first divorce, Willie used amphetamine and barbiturates, tried nasal inhalants, and experimented with polydrug mixtures of amphetamine and barbiturates as well as of heroin and cocaine. In his later thirties, Willie began intermittent use of tranquilizers, Valium, Librium, etc., to help him manage tensions in living.

Willie indicated that calculating the daily cost of drugs is difficult because his cost actually decreased as he grew older. Until he was in his early thirties, his habit cost from $100 to $125 per day. As he became more active in dealing, his daily costs dropped below the $60-65 level. This was because he could now trade cocaine for heroin and could purchase in large quantities to obtain a better price.

Willie said he only overdosed once, with heroin in his mid-twenties. "Everything started getting dark. I started to faint. Some friends got some milk down me and kept me on my feet, walking me around until I began to feel OK again."

The two longest periods in which he has been drug-free were for two or three years when married to Agatha and during the last two years. "Sometimes I will go for a month or more and not touch any drug except tranquilizers to help me sleep nights."

TABLE 9.3. Genealogy and Pattern of Drug Use and Abuse: Willie M.

Drug Substances	Age 13 14 15 16 17 18 19 20 21 22 23 24 25 26 27 28 29 30 31 32 33 34 35 36 37 38 39 40 41 42 43 44	Frequency of Drug Usage	Comments
1. Marijuana		Daily	It relaxes me.
2. Alcohol		Several times a week	I drink Scotch and some light wine on occasion.
3. Heroin		Daily	For years I was into that.
4. Other opiates Morphine Dilaudid Opium		Occasionally	I would use them when heroin was not available.
5. Cocaine		Daily	I was doing about a quarter-ounce per day on the average.
6. Amphetamine*		Less than once per week	I tried them a while but don't like the feeling they give you.
7. Barbiturates* (T-Birds, Seconal)			Same as amphetamine.
8. Inhalants* (nasal spray)		Infrequent	I tried nasal inhalants a while, that's all.

318

9. Polydrug mixtures* (barbiturates/amphetamine, heroin/coke)	Occasionally	Mostly "boy" and "girl." Heroin is the best way to get off coke.
10. Psychotropics (Librium, Valium, etc.)	Occasionally	I use Valium and Librium to help me relax and sleep.
11. Illegal methadone	Never	I just never got into it.
12. Hallucinogens (psychedelics)	Never	Most blacks don't do psychedelics. It's a middle-class white thing.
13. Non-prescription, over-the-counter drugs	Never	A lot of addicts do over-the-counter drugs, but I never did.
14. Others		

*When my first wife divorced me I was into everything for a while.

Legend

――― Denotes regular usage

‒ ‒ ‒ Denotes intermittent usage

Preference Rankings

Table 9.4 verifies Willie's preference for heroin, cocaine, and speedball mixtures of the two drugs. Marijuana, beer, and amphetamine occupy the mid-range of his preference rankings while hard liquor and barbiturates are less desirable. Though he dislikes amphetamine, this energizing drug is somewhat more desirable for him than hard liquor. LSD is in a class by itself as the drug he desires least of all.

TABLE 9.4. Drug Preference Rankings: Willie M.

Substance	First Assessment	First Reassessment	Second Reassessment	Mean	Composite Rank
Amphetamine	8	5	5	6.00	5.5
Barbiturates	7	8	8	7.67	8
Beer	5	7	6	6.00	5.5
Cocaine	2	2	3	2.33	2
Hard liquor	6	6	7	6.33	7
Heroin	1	1	2	1.33	1
LSD	9	9	9	9.00	9
Marijuana	3	4	4	3.67	4
Speedball	4	3	1	2.67	3

Ratings

Analysis of Willie's ratings of the ten drug-stimuli on the twenty-six scales of the semantic differential produced only two factors. Factor I is bipolar. At one end Willie included barbiturates, heroin, amphetamine, hard liquor, and LSD. These he described in negative terms as: bad, dangerous, unpleasant, wrong, hazardous, dull, sick, and negative. At the other end of this factor are two substances Willie contrasts with the above: beer and marijuana. The terms he used to describe beer and marijuana include: good, safe, pleasant, right, bright, healthy, weak, minor, tiny, soft, and clean. The stimulus "drugs in general" had a low loading on this first factor, so it appears that Willie does not consider the substances in this factor to be drugs. At one end of the dimension he seemed to be describing poisons; at the other, soft drinks.

Factor II is a cocaine factor, though it also includes (with somewhat lower loadings): drugs in general, heroin, and speedball. Substances in this factor are: good, active, pleasant, bright, beautiful, and soft.

Heroin occupies a unique position, being loaded somewhat on both the first and second factors. Willie seems to be ambivalent about it; On the one hand, it is dangerous and bad but on the other hand it is desirable. Willie's ambivalence is probably due to the fact that he has had trouble with heroin and is now cautious about its use.

Pattern of Use

Social Context

Willie took cocaine daily for four or five years. "I have only snorted cocaine once or twice in my life. I *shot* cocaine; I was not after the euphoria they talk about, I was after the flash or rush. It is kind of like coming in intercourse, only better and more sensational. However, it is very brief, you have to shoot up again in ten or fifteen minutes to get it back."

Commenting on the first time he took cocaine intravenously, Willie stated, "It happened a couple of years after I got out of the service. A friend took me to a hotel where a couple of guys had a batch of coke — they had knocked over a drugstore. I fired up with them. I didn't know what had happened! It made me nervous, it speeded me up something awful! I didn't get paranoid that time, I remember that (I usually get paranoid as hell). Anyway, I shot up a second time. I was talking a blue streak! I was sweating something awful, too. I remember later I went downstairs and out of the hotel. It was late fall and it was cold. However, I took my coat off and walked five miles home, feeling fine and talking to myself. I didn't know until the next morning, when my sister asked me about my car, that I walked right by my own car. Later, I had to get a friend to take me downtown and pick up my car; I had just walked off and left it."

Willie liked cocaine because of the high it provided. "It gave me a feeling of enjoyment that you can't describe, but as soon as I pulled the spike out it made me nervous and paranoid 100 percent of the time. I couldn't deal with people when I was on it; it made me want to withdraw and not be with anyone. I would only use it at home: I would lock up the house, pull down the blinds, shut the windows, and turn off the TV. I was afraid the police would be busting the door down at any minute. This feeling would last for an hour to an hour and a half after I had stopped shooting. It would throw me into a panic if I did cocaine all night and then went to work; it scared me to have to talk to people, I couldn't look them in the eye. I really panicked two or three times at work. I would have to get off away from everyone for a while to get myself together. Sometimes, I would call in sick; other times, I was almost unable to work. It was sheer hell!"

Willie stated that probably 80 percent of his total cocaine usage was at home with a woman living with him. The remaining 20 percent was with a close male friend; he never took cocaine with more than two people. "I was just too paranoid on cocaine and it made me angry and hostile. That's why I would stay home. I would never be on the street or in a car, just home and in a well-locked room. However, people react differently to coke. People's body makeup and chemistry are different. It affects different people different ways."

Willie's typical daily cocaine consumption was three or four grams (an eighth of an ounce) over a five-year period. "It is hard to nail it down like that, because there were times I would do more. A woman who lived with me and I did six or seven grams of Peruvian cocaine from 6:00 p.m. until 5:00 a.m. the next morning every day for over a year. We would spread that amount between us over the night. We did that every day for a year and every other day for three years, so I am not sure exactly how much I used over the five-year period. When I say four grams a day I am averaging it, but it may well be more than that. I would buy it by the ounce, half, or kilo; it would be about 50 to 60 percent pure, sometimes 40 percent pure. We'd cut it; I would keep the high quality cocaine and sell the rest. By the time it would get to the street, it would be about 8 to 10 percent pure; that is about the quality level you buy on the street if it is cocaine at all. A lot of what people buy on the street for cocaine is not cocaine but procaine. Most people can't tell the difference, though. About one-third of the coke on the street is procaine."

Willie stated that he had only been on two cocaine runs. "By 'run' I mean doing it for more than a twenty-four hour period without stopping. I did that twice, but there was really very little reason for me to do more than that. First, I knew I would go to work the next day, unless I was so paranoid that I couldn't do it. I needed my job to cover me; I have always tried to keep a regular job. Secondly, I always knew there was more cocaine available the next night if I wanted it — and I usually did — so there was no reason to go on an extended spree."

Willie took most of his cocaine during the evening hours. "It was because of my job; as paranoid as I would get on cocaine I wasn't about to do it during the day, but I would fire up after I got home in the evenings."

Ninety percent of the cocaine he used was Bolivian or Peruvian rock crystal; the remainder was street cocaine. When asked how he determined its quality Willie stated, "You can't tell by the looks; it is too easy to disguise cocaine. I would rely upon two things: one, who I was buying it from, and, two, by firing up a sample. If you know good cocaine, you can judge the quality by the rush or flash and the taste it leaves in your mouth. In addition a lot of high-grade cocaine has a peculiar alcoholic odor to it; in fact, I've seen some funny-looking pink cocaine with that smell recently. The pink is caused by the cut, probably vitamins or something. Prescription and rock crystal cocaine are strong. You can feel the difference quite clearly, your whole body reacts with high-quality cocaine.

"The person you do business with is also important. My original contacts dried up after three or four years. Then I developed contacts in the Midwest. The people I was doing business with really couldn't afford to rip you off because they knew it would only happen once. Consequently, they were usually quite honest about the quality of cocaine they were selling. It was good business and it was safer for them. Generally, they were very gentlemanly about the whole matter."

Willie was puzzled when questioned about development of tolerance to cocaine. "I don't think I ever developed any tolerance. It happens with heroin, but not cocaine. I would probably be doing more cocaine towards the end of the evening, but I don't call that tolerance. After four or five fixes you are pretty numb and you are not paying so close attention to how much you are using. However, I could take a pill of boy and two pills of girl doing a speedball and continue at that rate all night without increasing it. I can do two pills of girl over and over again and still get the same reaction all night. I have heard people saying they had to increase the size of their fixes, but it shouldn't happen with high-quality coke."

When asked what circumstances would trigger use of cocaine, Willie stated, "First, the availability of the drug and, secondly, I would use it if I was having personal problems. In the second case, I would get at coke indirectly, that is, personal problems usually drive me to boy and from boy would lead to girl. Then I would really get off into girl. However, there is an escape in heroin that you can't find in coke. Sometimes, I would use cocaine simply because I wanted to be high, though."

Though withdrawal from cocaine was uncomfortable, he did not perceive it as painful. "I would be tired and anxious as hell. I would be nervous, and couldn't sleep. Generally, I would take a pill — Dilaudid or Demerol — or shoot some heroin so I could get some rest; if I didn't take something, my mind would be racing and I would never get any sleep. It causes a strain on your heart; my chest hurt so bad that twice I went to my doctor to check it out. They say cocaine is nonaddictive but it can make you mentally addicted. I should know, I have been there. Cocaine can make people very psychotic. It's use should never be legalized. I think that if you shoot it long enough you have to have some kind of permanent mind or brain damage."

Reactions to Cocaine

Physiological Reactions

Table 9.5 indicates that for Willie physiological reactions were present either every time or not at all. Only one physiological reaction — ringing in his ears — occurred part of the time, and he attributed this to variations in the quality of the drug.

By and large, the physiological reactions Willie reported were those associated with stimulation of the central and autonomic nervous systems. He reported that 90-100 percent of the time he used cocaine, he experienced loss of appetite, loss of sensations of fatigue, sweating, dryness in the mouth and throat, sensitivity to light, visual anomalies, nausea, and marked increases in heart rate, pulse rate, and mental activity (but, surprisingly, no increase in respiration rate).

Willie never experienced dizziness with the rush, fainting, increased incidence of or sensitivity to allergies, hepatitis, tremors or muscle spasms, or convulsions. He reported that he might experience "loose bowels" or diarrhea the following

TABLE 9.5. Physiological Reactions to Cocaine Use and Abuse: Willie G.

Commonly Reported Reactions to Cocaine Use/Abuse	Reactions Observed Yes	Reactions Observed No	Percent/ Time Observed	Qualifying Comments and Observations
Dizziness – feeling of light-headedness		No		I have never had that reaction.
Sweating – perspiration or increases in temperature	Yes		100	My hands sweat and I perspire heavily.
Rhinorrhea – running nose		No		That's for people who snort cocaine.
Tremors – muscle spasms		No		Not that I know of.
Lacrimation – tears to eyes		No		Not that I ever noticed.
Mydriasis – dilation of pupils, light sensitivity	Yes		90	I guess so, because after I would shoot three or four hits I couldn't see so well. Sometimes, it would get so bad I would miss the vein.
Gooseflesh	Yes		5	It doesn't happen all the time.
Emesis – vomiting	Yes		100	I only vomited one or two times. However, cocaine makes you feel like you want to vomit 100 percent of the time. It's a rather weird, funny reaction.
Reactive hyperemia – clogging of nasal air passages		No		That's with snorting cocaine.
Anorexia – loss of appetite, sensation of hunger	Yes		100	You just lose all sensations of hunger.
Dryness of mouth and throat, lack of salivation	Yes		100	Your mouth is very dry.
Increased heart rate	Yes		100	Good cocaine makes your heart pound.
Tightness in chest or chest pains	Yes			It only happened three or four times. I thought there was something wrong with my heart.
Local anesthesia, numbness		No		If you miss a vein, the area around it will get numb.
Nosebleed		No		I have seen people who snort a lot of cocaine develop a nosebleed.
Elevation of pulse rate	Yes		100	Just like your heart, your pulse starts pounding.
Increased respiration rate		No		I have never noticed that. Sometimes a big hit will almost take your breath away.
Cellulitis – inflammation following administration		No		No.

324

Symptom	Yes/No	%	Comment
Infection of nasal mucous membrane	No		But sometimes you can get abscesses at the point of the hit. Anytime you miss a vein you can risk getting a burn. Coke causes bad burns.
Yawning	No		I don't think it happened with me.
Hyperphrenia — excessive mental activity	Yes	100	Your mind runs fast, almost like lightning.
Weight loss	Yes	20	If you do cocaine every day, you will certainly lose weight because you don't eat.
Fainting	No		Not for me.
Increased sensitivity to allergies	No		I never had allergies.
Diarrhea or explosive bowel movements	Yes		It only happened with me two or three times. Maybe it's the cut that does it. Sometimes, they cut the cocaine with epsom salts.
Hepatitis or liver infections	No		Never with cocaine. You have to use new spikes to avoid it though.
Headaches	Yes	100	When I quit shooting, I always get headaches "coming down."
Loss of fatigue	Yes	100	You have no sensation of fatigue at all.
Ringing in the ears	Yes	65	It depends on the quality of the cocaine.
Convulsions	No		Not for me.

morning, but attributed it to epsom salts in the cut. Occasionally he would experience numbness at the site of injection, particularly if he missed the vein. "The veins in my arms are gone, so I used the veins in my legs, and if I missed the vein the area of my leg would be numb." Willie noted that three or four times cocaine caused such intense chest pains that he subsequently saw his family physician; he thought he might be having a heart attack. Willie frequently experienced burns or abscesses at the site of injection: "I had a lot of abscesses on my legs. I probably developed an abscess or burn 30–40 percent of the time. When you do a lot of coke you get to where you can't see very well, and likely as not you will miss the vein. Any time you miss a vein it will cause a bad burn. The more coke you shoot, the chances for missing the vein increases."

Aside from the chest pains and profuse perspiration, and despite his heavy use, Willie did not report many of the classic toxic physiological reactions to cocaine: tremors or spasms of entire muscle groups, short, shallow respiration, convulsions, fainting, shortness of breath, labored respiration, and so on.

Psychological Reactions

Table 9.6 indicates that Willie did experience adverse psychological reactions. He reported that every time he used cocaine he experienced intense paranoid ideas — "as soon as I pulled the spike" — loss of self-control, anxiety and irrational fears, loss of interest in work and productive activities, insomnia and inability to relax, depression coming off the drug, increased excitement and restless activity — "I would just walk and pace around the house talking to my wife or myself." Willie reported that cocaine would prolong sexual intercourse when applied directly to the penis. "If you don't apply it directly, you won't last as long but it is more sensational when you come." In his opinion, cocaine always acts as an aphrodisiac, "but it seems to have more impact on women than men. I have seen women doing coke get carried away sexually. They might do eight or ten guys in a row and still be hot. Coke makes women easy prey for men."

Unlike the physiological reactions which occurred either always or never, there were some psychological reactions which occurred from 30–75 percent of the time. Cocaine seemed to increase Willie's thinking power and imagination about 75 percent of the time — "The hell of it was, sometimes my imagination would get away from me, get out of control." About 60 percent of the time cocaine would cause him to experience panic and terror. But Willie indicated that 50 percent of the time it would obliterate the experience of pain — "There have been times, particularly after I had been shooting a while, that I might have to stick the spike in twenty times to find the vein. I never felt any pain associated with that. Of course, it would be stiff and sore the next day." About 30 percent of the time cocaine would cause itching in his legs — "I never thought it was bugs or anything. I would just get this terrible itching sensation in my legs."

Willie reported that at no time did the drug make him feel or experience greater optimism, courage, or self-confidence — "It destroyed my self-confidence; it fucked me up" — sensations of increased physical strength or ability to do physical work, enduring euphoria — "It was gone as soon as I pulled the spike out" — an orgasm with the rush, believing that his mind was quicker than normal or that he was smarter than other people, changes in perceived reality, or visual, auditory, and olfactory hallucinations. At no time did cocaine cause Willie to carry a gun or run from imaginary enemies — "I panicked on occasion, but I never ran from imaginary things, and I was imagining police. I have never carried a gun, that's a good way to get in trouble with the police."

Willie reported that cocaine was not a trigger for violence for him. "It made me passive. I wouldn't go out of my house at all, I would just stay locked up at home I have seen guys get violent on coke, but they were violent men even when they were not doing coke; I am talking about killers. You hear stories that armed robbers use coke before they do a job, to jack up their courage. That's a lot of damn nonsense. I have lived with such men for years and I have never known a professional stick-up man or armed robber who would go on a dangerous job with a nervous, jittery dude high on cocaine. They would be crazy; the slightest sound would set him off. I have known guys to use heroin before a job like that, but never cocaine."

Integration

Use and dealing of cocaine met a variety of needs in Willie's life. First, since he is an ambitious man who has felt blocked from achievement, dealing in cocaine permitted him to achieve a level of financial success that he might not otherwise have enjoyed. It provided him the resources to slip out of town, travel, go to "Superbowls," and live an expensive life style in other cities. Second, his occupation as a dealer allowed him to capitalize on his considerable talents, whetted his intense competitiveness, and provided him with excitement, danger, and a method for expressing his contempt for society and its laws. Willie would probably have preferred achievement in a legally sanctioned occupation, had one presented itself. He certainly believed that, if he had been born ten years later we might be reading about his achievements in the newspapers and sports magazines. As Willie has indicated, however, he paid a high price for his temporary palliatives and chemical comforts.

LIFE ACTIVITIES AND EXPERIENCES: IN WILLIE'S OWN WORDS

Overview

The section that follows presents an hour-by-hour account of two days in Willie's life. They come from a period from late winter through early summer in

TABLE 9.6. Psychological Reactions to Cocaine Use and Abuse: Willie G.

Commonly Reported Reactions to Cocaine Use/Abuse	Reactions Observed Yes	Reactions Observed No	Percent/ Time Observed	Qualifying Comments and Observations
Increased feelings of self-control		No		No, I felt like I was losing my self-control.
Increased optimism, courage		No		It killed my self-confidence. I became highly paranoid on cocaine. I couldn't deal with people when I was on cocaine.
Increased activity, restlessness, excitement	Yes		100	Just the restlessness and excitement. You're walking and talking.
Feeling of increased physical strength or ability to do physical work		No		It gives you energy, but I didn't want to do anything. I would hardly go out of the room.
Intensified feelings of well-being, euphoria, "floating," etc.		No		It made me feel energetic and euphoric for a moment, but, strangely, once I pulled the spike out that vanished. I became nervous and very paranoid as soon as I pulled the spike.
Feeling that everything is perfect.		No		Heroin does that sometimes, not cocaine.
An exquisite "don't care about the world" attitude		No		Not at all!
A physical orgasm in the "rush"		No		I never had any reaction like than on cocaine.
Increased thinking power and imagination	Yes		75	My thinking power didn't increase, but my imagination would sometimes almost get out of control.
Feeling that the mind is quicker than normal, the feeling that one is smarter than everyone else		No		Never!
More talkative than usual, a stream of talk		No		I was more talkative, but cocaine makes me withdraw and not want to be with anyone.
Indifference to pain	Yes		50	Probably. I never noticed it much, but you're rather numb. It should.
Decreased interest in work, failure of ambition, loss of ambition for useful work	Yes		100	I didn't want to try to work on cocaine.
Insomnia	Yes		100	You can't relax. I would have to take something to relax me so I could sleep.
Depression, anxiety	Yes		100	I was always anxious on cocaine and depressed coming off.

Prolonged sexual intercourse	Yes	100	You can last longer if you don't do too much. If you do too much, you can't "get up," sometimes. If you can "get up," you can stay.
An aphrodisiac or sexual stimulant	Yes	100	It's an aphrodisiac. It seems to get women carried away sexually. I've seen it make women do a group of guys. It stimulates their sexual drive and makes women easy prey for men.
Better orgasm on coke	Yes	100	It's different. It's a more sensational orgasm.
Irrational fears	Yes	100	I would become very paranoid and afraid of everything.
Terror or panic	Yes	60	I was afraid to go to work after doing cocaine all night. It panicked me to talk to people. I couldn't look them in the eye. I felt that they could tell I had been doing cocaine.
Tactile hallucinations — the feeling that insects are crawling on or under the skin (particularly fingertips, palms of hands, etc.)	Yes	30	I felt tingling, creeping, itching sensations. I would be rubbing my face, shoulders, arms, and hands. My legs would itch.
Changes in reality or the way a room or objects look — the wall waving or in motion, etc.	No		Not for me. You don't see so well, but that's all.
Paranoid ideas — the feeling that people are after you. You believe you are being watched, talked about or threatened, a wife or girlfriend is unfaithful, untrustworthy, etc.	Yes	100	I felt like I was being watched or talked about. I was paranoid about everything. I would be locked up at home. I was afraid the police might break in any minute.
Causes one to carry a gun or run from imaginary enemies	No		Not for me.
Visual hallucinations	No		I never saw things that weren't there.
Auditory hallucinations — hearing voices talking about you, threatening, etc.	No		I never heard voices or anything like that.
Olfactory hallucinations — new odors, smells, etc.	No		But you are more sensitive to odors.
A trigger for violence	Yes	?	I don't know the percentage. It depends on the person's makeup. I have seen men get violent on coke, but they were violent men. It makes me very passive. I don't want to be on the street or in a car because cocaine makes me hostile!

1975. These days have been selected because they provide a reasonably accurate picture of Willie's life style and pattern of adjustment.

On the first day, in mid-February, Willie is in his apartment. He has moved away from his wife, this time for keeps. He had gone back and tried to live with her, but it did not work out.

After a visit with his parents he goes to get his annual physical. He runs into a white friend who he says feels black; Willie concludes that's OK it if makes the man happy.

Willie completes his physical and finds he is in good health. He is relieved, for he had been feeling down, thinking perhaps he had the flu.

This is his day off, so Willie is not pressed for time. After visiting acquaintances at the shoeshine parlor he visits Terry, his "main man." Terry is still an addict and would "burn anyone," Willie included, for heroin. Willie knows this, but he and Terry are almost like brothers.

At a health center an addict trying to get money to buy heroin crowds Willie. Willie does not like to be crowded, so he lays out a thinly veiled threat. The addict does not seem to know the risk he takes in persisting; Willie is simmering, but fortunately Terry intervenes and saves the situation. Willie is still angry.

His wife calls; she needs a ride. Even though he is separated from Betty, he tries to help her. He is still angry about the addict, and shares how he views people in the drug world and what steps he feels he must take to protect himself. He gets in a petty argument with Betty.

When Willie finally gets back to his apartment Terry comes by to visit. Willie is still angry at the addict; he all but tells Terry that if the man messes with him again, Willie will act. After Terry leaves, Willie goes to bed, but has trouble sleeping.

The second day, which occurred in the early summer of 1975, begins with Willie at Ann's house. Initially, he thought that she was the woman he had been searching for (a woman like his first wife, Agatha). However, recently he has had second thoughts, and has begun to back away. While Willie still maintains his own apartment, he sleeps at her place on a fairly regular basis. She wants to marry him, but Willie does not like the restraints Ann tries to place upon him; everything she does drives Willie further from her. Later during the day, she threatens Willie over the idea of sharing him with another woman. Willie handles the situation calmly; he has been threatened before by professionals.

At Ann's place Willie smokes some pot and reads the paper. He tells Ann about two addicts he knew who were executed in a drug slaying. Casually, he tells her about the drug world.

Willie goes to pick up his son; he has arranged a part-time job for the boy during the summer. He briefs his son on the job; Willie wants to be sure he does not have to learn some things about life the way Willie had to learn them. He wants to provide the direction, care, and guidance for his son that he never received himself.

Willie goes to work early, because he has made arrangements to get off early for a going-away party for Terry that evening. Terry is leaving town; Willie is sad to see Terry leave but feels it is best. He works diligently and has an interchange with a naive young man who owes him money. He tries to help the young man but gives up; he will not listen. Willie knows the youngster will be "taken" by his woman, but lets it pass; he tried.

After work, he goes by Ann's place. They have an argument; he faces her down on the threats she makes. Then he leaves and goes to the party. The people there chide him about what he will do now that his "main man" is leaving. Willie knows what he will do. It will just be lonelier with Terry gone.

Willie, Terry, and one of Willie's former girlfriends — she is now with Terry — have a quiet leisurely dinner and talk about old times. They decide to go for drinks, choosing a "brother's club" over a white place: Why spend money at a white place instead of at a brother's? Willie and Terry drink, laugh, tell lies and stories, and then it is over. Willie goes home to bed, but cannot sleep. He feels good about his son but is depressed over the quarrel with Ann. An up-and-down day.

Activity and Experience Audits

First Day: A Tuesday in February 1975

12:00 p.m.–12:30 a.m.
I was home reading the paper. The movie was coming off on TV; I had been watching Johnny Carson. I got off earlier that evening about 8:30, business had been slow. I was really physically beat. That's why, when the manager asked if someone wanted to get off early, I volunteered. I was just tired for two or three days. I felt kinda sickly, had been ill at work Sunday. I felt bad, was down. I wanted to go to sleep, I was alone, tired, and worn out. Didn't know what was the matter with me, maybe it was the damn flu.

12:30–9:00 a.m.
I went right to sleep, and rested well.

9:00–10:30 a.m.
I woke, dressed, made my bed, and cleaned up. I called my mother, I was feeling better that morning. Didn't have anything to do, just relax and take it easy, and I needed it.

I went to my mother's place, stopped and got a paper on the way. I was thinking about money and the fact that business was so damn slow.

10:30 a.m.–12:30 p.m.
I was at my folks' place, visited with my father. Mom fixed me a good breakfast. We talked about the rest of the family — my brother and sister and how

they were doing. She was talking about buying a new car. We also talked about my sons who live in Detroit and how they were getting along. It was a nice visit, I enjoyed it. I ate a good breakfast, read the paper, and chatted some more with dad about baseball and basketball. Dad is getting interested in basketball now that the Kansas City Kings might make it to the finals.

12:30–2:30 p.m.

I drove down to the clinic to get my annual physical. While I was there I ran into an old friend. I hadn't seen Dick for six to eight months; apparently, he had moved to Florida. He was talking about what the wages were like down there and things like that. He told me he and his wife were back in town looking for an apartment. I enjoyed visiting with him. He is a white dude but he wants to be considered black; he says he is black inside. I think it's kind of strange, but hell, I accepted it. That's what makes him happy.

I talked with a nurse about taking my physical. She wanted to draw blood, and I told her there were gonna be problems there because all my veins had collapsed. I told her I wanted someone who knew what the hell he was doing, and if she couldn't get it the first few times I didn't want a lot of holes punched in me. The doctor came in; he did it. It only took him a couple of minutes.

I waited for the doctor some more because he had someone in his office. Then he gave me my physical. They had the lab report and he said I'm OK, so I was relieved and happy. I wasn't sure, because I had been sick earlier in the week.

2:30–5:30 p.m.

I drove from the doctor's office to a hangout, really a shoeshine parlor. Everyone meets there. I stayed there till about 4:00. It is a place where you get all the news, information, or whatever else you might be interested in. There were four or five guys in there ranging from thirty to fifty years of age, all friends; some of them I had grown up with. We visited around about everything from women to why John Rutlin is retiring as coach this year. Then I drove to a neighborhood health center and visited with a dentist friend of mine till about 4:30. He and I grew up together. He is leaving the health center and going into private practice. I enjoyed visiting with him.

Then I went over to see a special guy. His name is Terry. He works in the daytime and I work at night, so we never get to see each other except on days off. We have been buddies since we were both fifteen. He is very personable, very bright, and aware of what is going on. On the negative side, he is still hung up on drugs; he'll burn anyone to get something in his arm. He's an extravagant dude. He is a teacher dedicated to his job and his philosophy of what kids should be learning in school, and I'm told he is pretty good. It kinda depresses me that he is still stuck in the drug thing.

I got into a hassle with another guy there I know. He and some other dudes were trying to put a drug act together. They needed a hundred dollars and were twenty-five dollars short. So this dude, he wanted me to come in on it. I told him no. The bastard kept insisting and kept crowding me. I told him what I did with my money was my business and what he did with his money was his business! He started getting hot-headed about it. I told him, "Get off my back or your ass will really be in trouble. I am not interested!" I told him he was going to have a hell of a lot of problems if he didn't leave me alone. He finally walked off because Terry came over and pulled him away.

5:30–7:00 p.m.

A phone call came from my wife; she said her brakes were out on her car and she needed some help. I drove over to her place still thinking about the guy who was crowding me. You always have to keep your guard up with people, because they're always going to try to get you for money; they'll snitch on you or get your ass in trouble, and I'm mad and pissed at the son of a bitch!

I blew the horn! My wife comes out. She's got my son with her, and another boy about his age. I drove the boys to the boys' club. I told my son we would go buy him some baseball shoes the next day; he was very happy about it.

Then I drove my wife to the clinic. She was talking about me doing her favors, and she wanted to return them. She told me her car was not working, and asked me if I would take her to the store. I said yes, but then she started stacking shit on me for being late. I was already angry, and she said she was not going to ask for any more help from me and I said, "Cool!" I guess it was just a marital spat.

She went into the store, but said she would be right back. I decided I wanted some cigarettes; I went in after them. Then I decided, hell, I'm here, I'll buy some groceries. I bought fifteen dollars worth of groceries and looked at them and didn't have nothing!

After that, I dropped my wife off. She had cooled off some; the woman never did ask me why I was late, so to hell with it. Then I drove home, and I was thinking about cleaning up my kitchen, like putting my dishes away. The whole place is straightened up except for the kitchen.

7:00–8:00 p.m.

Terry was in the neighborhood so he came up to see me. We smoked a few joints; he talked about what the guys on the streets were doing. He complimented me on the apartment, and said he wanted to get himself an apartment. He made some remark about the altercation between me and the dude at the clinic. I told him if that damn dude didn't mind his own business he would have trouble, *real trouble!* He apologized for the guy; he said the guy was mixed up. I said I didn't want him on my ass! He said he understood. I feel free with him and can talk with him about most anything. We have done a lot of traveling together and a lot of hustling together. He is a little younger than me, but we're very close. He is more like a brother, really, than a friend. We arranged to meet again later and he left.

8:00–12:00 p.m.

I started working on the kitchen, fixing some TV dinners, washing shelves, and cleaning the place out. I was thinking, well, when I get this done, I am gonna take a bath and go to bed and lie down when the basketball game comes on and read the paper. I had it all done except the stove by 9:30, so I quit. Took a bath, a real relaxing bath. I took my time resting, I wanted to relax.

Then I listened to the basketball game on the radio and smoked a joint.

12:00 p.m.–1:00 a.m.

I guess I stayed up till one. Turned the TV off and went right to sleep.

1:00–7:00 a.m.

I slept. About 2:30 I woke up, and ate a roll. I had to get up the next day. I wasn't sure the alarm clock would work. I couldn't relax; I was afraid I might never sleep. Back to sleep, woke up at 3:45! Back to sleep, woke up again at 5:30! Back to sleep! The alarm went off at 7:10, but I had gotten up at 6:50. I don't know why I was so restless, but I guess it was the fact that my wife had asked me to take her to work and I wanted to get her there on time.

The Day: A particularly good day: Physically, I was feeling better. It was good talking with the dentist, my old friend, and then with Terry, and visiting with my friends in the shoe shine parlor. I just tried to forget about the son of a bitch who crowded me in the clinic. He probably should leave me alone.

Second Day: Wednesday

12:00 p.m.–1:00 a.m.

Ann, the woman I've been dating, and I had been to a movie; I had been off Tuesday, so we went to a movie Tuesday night. By midnight I was at Ann's place. Ann and I were discussing something in the news; two addicts I knew were killed. It was a kind of a personal thing, I guess. I felt that one guy (Al G.) was a victim. However, it had to happen to the other guy sooner or later. Considering all the things he had done over twenty years, it was a fitting way for him to die. I understood why he had died. The other guy, I guess, just happened to be at the wrong place at the wrong time. He was a nice guy; I had known him a long time. Maybe I was a bit upset, but I didn't take it personal at all. It made me think how easy it was to get offed in the drug game. I explained to Ann how drugs and murder go hand in hand; you have to be prepared to be murdered or murder someone else. You can get rich overnight if you can survive the police and people. We discussed the movie a bit, then went to bed.

7:30–10:30 a.m.

I got up, cleaned up, and got ready to take Ann to work. I felt kind of tired and would have like to have stayed in bed, but I couldn't.

Then I drove to my wife's place to pick up my son. I was thinking about Terry's party coming up that evening; it was starting in the afternoon, but I couldn't go until in the evening. I was thinking of Terry; the party was for him, he's going to New York. I was thinking about how tight as friends we had been over the years. I was going to split the expenses of the party with some other people; I concluded that while it might set me back a bit he was worth it.

Then I got to thinking about my son. I had gotten him a job to keep him busy five or six hours a day during the summer. It is really necessary for him, and he wants to do it. I want to instill in him the fact that you have to work for what you get, and he wants to work. I am proud of that. He can work a few hours a day and play in the baseball league. A lot of the kids that live around him are doing all kinds of things that they shouldn't be doing, like smoking weed at age twelve and all, and I don't want him to be part of it.

When I got to his mother's place he had just gotten out of bed. I asked him why he wasn't ready; I had called him the night before and told him to be ready. He gave me some kid explanation and began hurrying around the house getting ready. I chatted with his mother a few minutes. She seems to be doing OK. I really think she has begun accepting the fact that I won't be there any more. She left to run some errands or something.

I tried to get my son to hurry. While I waited I sat down, drank a glass of milk, and ate a donut.

I drove him down to his new job. I was talking on the way with him about the job; I explained that he would start at such-and-such an hour and quit at such-and-such an hour, how much money he would make hourly and weekly — all. I told him that the manager will pay half of his salary and I will pay the other half. I told him that after his boss sees how he works he might want to commit some money to it, too. He seemed to understand what I told him. I dropped him at the apartments, and he went to start his first day at work.

I started to drive to my apartment, but changed my mind and drove over to Ann's place. I went in; no one was there. I had planned to go there, lay down, and try to get some rest and just relax till I had to go to work. I read the paper and rolled a couple of joints. I had intended to get an hour or so of sleep, but didn't.

I wanted to be off work, but I knew I would be out at seven. I had spoken with the manager of the restaurant about my friend leaving town, the going-away party and all, and he made arrangements so I could go in earlier and still get most of a day's work in. It was very nice of him.

10:30 a.m.–12:00 m.

I drove to work; I wasn't thinking about much.

I changed clothes in the dressing room; no one else was there. Then I went out and started work. I went upstairs to help set up a big luncheon. My idea was to just kind of stand around and let the others do the work, but it didn't happen that way, I had to help set up the luncheon. I thought I would take a break and get something to eat, but I never had the chance. The other two waiters and I worked like hell setting up for sixty people.

12:00 m.–2:30 p.m.
We served the guests; they were pretty nice. Then we hustled into one of the other rooms and set up for another luncheon. Then the manager asked me to go out to the restaurant and work the rest of my shift.

2:30–5:00 p.m.
I worked in the restaurant. It wasn't too busy — mostly serving people eating a late lunch. I stood around a lot, thinking I wished my shift were finished so I could get to the party. The waiters on my regular shift came on, and I chatted with them a while. Business began to pick up around 5:00.

5:00–5:30 p.m.
I took my lunch break. I talked with Mark, one of the waiters who had been working the luncheons. He is an extra waiter who helps us when we get in an overload situation. He's trying to get on full-time. We ate together. While we were eating another waiter, Joe, came up. Joe is a quiet guy. He owed me some money; he was trying to apologize about not paying me back yet. I told him he was an example of why I don't like square dudes, because a man's word is his bond. I told him I didn't want any bullshit, I just wanted my money. He got off into this thing about his chick getting busted for shoplifting. He claimed her as his woman — hell, I know the broad, and her husband, too, who is in the joint, but I didn't tell Joe that. Joe was saying he was trying to get bond for the woman. I told him she would probably be back in jail within a few days; I told him if it was really his woman that was one thing, but if not he should forget it. He is very young, he will get abused in the end by the gal. I was trying to help him, to enlighten him that he might be taken, but I doubt if he really listened to what I said.

5:30–7:00 p.m.
I went back to work waiting tables. We were real busy all evening. I made my quota; must have served thirty or forty customers during the period. We were hustling trying to keep up with the customers; it was a good night. Things have been better the last few weeks, in fact, they have been good enough that I raised my quota.

7:00–8:45 p.m.
I checked out, changed clothes, and left. I was thinking about getting to Terry's party.

Then I drove over to Ann's place. I was still thinking about the party which had been in progress since 4:00 p.m. I was getting myself together so I wouldn't get tied up with that woman, Ann.

When I got to Ann's place and told her where I was going, she wanted to go too. I told her it was OK. Then she said she really didn't feel like going. She said she wanted me to be careful with chicks, because she wouldn't share me with another woman. I told her the reason she was not "sharing" me with another woman was because I didn't want to share, but if I did want to I would. She said she would have to kill me if I did. I told her she wouldn't be justified in doing something like that. I explained to her that one has to accept things the way they are, that one has to accept the good things while they are available, and not worry about tomorrow. When I left she was in a pretty fair mood. I guess she was wondering if I was going out with some other woman.

I drove to my apartment. I was thinking about the conversation; I guess she thought she could run a game on me with the threats, but she couldn't. I didn't get hostile or overbearing, but I left her wondering what sort of man this guy is.

I got to my apartment, turned on the radio, showered, shaved, and changed clothes in a hurry. Then I left.

8:45 p.m. – 1:00 a.m.

Of all things, I got to the lobby and there was this guy and a lady sitting there. The guy I knew; he is a waiter, too, but not where I work. He came up and began talking with me about the different restaurants he had worked at in the city; he said he was out of work. I told him I had worked hard all day and had an appointment to make. He continued to ramble on and hold me up. I told him I would talk to him some other time and broke away. Damn!

I drove down to the club where the party was going on. Everyone was glad to see me. Terry is my main man and he was glad to see me. People kept saying, "This is your main man. He's leaving. What are you going to do now?" Terry had a chick, Grace, with him. She used to be a chick of mine; she was kind of nervous, but it was no problem for Terry and I. We partied and just talked, drank, and visited with the people who were there. He had waited mainly for me. We stayed about half an hour and then left. The party had begun to break up.

Terry, his chick, and I left. We went by my apartment. He went up to my place a few minutes, came back, and he, Grace, and I drove on over to the Plaza for dinner. Grace is a nice-looking chick. She is a kind of nympho, but all in all she is a pretty nice person.

We got to the restaurant. I let Terry and Grace out, then parked the car and came back. We ordered some drinks, then dinner, and just chatted and relaxed. We talked about a lot of funny things that have happened — nothing heavy — in our lifetime. Terry said there was no better way to close up his town than to be with his main man and his old lady. We had done some drinking. I was glad to be with Terry; I hated to see him go. However, it will be better for him to start somewhere else; he would only be killed if he stayed. I never got to the point where I felt depressed about his leaving. We paid the waitress and left.

We decided to go to a couple of places to drink. They were white places. Then we changed our minds and decided to go into the ghetto to a brother's club. We asked ourselves, who are we going to spend our money with, a brother or a white man? We went to a brother's club to drink; when we got there the place was just closing. We sat a minute in the parking lot, then drove to another brother's club.

We went in, sat down, got our drinks, and chatted and visited. There were maybe six to eight other people in the club. We talked and laughed and told big lies and stories. But I was kind of looking forward to ending the partying and cutting it off for the night; my relationship with Terry is set in concrete and it doesn't make any difference whether we party or not.

The Day: Part of the day was OK. Getting my son to work and started on a job was good. I enjoyed making the money I made that day. The thing I went through with this woman, Ann, was depressing; it was something that I thought about the whole evening. All in all, after the party, the goodbyes, and all, the day was up and down. It was hard to go to sleep, I was depressed about it all, I guess. The day didn't leave me too well. It was a lot of up and down.

10

Fred S.

LIFE THEMES

Fred S. is a lonely and unhappy young man much of whose life has been devoted to playing the role of the scapegoat in a wealthy, conflicted, and stalemated family. Five central themes are interwoven into the fabric of this man's existence:

- My father thinks only of his own success; he does not love me, so I hate him.
- I must destroy my father — not quickly, but by slow torture.
- To do this, I must become like my mother, whose alcoholism is hurting my father.
- But the idea of being like my mother is repulsive; so I hate myself, too.
- The situation is impossible; I am slowly destroying myself.

Cocaine Use in Relation to Life Themes

Fred is an intravenous, daily, intermediate-dosage cocaine user. He uses cocaine because it

- provides for brief moments an orgastic sense of well-being,
- helps him manage the disappointments he encounters in life,
- provides him a position of status in the local drug community,
- allows him to continue to play his role as the family scapegoat,

- allows him to punish himself because he must endure the fears, hallucinations, and suicidal thoughts that for him are sequelae to cocaine usage,
- allows him to punish his parents, in particular his father, and
- forces his parents to pay for that instrument — cocaine — which punishes all principals in the family.

EVOLUTION OF LIFE STYLE

Introduction

Fred is a small, reserved, twenty-one-year-old Caucasian male. He is slender, with high cheekbones, an angular face, large sad eyes, and almost shoulder-length hair. He typically wears "street clothes" — a wrinkled denim work shirt, crumpled corduroy slacks, a short gym jacket, and high-top work shoes. Fred is courteous, alert, and watchful; he misses very little. One gets the impression of a quiet David plotting his next move in a world of Goliaths. He is articulate and knowledgeable, with considerable psychological sophistication; that is hardly surprising, because Fred has been in and out of psychotherapy and treatment settings since he was thirteen years old. In our sessions he answered questions in a direct and straightforward fashion. However, he rarely smiled, and was never seen to laugh or joke. He would on occasion become animated, particularly when discussing himself, his parents, and the frightening world he lives in.

Developmental Experiences

Fred is the youngest son in a wealthy family, one of the wealthier ones in Kansas City. He has an older brother, age thirty-eight, and two older sisters of ages thirty and twenty-eight. There is so much difference between his and his siblings' ages that for all practical purposes he is an only child.

"My father is fifty-five years old. He's president of a large manufacturing company. In addition to the income from his business, he inherited several million dollars from my grandfather. My dad is a gutless wonder; I love him, but I don't respect him at all. That's changing a little now. I am beginning to understand him a little better, but he is so damn weak! He is very hard in business, but all he can do is compromise with the people that are close to him.

"My mother is dominant in our family. She has a problem with alcohol; She drinks more than a fifth a day, but my father would never correct her for the crazy shit she pulls on everyone. When mother and I would fight he wouldn't stop it. He would just be the referee! He has always tried to manipulate me into doing what my mother wanted, and some of the shit she wanted was absolutely crazy! Why didn't he step in like a man and stop that crazy shit?

He is very successful at making money and watching TV, but he is a weak, superficial man, an emotional cop-out!

"My dad always tried to be a buddy rather than my father. From the time I was eight to when I was thirteen, we would go quail and duck hunting together, but hell, he always brought a professional hunter along to teach me how to shoot. He said he wanted me to develop my killer instinct. Why didn't he take the damn lessons and develop *his* killer instinct? If we didn't kill our limit he would get all upset and worry about whether the hunting trip was a disappointment for me."

When asked how he might change his father if he had his life to live over, Fred said, "I would want him to be stronger and more discipline-oriented. I would want him to learn how to say no. I would want him to put his foot down with my mother, make her be less crazy and make her be a mother!

"My mother is a fifty-year-old, hostile, vindictive woman. My parents had separate bedrooms. At nights my mother would fix dinner for my dad and I; then she would go upstairs to watch TV and drink. She would only come back down for ice cubes. When she drank, which was every day, she would get very hostile and angry. My mother would like to be a socialite — have her name in the paper and everything. Thrill and status are important for her but she never socializes. She blames my father for anything that goes wrong in her life." Fred noted proudly that on one occasion his father "told my mother he was going to divorce her. Shit, man, she got her act together quick! She stopped drinking and was sweet as could be for a while. I could never figure out why he didn't learn something from that!

"My mother is not an affectionate woman. She is cold, hostile, or at best impersonal with me. When I was little she would give me a lot of material objects like a roomful of toys, substitutes for love. My father made good money; he would give me things, too. He was tight with my sisters, though. When I grew up I was still expecting those material things, the substitutes. It was all I had."

Fred describes his mother as manipulative and tyrannical. "She was demanding as hell. I don't like Christmas because we always had fights at Christmas time; my mother would get uptight because she didn't get what she wanted. It wasn't long before the family learned that if Christmas was to be at all happy for anyone, mother always had to get a very expensive gift. For a while, mother always got a new custom Cadillac for Christmas. She liked that!

"My mother did some hostile things to me, like shoving me down a flight of stairs with my arms full of water glasses. I got all cut up, you can still see the scars here. She would order my friends out of the house and tell them never to come back. My friends called her 'Queen Sauce.' My father always tried to talk me out of feeling angry with my mother. He said it was because of her hysterectomy. Shit, he tried to put all the blame for her behavior on the operation. That's a lot of shit!"

Fred's developmental years were characterized by constant fighting between his mother, father, and himself. "My mother would get to drinking and pitch a bitch. My father would try to rationalize it all with her, but it wouldn't work. She would tell him he was weak and no good. Then she would start talking about how stupid and fucked up I was, and then tell him she wished she had never married him. She would tell me I was stupid and no good and that I would never make it like my father did. My self-respect and self-esteem are still pretty low, but I am trying to work it through in therapy with my shrink." Despite the constant conflict and tension, Fred never ran away from home. "I didn't run away because it was all I had, and I was too scared."

When asked if his mother loved him, Fred said he really didn't know. "She had told me she loved me, but it's hard to reconcile a mother telling you she loves you one minute, then pushing you down a flight of stairs the next. Once in a while she was tender and loving. Then she would turn into this witch — I mean bitch — again. I have often had fantasies of having her tied to a whipping post! She gives me these terrible angry feelings that I have a hard time dealing with. Then my father comes along and tells me to rationalize them away. How the hell do you do that?

"My father was very inclined to call in a professional whenever he had problems with me. He has a psychologist on his staff; he would always call him to the house when trouble developed. When I was about thirteen years old, I started being rebellious. He called this psychologist. He and my father got their heads together; then my father came in and said, 'Son, I have decided you are going to military school.' I said, 'Like hell I am going to military school!' I started shouting and throwing stuff around the house. All hell broke loose! I refused to go. I thought he was trying to get rid of me, and I wasn't about to put up with that! The upshot was that I had to start seeing a psychiatrist. I didn't mind going to see my shrink every week; it was a helluva lot better than being shipped off to military school!"

Fred attended a private school. He made poor grades and had reading difficulties. "I made mostly Cs and Ds. What the hell did they expect? You stay on someone's ass all the time and keep telling them how stupid they are, and after a while you get to believing it! I really didn't like studying, but I am not certain the poor grades were not just a way to get back at my parents. In therapy I learned that, crazy as it sounds, my mother and father need me to be the family fuck-up. I guess I have played the fuck-up role all my life."

Fred reports he was a good athlete in grade school and junior high school. "Then I was good in football, basketball, and kickball, because I was big for my age. However, *now* I am little for my age. I took guitar lessons from the time I was eight till I was about fourteen; I liked it very much. I was into the Beatles, and would practice three or four hours a day in the basement. Of course, I had the best instructors money could buy. My father would praise me about my music, but my mother would say it was a waste of money. However, I liked it down there in the basement. My mother would never come down, and nobody would bother me."

Fred stayed in school until he was sixteen years of age. "I ditched classes a lot. But I finally just said to hell with it and dropped out when I was a sophomore in high school. My folks didn't like it, but I was playing the fuck-up, and by then I was turned off by education in the formal manner." Since high school, Fred has worked in a variety of menial positions, such as lot boy in a used-car lot, apprentice carpenter, delivery boy, and clerk (in his father's company). When he began participating in our research Fred was living in an apartment and was unemployed. He later obtained a job as a fry cook in a local drive-in, and, still later, a second job as an inventory clerk. "I was fired from the used-car lot because I was a cough-syrup freak then; they thought I was drunk. I was fired from the carpenter's apprentice job because the work was too heavy for me. I never have figured out why I was fired from the job in the drive-in."

Fred says he would like to become a computer operator or professional musician. "I never tried to join the musician's union because I don't have much confidence in myself. I have jammed a lot with musicians; they always said I was very good. However, I don't really like rock music that much."

At age eighteen, Fred was hospitalized by his father for drug addiction. "I was really strung out on coke and heroin. My father had me put away at this mental hospital in New England. I was there eight months. I developed some skill in group psychotherapy, psychodrama, and stuff like that. I tried to run a lot of games and cons on them, but it didn't work; they were hip to that kind of stuff. After I was detoxed from the heroin I spent the rest of the eight months plotting — day and night — trying to figure a con, the angles to give those people what they wanted so I could get the fuck out of there. It was a challenge. I finally wormed my way out of the place."

Fred has a record of five or six traffic arrests, one misdemeanor arrest for driving while intoxicated, and one felony arrest at age eighteen for possession of cocaine. Though convicted on the possession charge, Fred was placed on parole because he was a minor. The felony conviction prevented him from going into military service.

Fred is a nominal Protestant, but he never goes to church. He is a liberal in his political orientation, but wanted nothing to do with politics. "My father is interested in politics, but I don't want to be involved in that shit. I have enough problems of my own."

Interpretive Integration

At least seven characteristics of the family environment have shaped Fred's life style:

• An abundance of material wealth
• Overt rejection and hostility from a cold and domineering mother
• Indirect, partial acceptance from a successful, but aloof and ineffectual father

- Ongoing quarrels among mother, father, and son, with the mother using alcohol to vent her resentment against the other two members of the family
- A tense and emotionally unstable family where disagreements or misunderstandings were resolved by manipulative strategies, subterfuge, and denial
- A family in which parental communications created contradictory, "double-bind" situations
- A family environment characterized by a cornucopian abundance of material comfort but the absence of love, acceptance, and rational discipline

This kind of family environment depicts an almost classic picture of what has been described as, at worst, the breeding ground for a schizophrenic adjustment or, at best, the source of a schizoid or neurotic pattern of functioning. Reared in such a family environment, Fred developed a life style characterized by the following:

- Pervasive feelings of depression, unhappiness, and malaise
- Feelings of inadequacy combined with self-doubts and self-hatred
- Anger and resentment toward parental figures accompanying these inadequacy-feelings
- A crippling and unresolved Oedipal conflict with a repetitive internal struggle in which he cannot accept his parents' rejection and indifference; yet he cannot leave them alone, cannot change them, or force them to be other than they are
- Fear and hatred of women
- Somewhat easier access to closeness with men, with associated homosexual fears and fantasies
- Lack of a sense of moral or emotional obligations to other people
- A high level of tension and anxiety in all areas of living
- Rejection of traditional social values (hard work, success, achievement) and a search for a world where people are direct and straightforward yet nondemanding and nonaggressive
- Easy discouragement and a tendency to give up pursuit of long-range goals in the face of obstacles
- Periodic, paroxysmal episodes of ego breakdown characterized by confused thinking with strong paranoid overtones
- A pattern of personal functioning in which he feels he can attain desired goals only by devious plots, subterfuges, and manipulative ploys

Powerful motifs of depression, self-deprecation, discouragement, and loneliness permeate this young man's life. They are highlighted in the repetitive conflict between mother, father, and son: Fred commits a variety of legal and illegal acts — some of which cannot be reported here — which hurt, embarrass, and punish his parents. These intensify parental rejection, particularly by his mother. Increased parental rejection intensifies Fred's anger; he feels compelled to strike out again in reprisal. Despite the father's efforts at mediation, it remains a conflict in which everyone loses.

Fred's efforts to free himself from his family have been unsuccessful. Though he does live on his own, he has limited work skills and has been unable to maintain regular employment. When he was fired from his job as a fry cook, he was forced to turn to his father for help again. "My psychiatrist got mad as hell about it. He wanted me to be more independent and not ask them for help, but I owed this dealer a lot of money, and I couldn't find another job!" Fred's inability to resolve this struggle is a constant source of self-reproach. Once when tempted to overdose, he decided not to: "I know I don't have the guts to do it, but sometimes I get so depressed that I would just like to turn the projector off and leave."

When asked what kind of car he would be, Fred stated, "I would like to be a Ferrari. They're fast and beat all the others; but the fact is, I am a Ford LTD with a blown-out motor. I need an overhaul, a ring-and-valve job." When asked to compose his own epitaph, he said it would be: "I lived in a dead world. No matter how hard I tried, I would fail. No matter how hard this man tried, the people around him were dead and unfeeling."

He indicates he is moderately happy living alone in his apartment, but adds that sometimes it is lonely. "I have one buddy, Hartford, who lives down the hall from me; we're close. He's thirty-five; I seem to make better friends with older guys than guys my age. Hartford is probably the only real friend I have. He's gentle like me, not aggressive."

Fred readily admits he hates his mother, resents his father, and fears women, finding it easier to establish relations with men. "When I was in the mental hospital back East they told me I hated women. I don't think I hate women. I am afraid of them, I am deathly afraid of getting a woman like my father got. When I was sixteen years old, I dated this gal Linda. We got along good. She was not at all like my mother, and she thought I was smart in everything. Then the dealer cut me out. I tried to get back with her when I came back from New England, but it was impossible. It was the only decent relationship I have ever had with a chick, and the dealer destroyed it. I have laid other women since then. Some were prostitutes. Some were just acquaintances, but I don't want them close."

Fred made efforts to develop relationships with some of the young women he worked with in the restaurant. However, his efforts were so artless – or, perhaps, artful – that they rejected his advances. Yet Fred prides himself on being a manipulator. "I am good with a con or scam. I have to be in the world I live in; I am small and not too strong physically – if I make one mistake I end up in jail, or get hurt or killed. I have to be cunning and devious to get by." When asked what kind of animal he would be, he said, "When I was a kid I guess you could say I was a snake, kind of devious. Now I guess I am a fox, because that captures my cunning and the manipulative part of me."

Data not reported in detail here suggest that Fred is vulnerable to periodic psychological outbursts and disturbances. However, he does not display a fully psychotic adjustment. As of now Fred has not given up or withdrawn from his struggle. He is tense and anxious about: the rage and destructiveness he feels, the depression and malaise, ways in which to obtain cocaine, possible sources of money to pay his dealer, possible sources of general financial support, the next move his parents will make in the deadly game they all play, ways to survive the paranoia, hallucinations, and suicidal ideas he endures when using cocaine, whether he will ever find adequate love, acceptance, and peace, and what will ultimately become of him. Despite these fears Fred has remained in the arena and continues his struggle — a lonely David fighting giant shadows.

FORMAL PSYCHOLOGICAL ASSESSMENT

Dimensional Test Findings

Intelligence Tests

Fred functions in the Average intellectual range. Given the cultural enrichment and specialized educational experiences his family was able to provide, this assessment can probably be taken as an accurate measure of his intellectual capacity.

MMPI

Scores on the MMPI reveal that Fred is an anxious, agitated, and disturbed individual whose life is dominated by depression, chronic anxiety, somatic and hypochondriacal complaints, and disturbances in thinking and behavior (figure 10.1). The remarkably high F score could indicate, however, that Fred's MMPI is invalid. A second, more likely explanation is that his emotional disturbance is sufficiently severe for him to respond with a long list of bizarre, peculiar, and atypical experiences. Several months after he was administered this MMPI he completed a second one; The profile was essentially the same, but the F scale was within normal limits and the others scores ($D, Pd, Pa, Pt,$ and Sc) had declined to values within the 70–80 T-Score range.

The MMPI profile presents a picture of a deeply depressed, agitated, and disturbed man who has difficulty maintaining effective control over his feelings and impulses. Tense and restless, he has a high level of nervous energy. He is subject to rapid mood shifts, and consequently may be seen by others as unpredictable. Fred shows a cyclic pattern in his efforts to control himself: He experiences failure or reversal, becomes agitated and depressed, and acts out

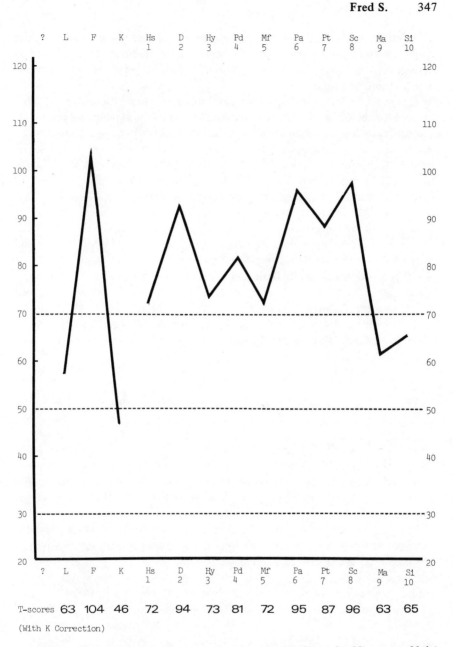

| T-scores | 63 | 104 | 46 | 72 | 94 | 73 | 81 | 72 | 95 | 87 | 96 | 63 | 65 |

(With K Correction)

FIGURE 10.1. MMPI Profile: Fred S. *Reproduced from the Minnesota Multiphasic Personality Inventory Profile and Case Summary form, by permission. Copyright 1948 by the Psychological Corporation, New York, N.Y. All rights reserved.*

his frustration in inappropriate ways; he then experiences new guilt and acts out again. He expects punishment and feels he deserves it. Fred admits to feelings of unreality, delusional thoughts, and strange experiences which are characteristic of disordered thinking.

Life generally holds little pleasure for Fred and he has difficulty maintaining his interest in day-to-day responsibilities. He experiences feelings of personal inadequacy and has a low sense of personal worth. Though he recognizes that he needs other people, he feels isolated from them. He is sensitive to slights, frequently feels misunderstood, and is concerned about offending others. Though he is socially perceptive, he tends to be cautious, reticent, and reserved; he avoids expressing his opinions or letting others know much about him.

On the MMPI Fred expressed alienation from his family, and showed that he receives little love or affection in his home. He perceives his parents as critical, unreasonable, temperamental, even frightening. In general, Fred is cynical and distrustful; he lives in an unstable world where he expects others to exploit and take advantage of him. Given these expectations, he feels justified in doing whatever is necessary to protect himself. He maintains a courteous facade, but his resentment and hostility are always close to the surface. Fred frequently finds himself in situations where he experiences more anger than he can effectively manage — then he withdraws.

Sixteen PF

The Sixteen PF Test (table 10.1) presents a markedly different picture from the MMPI. That is, the Sixteen PF presents a picture of an outgoing young man who faces the normal stresses of life with calmness and security; is neither overly submissive nor domineering with others, and is happy, self-reliant, relaxed, and trusting of other people. Peculiarly, none of the labile anxiety, frustration, and inner turmoil that appeared in the Life History Interview, Daily Activity and Experience Audit, drug experience data, and MMPI surfaced on the Sixteen PF.

The only aspects of his behavior revealed on the other measures that also emerged on the Sixteen PF Test are indications of Fred's concrete approach to life problems, tendencies to manipulate, exploit, and do what is expedient in relationships with others, disregard for or rejection of social convention, inability to pursue goals in the face of obstacles, desire for self-sufficiency, and a rather pragmatic, non-moralistic approach to problem solving.

Other Dimensional Measures

Fred obtained low scores on all but two scales of the Sensation-Seeking measure. Although his score on general Sensation-Seeking was depressed, Fred obtained very high scores on the Experience-Seeking and Disinhibition subscales. He therefore described himself as a man who seeks sensuous experiences and lives an unconventional life. He is a nonconformist who rejects the superficiality and dishonesty which he thinks characterize parental values. To this extent, the subscale scores are consistent with Fred's pattern of functioning.

Averaged over the three-month assessment periods, Fred's scores on the Novelty Experiencing Scales are similar to scores obtained by airmen and college males, he showed no greater need to seek new or novel life experiences than do these comparison groups. Fred obtained a Change Seeker Index score that is lower than the mean scores of college males or army men. These data indicate that Fred has no greater need for change than other young men.

Fred obtained scores of 5, 14, and 0 on the Eysenck Extraversion-Introversion, Neuroticism, and Lie Scales. When compared with adult industrial norms, these scores fell into the twelfth, eighty-first, and ninth percentiles, respectively. These findings would indicate that Fred is a shy and introverted young man with severe, even disabling, neurotic problems.

Integration

The general picture which emerges from the dimensional measures is of a shy, anxious, emotionally disturbed young man with average intellect and low self-confidence, who is lost in a labyrinth where he is fighting a seemingly losing battle to find his way. He struggles with anger, depression, and dysphoria, resentment and fear of parental authorities, a pattern of socially inappropriate — even self-destructive — behavior, pessimism and doubt about the future, and distress at his failure to achieve his goals.

Findings From Morphogenic Measures

Overview

In his Q-Sort descriptions Fred tried to present himself as self-controlled, friendly, and kind, but also lonely and somewhat sad. However, he also said that when under the influence of drugs he becomes anxious, self-centered, and feels potentially violent. Because he does not enjoy drugs or the states they induce, one must ask why he takes them. The morphogenic findings suggest that he takes them partly because the highly charged state produced by drugs like cocaine helps him release the tension of his submerged rage. At the same time, the relief offered by drugs is not satisfactory, for it is not always possible for Fred to control their effects; when their action gets out of hand, dangerous thoughts arise, and he panics because he cannot handle them. Yet he keeps going back for more.

On the Rep Test, Fred described his father as a nice person, but one interested only in making money and who lets himself get kicked around — indeed, he invites abuse. Fred described his mother as a hopeless, helpless alcoholic.

TABLE 10.1. Cattell 16PF Profile: Fred S.

Standard Score	Low Score Description	Factor	Standard Ten Score (Sten) 1–10	High Score Description
6	Reserved, detached, critical, cool, aloof, stiff, precise, objective	A		Outgoing, warm-hearted, easygoing, trustful, good-natured, participating
4	Less intelligent, concretistic thinking, less well-organized, poor judgment	B		More intelligent, abstract thinking, bright, insightful, fast-learning, better judgment
7	Affected by feelings, emotionally less stable, worrying, easily upset, changeable	C		Emotionally stable, mature, unruffled, faces reality, calm (higher ego strength)
6	Humble, mild, easily led, docile, accomodating, submissive, conforming	E		Assertive, aggressive, stubborn, headstrong, competitive, dominant, rebellious
6	Sober, taciturn, serious, introspective, reflective, slow, cautious	F		Happy-go-lucky, enthusiastic, talkative, cheerful, frank, quick, alert
2	Expedient, disregards rules, social conventions and obligations to people (weaker superego strength)	G		Conscientious, persistent, moralistic, persevering, well-disciplined (stronger superego strength)
5	Shy, timid, withdrawn, threat-sensitive	H		Venturesome, uninhibited, socially bold, active, impulsive
6	Tough-minded, self-reliant, cynical, realistic	I		Tender-minded, sensitive, dependent, seeking help and sympathy
6	Trusting, accepting conditions, understanding, tolerant, permissive	L		Suspicious, hard to fool, dogmatic

Score	Low description	Factor	High description
		L	
4	Practical, "down-to-earth" concerns, guided by objective reality	M	Imaginative, bohemian, absent-minded, unconventional, easily seduced from practical judgment
5	Forthright, unpretentious, genuine, spontaneous, natural, artless, socially clumsy	N	Astute, polished, socially aware, shrewd, smart, "cuts corners"
6	Self-assured, placid, secure, self-confident, complacent, serene	O	Apprehensive, self-reproaching, insecure, worrying, troubled, guilt-prone
8	Conservative, respectful of established, traditional ideas	Q₁	Experimenting, liberal, free-thinking, non-moralistic, experiments with problem-solutions
8	Group-dependent, depends on social approval, a "joiner" and sound follower	Q₂	Self-sufficient, resourceful, prefers to make own decisions
3	Undisciplined self-conflict, lax, follows own urges, careless of social rules	Q₃	Controlled, exacting, willpower, socially precise, compulsive, persistent, foresighted
5	Relaxed, tranquil, torpid, unfrustrated, composed, low ergic tension	Q₄	Tense, frustrated, driven, overwrought, high ergic tension

Average

He said that at his worst he himself is a lazy, sociopathic manipulator of others. Fred is entangled in unhealthy relationships with both parents. The data suggest that he identifies with his mother, despite his proclaimed dislike for her. Like that of his mother, his style is to seek release without anticipating the cost; like her, he uses drugs to injure his father. Fred constantly and fearfully faces the possibility that he also resembles his mother by being helpless, hopeless, and hateful; he consciously rejects this identity. However, he also rejects identification with his father; Fred will not strive for conventional success and achievement. Therefore, he feels — and for the moment is — blocked at every turn in a situation that seems destined to destroy everyone involved.

Q-Sorts

Standard Items

Fred's descriptions of his usual self were moderately consistent within assessment sessions, the overall median correlation coefficient being .618. The median correlation of these descriptions between assessment sessions was somewhat lower (median = .512) but still sufficient to show similarity. In fact, that applies to virtually all descriptions Fred provided with the standard items: Consistency was not high but was not so low as to cast doubt on Fred's sortings. Fred's data suggest that instability in his sortings occurred because Fred himself is unstable.

The correlations between Fred's descriptions of his usual self and his ideal self were low (median = .326), indicating lack of satisfaction with himself. However, there was a time-trend indicating that Fred's self-satisfaction increased; at the second reassessment session it reached .546. This finding seems to indicate modest improvement.

Factor analysis. Despite the somewhat low reliability of Fred's sortings, the outcome of the factor-analytic procedure was clear. Three factors were identified: The first is a concept of a General Self; it contains heavy loadings on all descriptions of the usual self. The second is a Drug Self, showing heavy loadings on all descriptions of the typical cocaine user and of the self during a cocaine high. The third is an Ideal Self, with heaviest loadings on all descriptions of the ideal self.

Items at the high end of the first factor — that is, similar to the factor-concept — reveal that Fred presents his usual self as being controlled, restrained, and logical. Although he says he is pleasant, friendly, and kind, nevertheless he describes himself as lonely. Items at the low end of the factor (dissimilar) show that Fred rejects the ideas that he is cruel, violent or explosive, and self-centered or boring. He does not think of himself as a work addict or as so devoted to success that winning is more important than how the game is played. Taken as a whole, this description could be said to represent Fred's Dr. Jekyll self.

Items at the high end of the Drug Self factor (Factor II) show that we are dealing here with Fred's Mr. Hyde. This self is anxious, nervous, believes winning is more important than how the game is played, and is violent, explosive, impulsive, hostile, and self-centered. Items at the low end of the factor reveal that this self is not pleasant, friendly, or humble, is no work addict, and is not slow, dragging, or boring.

Fred's Ideal Self (Factor III) differs from his usual self in that it is not lonely — indeed, it is respected by others. Also, his ideal self is happy and wise, as opposed to merely logical. Except for these discrepancies, however, the two descriptions do not differ greatly.

To summarize, Fred feels he is two different persons. Neither is happy. The first person is logical, controlled and restrained, and rejecting of hostility; he tries to be nice, but is lonely in spite of that. The picture is of a repressed, held-in person, who is prone to intellectualization and feels rejected by others but cannot understand why. The second person emerges when Fred takes drugs; it is the unrepressed personality. Evidently, expressing it prevents the first personality from exploding under the pressure of upsurging, unrepressable hostility. It does not bring Fred closer to his ideal; it only releases energy. One cannot say that Fred likes drugs, that he seeks happiness in the reactions they produce, or that they fit neatly into his self-concept; rather, he seems to need them to achieve temporary release from a deeply hidden, destructive personality which he cannot otherwise keep under control.

Individualized Items

None of the descriptions Fred provided with individualized items (table 10.2) reached an impressive level of consistency, either within or between assessment sessions. Most correlations were in the same range as that for the standard-item descriptions (about .500), though some were especially low. Fred was remarkably inconsistent in his descriptions of what most nonusers are like (median = .172). He was almost equally inconsistent in describing himself during a cocaine high (median = .206) and after the effects of cocaine wear off (median = .305). Fred was not trying to conceal anything; his thinking is simply not stable enough to produce consistent data.

The correlations between Fred's descriptions of his usual self and his ideal self were no higher with individualized items than with standard items (median = .284). In fact, few correlations among specific sortings reached levels worth mentioning. Results like these are to be expected when reliabilities of specific sortings are as low as they are in Fred's case.

Factor analysis. Factor-analytic procedures yielded seven independent factors, of which four were coherent enough to justify interpretation. The first factor contains all Fred's descriptions of his ideal self (positive loading) and all his descriptions of his bad self (negative loading). This factor we called his Bipolar Ideal. The second factor contains all Fred's descriptions of himself when wanting cocaine, when on a cocaine high, and when on an amphetamine high; it is termed his Drug Self. The third factor contains all Fred's descriptions of his usual self, so the appropriateness of assigning that name to it is obvious. The fourth factor contains only two heavily loaded Q-sortings, both describing

TABLE 10.2. Individualized Q-Sort Items: Fred S.

Achievement
Positive
*1. Reaching his goal
*2. Accomplishing
Negative
*3. Believe winning is more important than how the game is played
4. Running a con

Affect
Positive
*5. Happy
6. Glad
Negative
*7. Sad
8. Down

Anxiety
Positive
9. Relaxed
10. Content, not anxious
Negative
*11. Anxious
12. Uptight

Chastity
Positive
13. Virgin
14. Not doing sex when confined
Negative
15. Impotent
16. Can not get it up

Dependence
Positive
17. Needs help because of injury
18. Needs people
Negative
*19. Clings to apron strings
20. Dependent and does not need to be

Dominance
Positive
*21. Strong
22. Motivated
Negative
23. Weak
24. Meek

Excitement
Positive
25. Naturally excited
*26. Adventurous
Negative
*27. Explosive
28. Hostile

Humility
Positive
29. Doesn't show off
*30. Modest
Negative
*31. Ignored
*32. Lonely

Independence
Positive
*33. Independent
*34. Stand on your own two feet
Negative
35. Too sure of himself

36. Overconfident

Knowledge
Positive
37. Smart
38. Clever
Negative
39. Dumb
40. Stupid

Restraint
Positive
41. Controlled
42. Restrained
Negative
*43. Slow
44. Unsure

Self-satisfaction (Stasis)
Positive
*45. Satisfied
46. Content, not ambitious

Negative
*47. Lazy
48. Sociopath

Sexuality
Positive
*49. Romantic
*50 Sexually stimulating
Negative
51. Rapist

52. Does forcible sex

Interpersonal Relations
Positive
*53. Kind
54. Warm
Negative
55. Mean
*56. Cruel

Social Recognition
Positive
57. Politician
58. Admired
Negative
59. Slandered
*60. Laughed at

Note: Items marked with an asterisk (*) are not significantly altered from their original (standard) wording.

354

how Fred feels after the effects of cocaine have worn off; this is his After-Drug Self.

Fred's Bipolar ideal (Factor I) is a person strong and motivated, adventurous and naturally excited, and happy and glad. Traits characteristic of the other pole of this ideal — i.e., traits of the bad self — are being lazy, sociopathic, mean and cruel, and sexually impotent or incompetent. The appearance of sexual inadequacy as a characteristic of the bad self indicates that this is a problem for Fred. Considering his background, one would be surprised if it were not.

Fred's Drug Self (Factor II), is not as much like Mr. Hyde as is that which he described with the standard items. Nevertheless, it is clear that this drug self is not happy and does not use cocaine to increase pleasure or enjoyable sensations. The Drug Self is strong and motivated — in fact, too much so, to the point of being too sure of itself and overconfident. Traits which are the opposite of the Drug Self are: being relaxed and content, dumb, stupid, weak, meek, slow, and unsure; these traits are all strongly rejected. This description may provide a more accurate picture of what Fred seeks from drugs than do the standard Q-Sort items. He appears to obtain equivalent results from amphetamine and cocaine; both load heavily in the same factor. He wants from both strength, sureness of purpose, determination, confidence, and potency. However, they give him more than he can handle.

Fred's Usual Self (Factor III) does not differ greatly from that he described with the standard items. With the individualized items, however, he emphasized anxiety and sadness more and loneliness less. His sorting of the items again contained more than a hint of repressed hostility, but its sexual character was more obvious here.

The fourth factor reveals that after the effects of drugs wear off Fred enters another unhappy state. With his After-Drug Self control, restraint, independence, relaxation, and contentment have been lost. Instead, Fred becomes sad, "down," anxious, and uptight; he becomes a lazy sociopath. Fred's description does not make clear why this factor contains a component related to winning at any cost and running a con game. However, other material suggests that Fred is referring to his use of his identity as an addict to defeat his father; it is the pressure to win this contest with his father that has most likely kept Fred using drugs. Apparently, the conflict comes to the fore in his mind mainly after the drugs' effects have worn off.

Rep Test

Role Groups

Fred's descriptions of the people on this test were no more consistent than were his Q-Sorts; the median correlation coefficient in all testing sessions was .498. He was most consistent in describing his ideal self (median r = .806), the person he dislikes most (median r = .742), and a person who behaves strangely (median r = .730), but none of these people, oddly enough, appear strongly in any of his role-group factors. He was least consistent in describing the person who needs him most (median r = .069) and his father (median r = .192); these appear together as the strongest members of Factor III, described below.

The interpersonal constructs created by Fred are as follows:

Interpersonal Constructs

1. Aggressive
2. Don't trust me
3. Plays "kick me" game
4. Trying to escape
5. Trying to be happy
6. Likes to have a good time
7. An achiever – money conscious
8. Straight thinking – practical
9. Can control their "parent"; can turn off and on
10. Foremost concern is money
11. Sure of themselves
12. Can take care of themselves
13. Can stay on top of things
14. Is out of it – cannot function
15. Enjoys music

Factor analysis. Fred's data yield five factors, of which four can be interpreted. The dominant members of Factor I are a strange group: person of the other sex with whom you take cocaine, person who dislikes you, wife or girlfriend, person you would most like to help, and your usual self. The contents of this factor imply that Fred feels a need for help, dislikes himself, and expects others, especially women, to feel the same toward him. People in this group are described as sexy, liking to have a good time, enjoying music, and trying to be happy, but also as being selfish and trying to escape. The factor suggests a modern version of the roaring twenties (when cocaine first became popular).

Factor II contains Fred's self on cocaine and his worst self. Though these persons like music and are trying to escape, they are mean and selfish. They are also out of it, they cannot function, are not practical, and cannot stay on top of things.

Factor III clearly depicts Fred's father as the person who needs Fred most. Fred sees this man as kind, wise, and someone who likes to have a good time. His father can take care of himself, but his foremost concerns are money and achievement. He also plays the "kick me" game, and Fred is doubtless his willing accomplice.

Factor IV describes an alcoholic mother who is mean and selfish and does not trust Fred. She, too, likes to have a good time and is trying to escape, but unlike the father she is out of it – she cannot function. His mother seems to provide the model for Fred's drug-related behavior.

Construct Groups

Factor analysis produced five sets of interpersonal constructs. Each represents a dimension upon which Fred judges people. Factor I is bipolar. At one end it contains the traits: aggressive, strong, and sure of themselves. At the other end it contains the traits: selfish and trying to escape. People rated high on this trait are also realistic; while they may not be generous, at least they are not niggardly. Factor II seems to be a measure of how heavily a person will allow Fred to lean upon him. It includes the traits of kindness, helpfulness, and wisdom. To be high on this trait also implies that a person is not mean and does not distrust Fred. Factor III is a sensual-pleasure factor. People high on this trait combine the desirable characteristics of being sexy, seeking happiness, and of being on top of things. Factor IV is the trait of money consciousness. Factor V is the ability to manipulate authority figures by "turning off and on," presumably by being as pleasant or unpleasant as necessary to get what one wants.

Taken together, these factors suggest that Fred is sophisticated in his conceptions of people. He judges them by their toughness, kindness toward him, sensuality, interest in money, and ability to manipulate others. All these traits are important in Fred's own personality, and it is apparent that he projects them onto other people. How accurately he does so cannot be ascertained, but the constructs should be serviceable in the kind of life style Fred has adopted.

Setting Survey

This is the only source of morphogenic data in which Fred displayed consistency. The overall median correlation coefficient was .865, and values for all four scores considered separately were also quite impressive. Apparently, Fred has an action pattern that is consistent, despite his inner psychological turmoil. He therefore seems to be one of the many psychologically disturbed people who appear upon close examination to be desperately in need of help but who are nevertheless capable of continuing to function; such persons can sometimes continue their borderline existences indefinitely, so long as no serious crises are encountered.

Nothing unusual turns up in Fred's Setting Survey. He works steadily and engages in a large amount of social-recreational activity, but this is not uncommon for an unmarried person. There is, perhaps, a hint of hypochondria or dependency in his continued entering into physical and mental health settings. This is also suggested by the fact that physical health settings are described by him as most satisfying of all.

Integration

The organizing themes in Fred's life style concern his relations with his parents and the resulting impulses of hostility and destructiveness that trouble him so greatly. Throughout the morphogenic data the picture of Fred that comes across is that of a person living on the knife edge of existence. So much of his life is tied up with anger and potential destructiveness that he is almost always tense, nervous, and anxious. As a result he is always ready to seek escape by surrendering to drug-exaggerated, immediate sensory experiences. Fred would like to be calm, logical, and self-controlled, but that is impossible for him over any extended period of time.

Fred uses drugs partly to release pent-up tension, partly to enhance sensory experience in an attempt to escape, and partly to make himself feel self-assertive and competent. Unfortunately, the effects are not pleasurable. Instead of carrying him passively to nirvana, the drugs release a stream of repressed emotion that threatens to go out of control altogether.

Fred's attitudes toward his parents show clearly on the Rep Test. Other data indicate that Fred cannot tolerate becoming like his father, though he knows he is expected to by others — and even by himself. He finds little in his father that he regards as worth emulating. Despite her addiction to alcohol, his mother's identity appeals more directly to Fred; like him, she is trying to enjoy herself and escape harsh realities. But her solution can lead to disintegration of the self, a possibility Fred finds intolerable.

STYLE OF DRUG USE

General Pattern

As indicated in Table 10.3, Fred has used most major legal and illegal drugs. The only exceptions are barbiturates — "I tried that once; I don't like the barb feeling at all" — and inhalants. Fred began drug use at age thirteen with marijuana and the hallucinogens. He has used marijuana daily since then because, as he says, "Good grass relaxes me. It's a kind of tranquilizer. I have done a fantastic amount of grass." Regarding hallucinogens, Fred states his usage was just part of growing up: "I have done MDA and the speed form of THC [probably phencyclidine] at work. I loathe THC because it gives you tunnel vision. I also tried peyote and organic mescaline; I tried them till I was about sixteen years old but I am beyond that kid stuff now. I don't need to sit around and talk metaphysical shit anymore." He reported fairly regular consumption of alcohol (two or three times per week) but indicates it was confined mostly to beer.

It was at about age sixteen that Fred began using amphetamine, alcohol, and cocaine. He gave up amphetamine after a year because he did not like "the speed feeling. Speed wore me down and made me feel bad. It's bad enough going up but I felt even worse coming down." Fred snorted cocaine for a year and then began intravenous cocaine use, which has continued on a several-times-weekly to daily basis. He reports that snorting cocaine was OK, but he did not do much cocaine until he began intravenous use. Cocaine is his drug because it gives him, briefly, "a fantastic feeling of well-being that you wouldn't believe."

At age seventeen Fred began taking heroin intravenously. "I started at the top with Vietnamese heroin that was 80 percent pure. It wasn't available too long, but it was the best shit I have ever done!" By the time he was eighteen, Fred was addicted to heroin. He broke this addiction with cocaine, though he later became addicted to heroin again. "Coke is good to help you kick the heroin habit, if you have a lot of coke. The coke will keep the pain down. You stay high on a load of coke and it will carry you through withdrawal. Of course, you are high as hell for a couple of weeks." For the last three years, however, he has used heroin to "come down" from the cocaine high. He notes that with this procedure he runs the risk of becoming addicted to heroin again. Consequently, he will use tranquilizers, alcohol, or other downers to get off cocaine if he is only on a run of one or two days.

From age eighteen to twenty-two, Fred expanded his drug-use to include other opiates (codeine), tranquilizers, nonprescription drugs (Robitussin), cough syrup, illegal methadone, and polydrug mixtures of cocaine and heroin (speedballing) taken intravenously. He took tranquilizers orally to relax and "come off" cocaine, and he would use Robitussin when nothing else was available.

Fred's use of drugs was quite expensive. His pattern of three grams of cocaine per day cost approximately $160-180. (At the time he was interviewed, street rates for cocaine were $60-100 per gram.) Fred indicates that he was able to obtain high-grade cocaine at a lower price by purchasing it in half- and one-ounce quantities.

Fred thinks he experienced a cocaine overdose once. "I felt like my heart was stopping. It was terrible; it felt like I was being stabbed again and again with a knife in my heart. I was scared! I quickly fired some heroin right behind the coke, and began to feel better after a while. But it scared me bad." Fred also describes a heroin overdose: "I just passed out. My friend got me up, walked me — more like drug me — around, got some milk down me, and kept me moving. I finally came around."

Since age sixteen the longest time he has stopped taking drugs of his own volition was for one month. "Of course, that doesn't include the time I was in the mental hospital. I was off drugs for eight months there, but I was locked up."

Preference Rankings

Fred's preference rankings (table 10.4) indicate that cocaine, heroin, and speedball mixtures are his drugs of choice. These are followed closely by mari-

TABLE 10.3. Genealogy and Pattern of Drug Use and Abuse: Fred S.

Drug Substances	13	14	15	16	17	18	19	20	21	22	Frequency of Drug Usage	Comments
				Age								
1. Hallucinogens (psychedelics, THC, MDA, peyote, organic mescaline)											Regular	I tried them all as a kid.
2. Marijuana											Daily	I like good grass. It relaxes me. I would do it every-day if good stuff were available.
3. Amphetamine											Intermittent	I didn't really like it. It's bad enough "going up" but I felt worse "coming down." It wore me down.
4. Cocaine											Daily	Shit, I love co-caine. It gives you feelings you wouldn't believe. I would do it everyday if I could.

	Usage	Comment
5. Heroin	Regular	It's the best downer for co-caine you can get.
6. Other opiates Codeine	Regular	I tried codeine.
7. Psychotropics (librium, Valiums, etc.)	Intermittent	I use them if I am too tense to relax.
8. Alcohol	Fairly regular	I drink some beer fairly regularly and occasionally some hard stuff.
9. Non-prescription, over-the-counter drugs, cough syrup	Regular	I was a cough-syrup freak for a while.
10. Polydrug (cocaine/heroin)	Daily	When they were available.
11. Illegal methadone	Regular	I tried it awhile.
12. Barbiturates	None	I tried them once. I don't like the barb feeling at all.
13. Inhalants	Never	I never did it.
14. Other		

Legend

— Denotes regular usage

- - - Denotes intermittent usage

juana. Beer and hard liquor occupy intermediate preference positions. His high preference for speedballs (higher than for cocaine and heroin separately) is not surprising when one takes into account that cocaine creates not only a brief sense of well-being but frightening delusions and hallucinations in Fred; he needs the buffering that heroin provides. As Fred states, "You don't control cocaine; it controls you!"

TABLE 10.4. Drug Preference Rankings: Fred S.

Substance	First Assessment	First Reassessment	Second Reassessment	Mean	Composite Rank
Amphetamine	9	7	9	8.3	9
Barbiturates	7	8	5	6.7	6.5
Beer	5	5	6	5.3	5
Cocaine	2	2	2	2.0	2
Hard liquor	6	6	8	6.7	6.5
Heroin	3	3	3	3.0	3
LSD	8	9	7	8.0	8
Marijuana	4	4	4	4.0	4
Speedball	1	1	1	1.0	1

Another surprising fact is that although cocaine has a high preference value, the other "upper," amphetamine, has the lowest preference rank. For Fred, these two drugs are poles apart.

Ratings

On the semantic differential Fred described a complex set of relationships among drugs. His data yield three independent factors. However, these do not include all the substances, several of which have no high loadings on any factor. Factor I contains the "real" drugs: speedball, heroin, and drugs in general. These Fred described as being potent and dangerous. Factor II contains only beer and marijuana, which he described as pleasant, weak, and safe. Factor III contains mainly the barbiturates, which are not pleasant — in fact, as far as Fred is concerned they are worthless.

Cocaine does not appear uniquely in any factor. As a component of the speedball it has a modest loading in Factor I. It also loads slightly negatively in the other two factors, indicating that he regards it as somewhat the opposite of beer, marijuana, and the barbiturates. Amphetamine is in a class by itself, with no high loadings on any factor. He says it is the most potent of all, being dangerous, hazardous, and mighty; it is also wrong and worthless. It is too harsh for Fred.

Hard liquor is also not loaded strongly on any factor. It is strong, but trite and sick; it is also wrong, weary, and hazardous. Undoubtedly, these ratings were influenced by Fred's perception of his mother's difficulties. Finally, LSD was given a unique, though largely favorable, description. It is dangerous, but it is also beautiful, exciting, and creative. One might think such a drug would appeal to Fred, but to him LSD is soft (i.e., it is not a hard drug) and, as other data have shown, he regards it as juvenile.

Pattern of Use

Social Context

As stated above, Fred has used cocaine since age sixteen, snorting off and on for a year or so and then taking it intravenously. He was introduced to it by an acquaintance who told him that cocaine was a nice "upper," an expensive but nonaddictive amphetamine. "I tried it. It gave me a warm feeling inside. Colors got richer. It was nice, but that was about all there was to it."

When Fred was seventeen, a friend taught him how to take drugs intravenously. His experiences shooting cocaine were so different from snorting that he felt as if he were doing different drugs. Regarding intravenous cocaine use Fred states, "You get a feeling which I can't describe and which you wouldn't believe. It's an orgastic feeling; for me, it's a quick up and a quick down. You get a fume, a taste in your mouth that goes with it. It's exquisite, a good feeling, a kick. I don't like me when I am on it, because I can't be around people. I get anxious as hell; I get paranoid and I am afraid I will be jumped on or followed any moment! I am afraid the cops are going to get me. It takes about a gram for me to start getting paranoid; I snorted as much as a gram of coke and never got paranoid, but shooting I sure do. Afterwards, you have this incredible craving for more. It's not a physical thing, but I have traded and sold my TVs, my tape recorder, anything, to get more."

Despite the adverse reactions, cocaine is Fred's drug because it helps him cope with depression and discouragement. He indicates that speedballing cocaine and heroin is the best way to take coke if one can afford it, but added that he had never done a run speedballing. "I sort of mix snorting and shooting. I snort the first hit, then shoot the rest. That way I don't come down so hard."

Fred never took cocaine intravenously with more than one other male. "I have this guy who usually brings or sells to me. We fix and shoot, and I have one guy to talk to and share ecstatic ideas and delusions with." Fred estimates that 70 percent of his cocaine usage has been with one male companion; the remaining 30 percent has been alone, while doing extended cocaine runs. He never has shot cocaine with women. His extended runs have generally been done alone because he cannot tolerate the paranoia that goes with heavy cocaine use. "Hell, I would start hallucinating cops and federal agents in trees outside my apartment. At times I would get so scared that I would throw my rig away, flush my stuff down the stool, and run."

His typical usage pattern during the last eighteen months has been a regular three grams per day. He states that once he shot fourteen grams on a three-day run. The largest single hit he has had is a quarter ounce.

"When I did that fourteen grams in three days I was crazy as hell. That's when I was hallucinating federal agents in trees. However, the coke was only 40 percent pure; if it had been pharmaceutical cocaine — that's 98.3 percent pure — it probably would have killed me. I was sick as it was. My body was toxic, it was trying to reject the coke, so that I would shoot and vomit, shoot and vomit, but I couldn't stop till it was all gone. I was crazy and delusional as hell. My father put me away right after that!"

Like many other cocaine users, Fred engaged in frequent cocaine runs. He estimates he has done about fifteen runs of two or three days' duration. The longest run without sleep was the three-day one described above; the third day was "pure hell. You're not too tired physically, but you are crazy and strung out as hell the third day."

It has not been uncommon for him to do extended runs — interspersed with sleep — for several weeks. During one such run he stopped using cocaine for only three days during a period of three months: "I would do three or four grams of coke, shoot some heroin to get off and get some sleep, get up and start all over again. Of course, I got strung out on heroin on that run, too." During this year, Fred reports having had a two-month and a one-month run, using the strategy of taking three to four grams per day.

Fred states that, though he frequently had to "cop" cocaine during the day to keep a run going, all his runs began in the evening. "That's the way it usually works out, because late in the evening is the safest time; that's when people like to deal."

The bulk of cocaine he has used has been street cocaine, but "when they know you can pay, you can get the best. I had the money and could pay the price for good stuff." He feels his street coke has been better than that to which most people had access. "It was typically 40 percent pure, and sometimes 50 percent pure." Fred states that 70 percent of the cocaine he has used is street cocaine, 20 percent pharmaceutical, and the remaining 10 percent concentrated rock crystal.

There have been only two ways he can tell the difference between high- and low-grade cocaine: by the "rush" and the "fume." "There is no way to tell by how the stuff looks. You have to shoot some; fire it up and you can tell by the rush. You don't get much of a rush with cheap stuff. Also, you can tell by the fume; you can mix some with water and if it's good, you can smell the fume. Most of the time, you can tell cocaine from procaine by the rush, too. The procaine rush is harder, raw like an amphetamine rush. I don't think you can tell procaine if it is mixed with good coke; the coke will hide it."

Any life event that makes him depressed can trigger a cocaine run. "Things like getting fired from a job, losing a close girlfriend, having a big fight with my mother and father, anything that would get me depressed, any disappointment in life — and I have had a lot of them — would set me off on a run. I have to add, too, that doing coke is a way to fuck-up! Partly, I use it to help me deal with hurt and disappointment. However, it was also a way to get back at my mother and father, too!"

Fred's experience has been that on a run his body develops a tolerance to cocaine, up to a point. "After a gram of coke, I had to increase the size of the hits. It depends in part on the quality of cocaine you're shooting. On a run you never get back to the rush you get with the first hit, but it is still good. After three grams I start getting a toxic reaction; my body will try to repel the coke, and I will start vomiting more then."

Fred states that heavy coke users recommend staying away from cocaine for at least two days after a run, to get the cocaine out of the system. However, he says that frequently he would begin shooting again after twelve hours (including a good night's sleep) and still "get off" pretty good.

The withdrawal reaction is severe in coming off a run. "I was tired and worn out. I would get splitting headaches from the lactose in the cut; I am allergic to it. I would want more coke, and would be depressed as hell; I would get suicidal thoughts, and would just try to hang on till it ended. I wasn't hungry at all. Most of the time I would have to take something to help me get off: heroin, Dilaudid, tranquilizers. Any kind of downer would help." Fred thinks that heroin is the best drug to use to "get off" a cocaine run. Tranquilizers or even alcohol are not as effective as the opiates. Fred often has used tranquilizers however, because they are cheap and more easily accessible than opiates.

Reactions to Cocaine

Physiological Reactions

Table 10.5 shows some physiological reactions which occurred every time Fred used cocaine. They are sequelae to central nervous system stimulation: increased heart rate; elevation of pulse and respiration rate, dryness of the mouth and throat, increased urination and diarrhea, and loss of appetite or sensations of hunger.

A second cluster of physiological reactions which occurred with high frequency included accelerated mental activity, loss of fatigue, local anesthesia at the site of injection, sensitivity to light, visual anomalies (fog, snow, and whiteness of the room, which were in all probability visual hallucinations), nausea, sweating, a sensation of tightness across the chest, headaches, ringing in the ears, and what he described as a tightening or shrinking of the genitalia. Although Fred reports feeling nausea 80 percent of the time he has used cocaine, vomiting and muscle spasms have occurred only during 30 percent of his cocaine usage: "These reactions occurred only after heavy or prolonged usage when my body was becoming toxic to the coke." Fred often experienced gooseflesh, but states it was an anticipatory reaction to intravenous cocaine usage. Not surprisingly, Fred reports none of the reactions associated with snorting cocaine — i.e., rhinorrhea, lacrimation, reactive hyperemia, and nose-

TABLE 10.5. Physiological Reactions to Cocaine Use and Abuse: Fred S.

Commonly Reported Reaction to Cocaine Use/Abuse	Reactions Observed Yes	Reactions Observed No	Percent/ Time Observed	Qualifying Comments and Observations
Dizziness – feeling of light-headedness	Yes		30	Yeah, if the shot is bigger than you thought. You almost black out. The lights get dim, then come back up. It only comes on heavy hits. I don't like that feeling. It's like being close to death.
Sweating – perspiration or increases in temperature	Yes		60	You sweat pretty regular.
Rhinorrhea – running nose		No		You do that snorting.
Tremors – muscle spasms	Yes		30	I get "twitches" in my legs doing coke. I can't stop the twitching.
Lacrimation – tears to eyes		No		Snorting good coke will sometimes bring tears to your eyes.
Mydriasis – dilation of pupils, light sensitivity	Yes		50	If you do a lot, the room looks like a fog or snow-storm. It's hazy, misty, and white. It takes a lot of good coke to create that reaction. One shot won't do it; you have to do a gram or two of good stuff.
Gooseflesh	Yes		60	It's psychological. I get "gooseflesh" in anticipa-tion before I make the first hit.
Emesis – vomiting	Yes		30	After I shoot more than three grams of pharma-ceutical coke, I get toxic. Your body tries to reject the poison. I would shoot and throw up, shoot and throw up. You feel nausea, like you want to vomit about 80 percent of the time.
Reactive hyperemia – clogging of nasal air passages		No		You get some of that snorting, though. They un-clog if you snort, then shoot.
Anorexia – loss of appetite, sensation of hunger	Yes		100	You have no hunger at all.
Dryness of mouth and throat, lack of salivation	Yes		100	That's how it is.
Increased heart rate	Yes		100	It pounds like hell after the hit.
Tightness in chest or chest pains	Yes		70	I don't get pain, just a tightness across my chest.
Local anesthesia, numbness	Yes		70	You have to shoot more than a gram. If you snort enough coke, your head will feel numb.

Effect	Yes/No	%	Comment
Nosebleed	No		Some snorters get nosebleeds. I snort the first hit, then shoot the rest. You don't come down so hard.
Elevation of pulse rate	Yes	100	Your whole body is fired up.
Increased respiration rate	Yes	100	It increases as you shoot more coke.
Cellulitis – inflammation following administration	No		Not for me.
Infection of nasal mucous membrane	No		Heavy snorters get that, but I am a shooter.
Yawning	No		I never noticed anything like that.
Hyperphrenia – excessive mental activity	Yes	80	Your mind is moving. Thoughts come and go faster.
Weight loss	Yes	100	It is because you aren't hungry and don't eat when you do a lot of coke.
Fainting	No		I have never fainted but have been close to it; things get dark, the room gets dark, colors get dark.
Increased sensitivity to allergies	No		Not the coke. I am not allergic to coke even though I have done a lot!
Diarrhea or explosive bowel movements	Yes	100	I get diarrhea shooting. Sometimes I have to go right to the john after a hit right then.
Hepatitis or liver infections	No		I have never had hepatitis. It is surprising, as much shooting as I have done, but I am careful about the spikes I use.
Headaches	Yes	50	I get headaches from the cut. I am allergic to lactose. A high quantity of lactose in the cut will stop a run for me.
Loss of fatigue	Yes	100	You don't feel any sensation of being tired at all. That's good.
Ringing in the ears	Yes	40	If it is high grade, they ring.
Convulsions	No		I saw a guy have a seizure twice on coke in two days, but he would get up, didn't know anything about what had happened, and go right back to shooting again. It scared me at first, but maybe he was one of those people who are prone to having seizures.
Increased urination	Yes	100	It stimulates your whole system.
Abscesses	No	100	I have never had an abscess but have gotten big bumps on my arm when I miss the vein. This was usually towards the end of a run when all your veins are down about 10 percent.

bleed. He has never fainted — though he has been close on some occasions — or developed inflammation, infections, or abscesses at the site of injection — though he did report occasional burns. Fred said he has never had hepatitis — "I use new spikes." Nor has he experienced convulsions as a toxic reaction — "When I get toxic, I start vomiting and my body repels it as fast as I shoot it. That's OK because I still get the flash!"

Psychological Reactions

Table 10.6 indicates that psychological reactions are a "mixed bag" for Fred, with increases in feelings of well-being and euphoria accompanied simultaneously by increased anxiety, paranoid fears, and hallucinations. The psychological reactions that always occurred include increases in restlessness, excitement, psychomotor activity, a sense of optimism, well-being and euphoria — "so short-lived" — talkativeness, indifference to pain, insomnia, anxiety and irrational fears, and paranoid ideation.

A second cluster of psychological reactions which occurred with high frequency include increased feelings of physical strength or ability to work — accompanied however by decreased *motivation* for work ("You're not interested in work, just the next hit") — a brief sensation that everything is perfect, accelerated mental activity, terror and panic, and visual and auditory hallucinations accompanied by changes in perceived reality.

Fred reports that cocaine is not an aphrodisiac. "It is not sexually stimulating at all for me. I imagine it would be for snorters. I have never done sex with cocaine, I really don't know." For him cocaine does not prolong intercourse, nor does it produce a more spectacular orgasm with the rush. It does not generate olfactory or tactile hallucinations; Fred had heard about tactile hallucinations, but never experienced them. He does not feel intravenous use of cocaine is associated with greater self-control. "I feel like I am losing self-control. You don't control coke; it controls you!"

Though Fred describes himself as a gentle, nonaggressive person, it is his impression that extended use of cocaine could trigger violence. He notes that after one extended run, "My father had me at the police station. I was crazy as hell; I knocked this cop on his ass. Normally, I am not aggressive at all, except with my mother."

Integration

Fred's drug use serves complex functions in his personal adjustment: First, cocaine helps him manage recurrent bouts of depression and assists in mediating reversals in living. It increases his self-confidence and temporarily makes him feel strong. Fred overuses the drug and must therefore deal also with irrational fears, paranoid delusions, and hallucinations. To reestablish equilibrium Fred uses heroin, other opiates, tranquilizers, and even alcohol.

Although this young man has used cocaine heavily, he fears amphetamine. Apparently it is too harsh, and provides more stimulation than he can tolerate. The "crash" on withdrawal from amphetamine involves more physical exhaustion, depression, and stress than he can cope with.

Fred's drug usage provides him a position of status in the drug community. During one twelve-month period he spent more than $16,000 on cocaine; the bulk of this money came from bad checks which Fred wrote against his father's account and which his father subsequently covered. Fred is a legendary figure in the local drug community. As he put it, "In the dope world I have a name. They know who I am. I have a name as a junkie and a dealer. I am respected because they always know I have excellent stuff." This position of respect, which is very important to him, is also due to the fact that, despite his youth, Fred is viewed as an expert on drugs: He has tried many substances, studied them carefully (maintaining an extensive drug library), knows the chemical properties and clinical effects of the most frequently used ones, and is in effect a reasonably well-informed, self-taught pharmacist. The respect and visibility he thus enjoys has created some problems. "You can't buy that much coke without attracting the attention of every damn narcotic agent in town. They know me, but they can't prove anything yet. However, they are after my ass; unless I am damn careful — and I try to be — they will eventually catch me."

Fred admits that his cocaine usage is a way to get back at his parents. By allowing his dealer to front him cocaine and then writing bad checks against his father's account, he forces his parents into the position where they must either rescue their son or see him go to jail, be hurt, or killed. The family — particularly the father — is faced with a son who will play the confrontation game to the brink.

Finally, Fred's cocaine usage allows him to punish himself. He has vividly described his need to be isolated from other people, the fearful loss of control he experiences with cocaine, the frightening paranoid delusions, the visual and auditory hallucinations, and the depression and suicidal fantasies he experiences with withdrawal. Clearly, self-destructive impulses play a significant role in his pattern of drug use.

LIFE ACTIVITIES AND EXPERIENCES: IN FRED'S OWN WORDS

Overview

The section that follows presents hour-by-hour accounts of two days in Fred's life. They occurred in early March and late April, 1975.

The first day starts with Ralph, a friend and cocaine dealer, and Fred discussing the current price of cocaine — it has gone up. Fred is "blue" and discouraged

TABLE 10.6. Psychological Reactions to Cocaine Use and Abuse: Fred S.

Commonly Reported Reactions to Cocaine Use/Abuse	Reactions Observed		Percent/ Time Observed	Qualifying Comments and Observations
	Yes	No		
Increased feelings of self-control		No		I feel like I am losing control, if anything. You don't control it; it controls you. Snorting, you have the drug under control, but not shooting. It's almost like two different compounds.
Increased optimism, courage	Yes		90	You just feel so good.
Increased activity, restlessness, excitement	Yes		100	I get excited and hyper if I do just a gram. That's not much for me, but if I do three grams, I start getting anxious as hell.
Feeling of increased physical strength or ability to do physical work	Yes		60	You feel like you could do more work, you feel like you could do anything you wanted to do, but really all you are interested in is the next hit.
Intensified feelings of well-being, euphoria, "floating," etc.	Yes		100	It's indescribable, you feel so good, but the rush doesn't last but a few minutes. For me it is a quick up and a quick down. It's short-lived.
Feeling that everything is perfect	Yes		80	While it lasts, but the rush is not long.
An exquisite "don't care about the world" attitude		No		Heroin will give you that feeling sometimes.
A physical orgasm in the "rush"		No		I haven't had that reaction at all. There is an orgastic quality to coke though, in the "flash."
Increased thinking power and imagination	Yes		70	Yeah, for a short while. My imagination goes crazy though after a gram or two.
Feeling that the mind is quicker than normal, the feeling that one is smarter than everyone else	Yes		60	Snorters get it, too. Your mind is racing; sometimes it's hard to hold on to. It makes you think more. I don't know if it's the coke though. Coffee or amphetamines will do the same thing for me.

More talkative than usual, a stream of talk	Yes	100	I just talk my head off if I am shooting with another guy.
Indifference to pain	Yes	100	You don't notice pain.
Decreased interest in work, failure of ambition, loss of ambition for useful work	Yes	70	You don't want to work. You're just interested in the next hit.
Insomnia	Yes	100	It depends on how much you take. You can take one hit and sleep on it. If you go over a gram, you will have to have some kind of downer or you're in trouble.
Depression, anxiety	Yes	100	Quitting causes depression with me. I get depressed after I stop shooting. I start getting anxious as hell after a gram.
Prolonged sexual intercourse	No		I never wanted to fuck when I was shooting.
An aphrodisiac or sexual stimulant	No		Not for me. I've heard it's an aphrodisiac with women, but I don't know.
Better orgasm on coke	Yes	100	I don't have intercourse when I shoot! If you are shooting, that's all you're interested in. If you're on a run and have to be at work at 9:00 a.m. and can only cop more coke at 9:00 a.m. you cop coke!
Irrational fears	Yes	60	I get terrified. I am afraid the cops will bust in any moment.
Terror or panic	Yes	60	Same as above.
Tactile hallucinations — the feeling that insects are crawling on or under the skin (particularly fingertips, palms of hands, etc.)	No		I have heard of that but not sure I believe it. As much coke as I have done, I should have had that kind of reaction if there is one.
Changes in reality or the way a room or objects look — the wall waving or in motion, etc.	Yes	60	Colors get brighter sometimes, a room will get darker like someone turned the lights down.
Paranoid ideas — the feeling that people are after you. You believe you are being watched, talked about or threatened, a wife or girlfriend is unfaithful, untrustworthy, etc.	Yes	100	I get paranoid as hell. After one gram I start getting paranoid. I don't want to be around people. I have to be by myself. It is scary. I keep thinking the cops will bust in any moment. I get delusions of being jumped on or followed any second.

TABLE 10.6. Psychological Reactions in Cocaine Use and Abuse: Fred S. *(Continued)*

Commonly Reported Reactions to Cocaine Use/Abuse	Reactions Observed Yes No	Percent/ Time Observed	Qualifying Comments and Observations
Causes one to carry a gun or run from imaginary enemies	Yes	10	On one run I carried a gun. I thought people were after me.
Visual hallucinations	Yes	10	I hallucinated federal agents in a tree once. I hallucinated it. It was at night. I threw a gram of coke away and ran around the block.
Auditory hallucinations — hearing voices talking about you, threatening, etc.	Yes	60	You're scared and you misinterpret sounds. It sounds like people are talking about you in whispers or something, kind of in the distance. You can barely hear it.
Olfactory hallucinations — new odors, smells, etc.	No		I never noticed it.
A trigger for violence	Yes	20	You get out of your mind if you do a lot. They had to strap me down once. I had decked a cop. I floored him, and I am not a violent person, but I had been doing more than three grams a day for a couple of months, and I was out of it. I've seen others get violent on coke. They would hit people and things.

because a few days earlier he lost his job as a fry cook at a drive-in. He is worried about how he will survive (his mother refuses to let him live at home). He wishes he had some coke. He visits with an addict on methadone maintenance; the addict tells Fred how he sells his take-home medication. On the way home, he sees Mr. Crabtree, a black addict who owes him money. Fred attempts to collect from him because he owes money to his own dealer, Mr. Landis. He fails to get Mr. Crabtree to pay. When he arrives home, Fred "checks out" a drug for a friend in one of his reference books.

Fred visits with Hartford, an unemployed musician, age thirty-five, who is Fred's only real friend. Hartford is like Fred's grandmother, understanding but non-demanding. They visit. Fred then watches his favorite TV program, "Star Trek," until his friend Charlie comes by. Again, Fred is sought out as the expert, first on where good grass can be obtained, and, second, on the long-term effects of LSD abuse.

Fred describes how he lost his job and comes to the conclusion he may have fired himself. Fred then makes arrangements for a cocaine sale, and is briefly visited by Landis, who demands his money. Fred is afraid of Landis, whom he says is a big connection locally. He wonders how he could "score" some more cocaine, how he is going to pay for cocaine he has already used. Then he goes along on the cocaine sale with Hartford, and describes one way a cocaine sale is transacted. He goes to bed wishing he had some of the cocaine he helped sell.

On the second day Fred is depressed. He still owes Landis money; he is still unemployed; and he failed the entrance requirements for a trade school he had tried to enter. He leaves Hartford's apartment in the wee hours, goes to his own, and goes to bed. There, he is awakened by Landis, who demands $230 by 8 p.m. — or else. Fred is frightened because he doesn't have the money. At 3 p.m. he has an appointment with his psychiatrist, but he cannot talk to him about what is on his mind; he fears either he will make his psychiatrist feel depressed at Fred's lack of progress, or the psychiatrist might terminate his therapy. Fred's father then picks him up and they visit his mother in the hospital. The two then go on to the father's home. A bitter confrontation occurs between father and son in which both are badly hurt — but no resolution occurs. Both go to bed drained and exhausted. Fred wonders if life is worth it all.

Activity and Experience Audits

First Day: A Thursday in March

I slept from midnight till noon.

12:00 n. –3:00 p.m.

I was in my place alone cooking some soup. There was a knock at the door and a friend, Ralph, came in. He told me the prices — $2,000 an ounce. It has gone high as hell in the ghetto! There is a lot of high-grade coke in the suburbs now, but in the ghetto the dudes are making at least $800 to $1,000 profit per ounce. He offered me a 'tester'; I refused, but he fired up. I guess it was good. He said it was about 40 percent pure. It made him real uptight and nervous, so I gave him a Valium and he drank a bottle of paregoric. (It has opium in it; it doesn't hurt, and could help.)

I had a cigarette and sat rapping with him. I owe him some money. Ralph was telling me how poor he is and how bad he needs the money, and I thought, "Sure, you just said you moved two ounces of the stuff at $800 to $1,000 profit and you're real poor!" He said he was desolate. Shit!

He tried to front me some coke, and I gave him the same shit! I told him I had just lost my job — which was true; I told him what poor was really like! I told him he would have to get it in bits and pieces 'cause that is the only way I could repay him, and he just had to accept it. Shit, it was the truth!

He and I went to school together. He started talking about his new girlfriend. This cat is about my age, twenty-one, but he hangs around with a lot younger crowds than he is. I guess he's "the man" to them; maybe that is important for him. Ralph looks up to me but for the stupidest reasons — the fact that I have been strung out longer than him, and the fact that I know a hell of a lot more about dope than he does.

He starts talkin' about his new girlfriend. He seems to like her a lot because he fucks her a lot and she is good-looking. It seems to be a kinky kind of relationship. He lays her a lot, and she's pretty!

He talked about where he works and the products he's selling. I talked about losing my job and being unemployed. After a while he left.

I had Hartford's TV. Mine had been stolen a month or so ago. Hartford — I sometimes call him "H" — was at work. He lives down the hall from me, lends it to me all the time. I watched the box, and was just thinking how I could get some money together to buy some coke, what kind of con could I put on someone to get some money. I finally concluded it would put me even more behind financially than I already am. That would be trouble, and there was no legal way I could get the money. I crossed it off in my head. Also, I was trying to relax — I was feeling tense at seeing the coke.

About 1:30 another friend of mine, Jacob, came in. He's a couple of years older than I am. He is a real friend who I trust completely. He's just the kind of dude you can trust, even if he was an addict. He's on methadone now; he has been for some time and hasn't shot dope in a long time.

He said I looked tense. I told him why. He talked about the hassles coming down between him and the girl he lives with. I commented that he was the kind of person who had a high threshold of anger, he holds things in instead of dealing with it up-front; instead of pursuing a situation and winning it, he holds back — he folds! She never gives in but always puts it on him — he folds! I think he is too good for her and told him so. He said there were a lot of things about the relationship I did not know. I guess so.

He was also telling me how he gets "take-outs" on his methadone. He will hold them, and sell his another day — he tries to cut it down. He said the other day they made him take it right in front of their eyes, and he became high as hell taking his regular dose of methadone.

I went in and shaved and showered. (I am usually too tired to do it when I wake up.) I took Hartford's TV back. Then I went with Jacob to the place where he gets his methadone.

3:00–4:30 p.m.

I sat over there and visited with three or four friends in the recreation room. A nurse came in that I know. It's good to know nurses; they can often be very helpful. I asked her how much methadone a guy could take and still not get hooked. I told her about Ralph, didn't mention his name. She said it takes a couple of weeks using methadone daily to get hooked. Ralph has only taken it three or four days, so he is OK now.

I got a ride with a guy I know. Halfway home we went by a 7-11 store and I saw Mr. Crabtree, who owes me money. I said, 'Pull over!'

I went in and told him he owed me eighty dollars. He said I owed him ten dollars. I said, OK, pay me the seventy dollars. He tried to act like he didn't owe me anything. I was pissed, but went out and got in the car. The guy dropped me off at my place and he went home.

I went up to my place and looked through a new drug book I have. I was looking for a drug a friend had had prescribed for him; he wanted to know what it was. I found it and noted it.

4:30–6:30 p.m.

I went to Hartford's place. He was going to work. I was going to get his TV again and bring it to my pad. He asked me if I wanted to go for a walk. I said sure.

He doesn't usually talk a lot, but is an interesting guy. We did talk about a friend of ours who was caught in Mexico and charged with possession of marijuana. We were afraid they would throw away the key on him. We talked about others who had been busted in other countries, and how bad the busts are.

He went on to work. I enjoy being with H., I can talk freely with him. I got the TV and brought it to my place. I watched "Star Trek," one of my favorite programs. It is interesting, kinda exciting, and at the same time halfway believable. I watched it till 6:30.

6:30–12:00 p.m.

Right before the program was over Charlie — he's younger than me, but halfway a friend — came in. He's still into acid and LSD, things that I outgrew a long time ago. He asked me if I would cop him a pound of pot. I told Charlie the situation, and he said it was OK.

We smoked a couple of joints and watched TV. He talked about a friend who had done too much acid and had a toxic psychosis. Charlie said he was still strange-acting some time afterwards. He said since I knew a lot about dope was there anything he could do to help his friend? We talked some more, and I got the impression that the friend was partly in a toxic psychosis and was also using it to manipulate people. He asked if there would be permanent damage; would the dude stay freaked out? I told him he would probably come down; it takes time. I did tell him, however, that some dudes have permanent damage; I told him what my own shrink had told me about it. He borrowed a drug book and left.

I went on watching the box. I was thinking a little about my mother, who was in the hospital, and was wondering what was going on with her. Also, I thought about my job and wondered why I had gotten fired. I concluded it was mostly my attendance — I was late twice and the manager said that was something we don't do — and the fact that I owed this dude some money. Landis, my coke connection, would come by every evening and I would have to go out and shoo him away. That meant I was leaving my station. They didn't like that.

The way the manager had fired me was almost humorous. The manager and his assistant sat down with me after work and said, "We think maybe we will have to let you go." I said, "What do you mean maybe?" He said, "Well, we may have to let you go." I said, "You mean I am fired?" He said, "Yeah!" Shit! Maybe I fired myself. I started to ask for a second chance, or at least ask him why he was firing me, but hell, there was no sense in asking those things; he had already made his decision. It would have been like kicking a dead dog! I was both pissed and scared; I owe money to so many different people that aren't too trustworthy. It was a real setback for me! I was also thinking about the coke deal coming up and about how to get it together.

I went to the phone and made a call. I was told everything was set, but it would be late that night.

I borrowed some papers from Hartford's place to roll pot. I went back to my place and continued to watch TV. I was thinking of some ways I might get some money together, but finally gave it up. I was also thinking about a girl I had met two or three days earlier. I liked her. I was thinking about taking her out. However, she lives with a guy, and she said it was not safe to come over there; he might bust me up. She said she would come by some time. I was wondering when in the hell she was coming!

Then Landis came by. My wallet was laying on the table with money in it. He sat down and asked if I had any money for him! He could see my wallet. I told him no.

He picked up my wallet and said, "What the hell do you call this?" I told him, that's money I need, it's not mine. I was bullshitting him. I told him I couldn't afford to give it to him (the truth), and I was fronting for another guy (not the truth). He told me he would cross off my debt if I would go to the doctor's office and cop a bottle of coke for him. He left.

I've seen guys cop from doctor's offices. You go to an ear, nose, and throat doctor with some complaint. You have to be quick, though! I thought it might be easier than paying this dude his 230 bills, but my ass would really be in trouble if I was busted. I told him I would weigh it.

He left, not too happy. I am afraid of this guy; he's a big connection, the biggest I know. He is muscular and talks very demanding. You don't b.s. with that dude very often. He doesn't think twice about having someone hurt if they don't pay. He left me kind of shook. Yet it's strange, 'cause he can be diplomatic as hell when he sets his mind to it — smooth and oily. I got to thinking that maybe I could find some way to get dad to lend me some money. After I thought about it, I knew it wouldn't work. Moreover, I couldn't go cop cocaine from a doctor's office. I decided that I would simply have to pay it out in bits and pieces and take my chances.

The guy who was going to buy the coke threw some pebbles at my window. I opened it; I knew he was there. I said, "Hi!" He was with H. I unplugged the TV and brought it down to H.'s place; then the three of us walked to the other dude's place.

12:00 p.m. – 3:00 a.m.

There we were in the apartment watching TV — H., the guy who was going to cop, another guy, and I. Hartford is a very close friend even though he is ten years older than me. We used to cop cough syrup together. It was easy; you could cop a bottle of cough syrup every day at some stores. Well, Hartford is real, a real interesting guy. He graduated from college and is very intelligent. He doesn't get angry too much. He's a dude I can talk to when I'm in trouble — which seems to be often. I owe him some money, but he does not press me for it; he just says, "pay me when you can."

The other two guys were his friends. They are about Hartford's age. We watched TV and were talking; two of them were playing chess. We're smoking pot. The guy reads a lot of underground comic books. One he gets every month, I was looking at that evening. It publishes price lists on drugs in different parts of the country. It usually has a foldout; this month the foldout was a picture of a peyote cactus. H. thought it was cool. I'm feeling pretty good. I'm thinking about the guy who is coming out to sell the gram.

Ralph arrives with the stuff. He asks how we were doing and sat down and bullshit a few minutes. Then he shows the stuff. The dude tasted it and says great!

Ralph lays it on the table. Then the dude lays his money on the table. Then Ralph goes outside. The third dude picks up the money, goes outside the hall, and gives it to Ralph. I think if you do it this way, the guy who brings the stuff cannot be charged with selling it. He is protected; he could say he was giving it as a gift.

The dude with the gram snorts a bit while we all watch (my mouth was watering). He complimented us on the quality, and H. and I left. It was good quality — about 40 percent, he said. H. and I walked back to his place.

3:00–3:45 a.m.

Hartford and I played a game of Battleship. You set your ships up where the other guy can't see them and through a procedure try to sink the other guy's ships. He won, and I had fun that night.

I smoked a joint and went to bed thinking. I was a little nervous thinking about that coke going right under my nose. I wondered why I didn't try to set up a scam to rip them all off, but then I really wouldn't have done it to friends.

I went to sleep.

The Day: It was a kind of taxing day. There were a lot of points in the day where I was uptight, thinking about either coke or confronted with my debts in scary ways. I really never felt at ease all day long. I wasn't at peace with myself at all.

Second Day: A Monday in April

12:00 p.m.–2:00 a.m.

I was in Hartford's place, playing chess. He and I were alone. We were not saying much. The TV was on. I had told him earlier he would look good with a beard and damn if he didn't start growing one!

He asked if I was hungry. I said yes, so he cooked some pancakes — they were good.

At 2:00 I said goodnight. It had been a quiet evening with him, relaxing. I felt a bit inhibited that evening! Hadn't talked much.

I had taken some tests to get into a special school, and my scores had not been high enough to enroll. The woman had said I was rusty and needed to practice. So I have to take pre-school courses and pass them before I can get into the school. I felt like I had let my father and myself down by not getting a better score. I was feeling kinda blue about it all, feeling kind of down.

I went to my place and took a Val [Valium]. I was thinking about my financial obligations, where was I going to get a job, and so on. I had no luck in finding a job yet. I had to take those classes, too. I went to sleep thinking about things like this.

1:00 p.m.–2:30 p.m.

Someone knocking at the door woke me up. I opened it — there was Landis! He's about twenty-seven years old and the worst kind of dude you could cross! He has no heart. He's a high cat! He doesn't carry a gun, doesn't believe in it, but he doesn't have to. He's a strong, muscular dude, worked behind enemy lines some on a "killer team" in Vietnam. He wanted his 230 bills that I owed him. Those type dudes set you up; they front you stuff — "Shoot now and pay later" — then make you beholden to them.

I told him I had half of it owed to me. He said, "Fred, tell me who it is and

I will collect it!" Knowing his style of collection, I asked him to hold off a few days. He said, "Nope, I need it tonight." I told him I couldn't raise 230 by tonight. He said I would have to! He snorted some coke, then offered me a hit. He laughed and said, "Fred, if you take it, that may be the last hit you ever do!" I refused. He left.

It was weird. I was uptight, nervous, and scared at the same time. However, he knows I am good for it; I have made a lot of business for him. I turned about $10,000 last year to him when I was doing coke like crazy. I have never ripped Landis off. I am, frankly, afraid to.

Before he left, he asked me what time I wanted him to come by. I said I didn't know. He said he would see me at 8:00 p.m.; I should have the money. I decided not to be there at 8:00.

2:30–4:00 p.m.

I had an appointment with my shrink (Dad pays the bill) at 3:00 p.m. I took a bus to the shrink's place.

I had just had my life threatened. I didn't know what the hell to tell my shrink, so I didn't say anything. I didn't know how to tell him. He gets all angry and upset, so I didn't say anything. He said I was a bore! Any damn fool could tell I was scared, but not him. I never tell the dude the complete facts or truth, because he gets so damn upset and mad at me. He gets all depressed and down that I don't do so well. Then he makes me feel bad. I could tell the whole truth, but I'm afraid he'll get so angry he will throw me out of therapy or make me mad at myself; so I only tell him bits and pieces. I know it sounds a bit crazy, but that's how he and I work.

4:00–5:00 p.m.

My father picked me up. We were going to get a six-pack, have lunch, and talk about where I was at. He was in a bad mood; I guess my mother had not been feeling so well. Right off he started yelling at me in the car. Finally he settled down. I was scared; a six-pack and lunch?

We drove down and visited my mother. She was OK.

5:00–11:00 p.m.

We drove to his place. We were going to talk about my financial situation. My father said we couldn't get anyplace if I continued to lie to him. He said we had to get down to the truth if we were going to get anything done. He said he didn't want me to lie to him anymore. He said I should be truthful with him — even if it hurt.

He said he wanted the complete truth — so I gave it to him. At this, he really got mad!!! I thought he was going to have a heart attack! He really worked me over, man! Landis, the dude, had earlier let a contract on me — a year or so ago — but found out I had not ripped off his cocaine, and lifted it. My father — he knows Landis — said he did not give a damn what Landis did to me, it was my bill. He told me he was gonna let me live at home while my mother was in the hospital, but my bill with Landis was my problem. A real help! He was raising holy hell! I am thinking how nice it would be to overdose. I'm just fantasizing it; I don't have the guts to do it, but I was thinking how nice it might be to turn off the projector and leave.

He was shouting. He said he didn't give a fuck about me, didn't give a fuck about my mother, and didn't give a fuck if he died the next day!!! He was also feeling real sorry for himself. He told me he would let me stay at the house because of Landis. He had some work I could do around the house — he'd pay me for it, and if I could hold my act together, he'd help me find some temporary work till I could get a permanent job!!! I agreed to do that.

He worked me over; I cried. He kept asking me why I did this, why I did that. Shit!

We had dinner — I guess you could call it that. I had Jello and a beer. He had Jello. My stomach was so tied in knots that I couldn't eat anything else. I guess his was, too. Sometimes my stomach gets so tied up, I vomit when I do eat. I didn't tonight, though. I was drained and still tied in knots. I was wondering what Landis was going to do when he didn't find me at 8:00.

We sat watching the box. I was numb! We tried to chat — he started up again! He was really rubbing it into me about how much I have cost him in the last six years. Rubbing in how much I have put in my arm. He asked me if I wanted to look at the figures; I told him no. I didn't want to see the damn figures! I know them!

Finally, man, I unloaded on him. I didn't plan it that way, the tension just kept building up till finally I couldn't handle it. I told him to get off my back! He was partly responsible for my behavior; what the hell did he want me to do? I shouted at him, "Get off my back! Cool it!!! Shit, man, we both hit a lot of grief!" I cried. He almost cried, too, but finally got off my back!

We watched the news. He said it was a shame that they — the Israelis and Arabs — couldn't make peace in the Middle East. I didn't say much of anything.

Afterwards, I think he said he didn't know what to do with me. He said he didn't want to have to put me away, because he didn't want to spend the money on it. He did once before. He told me my shrink wasn't doing me no good. I told him I had really only fucked-up once in the last year, and things were not so bad as he thought they were. I thought about agreeing to be put away, but I couldn't really do that; it would be a waste of his money. I would just sit up nights thinking up ways to con people so I could get out. I had already increased my therapy sessions to twice a week. The only thing I could think of was to tell him I would try harder.

He wanted me to say something positive. He kept asking me why. I kept telling him I didn't know. He asked me if I was going to be a junkie the rest of my life. Of course, I told him no.

The news was over by then. He began trying to persuade me to go to bed. I told him I'm keyed up; I wanted to watch TV and relax if I could. He kept pressing me. He went and closed the house, and began pushing again and again, so finally I said, "OK, I'll go to bed!"

I had a beer with him. He offered me a sleeping pill; he said it would knock me right out. I refused it. He told me they were very good, he uses them. I said no!

He went to his room. I went to the old room I used to have. I rolled me a joint, and laid in bed smoking it.

Sure as hell, he came in and said, "Is that marijuana you're smoking?" I said, "Yeah." I told him I took that to relax me; it is better for me than his pills. He surprised me: He said, "OK, I can understand that," and he went back to bed.

I finished my beer and went to bed and went right to sleep. Wow!

The Day: Man, I was exhausted, drained, empty, and wore out! I had no trouble going to sleep. I had been through a lot of emotional shit during that day. I was *out of it.*

11

Rufus B.

LIFE THEMES

Rufus B. is a flamboyant, ebullient man who has been a highly successful pimp. He and his stable of "hustling ladies" have worked all the major cities — Chicago, Los Angeles, New York — going from one convention to the next, following the action wherever it may be. During the last two years Rufus has suffered serious reversals, which, however, he considers to be only temporary. The major themes in Rufus's life are as follows:

- I have to be on top, to be noticed; I must be somebody no one can ignore.
- I will be as ruthless as necessary to achieve this, because it is my only purpose in life.
- If I am not loved, respected, admired, feared, or even hated by others, I will be nothing.
- It may seem that now I have lost everything, but that is not so. Though I sometimes wonder whether it is worth the struggle, I am determined to regain the place on top that is rightfully mine.

Cocaine Use in Relation to Life Themes

Rufus is an intravenous, daily, intermediate-dosage cocaine user. Cocaine or speedball mixtures of heroin and cocaine are his drugs of choice because

- they permit this driven, sensuous man to stop, relax, and temporarily escape the specter of depression which follows him wherever he goes,
- cocaine enhances sex,
- cocaine allows Rufus to get high and feel mellow with friends, yet it does not diminish his cat-like alertness to events occurring around him, and
- like his El Dorado Cadillac, cocaine is a sign of the high status he has enjoyed and intends to regain.

EVOLUTION OF LIFE STYLE

Rufus is a lean but powerfully built, handsome thirty-five-year-old Negro male. By all standards, he is a fashionplate. His dress is "mod" and expensive, yet tasteful. His clothes are tailored to a perfect fit. Rufus usually wears slacks, a silk, floral shirt in contrasting but complementary colors, lift alligator shoes, an expensive hand-stitched leather jacket, and occasionally a snap-brim hat with a solid silver chain around the crown. On four different occasions he wore the same style leather jacket, but in each instance in a different color. When asked how many such jackets he owned, Rufus stated, "Shit man, I got six of them, all different colors and tailored for me. I wear the one that goes with my other clothes."

Rufus is socially alert and charming. He is cheerful, self-assured, and aggressive. He becomes animated talking about himself. He has a mobile face, and a warm smile, and wears a flashing, three-carat diamond in one ear. "I was the first pimp in the city to wear a diamond like that. People notice me because of that, man! People say, that dude, the one with the big diamond in his ear, sent me! There are two or three other dudes who wear diamonds now, but shit, they copied me. I did it first!"

Although Rufus is animated and verbal he maintains a relaxed physical looseness, at ease yet alert. He generally answered our questions in a direct and straightforward manner. On occasions when he felt the interviewer was probing into an inappropriate area, he either gracefully bent the discussion away from the topic or fabricated what he thought was a plausible tale, smiling all the while. If this failed, his demeanor could quickly change to belligerence: "That's none of your goddamn business!"

Rufus is proud of his physique and rugged good looks, his manliness and fearlessness, his style and street savvy, his ability to charm others, particularly women, and his past success as "the best pimp that ever came out of Kansas City." Yet, not all of Rufus's experiences have been happy. He has suffered serious setbacks in the last two years. However, Rufus retains his bravado. "Shit man, I've been in trouble before. They can't keep me off the street. That's my street! I'll make it like I always do!"

Developmental Experiences

Rufus was born in Houston, the eldest son of a maintenance engineer who is now fifty-five years old. Rufus has a brother, age thirty-two, and a sister, age twenty-six. Though the father was the primary family provider, Rufus indicates that both parents worked during his developmental years.

Rufus says his father was "a good man, a hard worker who took good care of his family. We all ate well, always had a roof over our heads, and slept well. My father was with Patton with the Redball Express during World War II. My mother moved to Kansas City while he was in the service to be near her parents. I was just a little baby then.

"After the war my father couldn't get a job in Kansas City. He always resented the fact we weren't back in Houston, but he took whatever jobs he could get. He went to night school on the GI Bill, but was never able to finish. Finally, he got this job as a maintenance engineer and has been with this company twenty-five years. He always had to get out and scrape to make a living for us kids."

Rufus was very close to his father. "I loved him, man. He was always tryin' to look out for us kids. He taught me and my brother how to defend ourselves and take no shit off anyone! He always told me to look after my brother. I tried, but it didn't work too well, I guess, 'cause he is in the joint now. My father said it didn't make any difference whether we won or lost a fight; he said if you had to lose, look good losing. When I was just a little kid, my father would set me up on his knee and we would talk 'man to man.' I remember him saying 'Big Son' this and 'Big Son' that. He treated me like I was important." Rufus learned how to manipulate his father: "My father would drink at home. If I wanted something, I would ask him when he had been drinking. I'd get it for sure!"

His father spent considerable time with the children. "We went fishing quite a bit, and he would play ball at nights with my brother and I. Sometimes he and I would just go for a walk. We were very close. I respected him.

"He wasn't afraid to discipline me. When I was little, he would make me stay in the house if I did something wrong, or whip my butt with his hands. When I got older he would hit me in the chest. The worst thing he ever did to me was when I was about eleven. He caught me smokin'. He gave me a cigar and made me smoke it. Man, I have never been so sick in my life. I never smoked again till I was twenty-three years old."

When asked what he would change about his father, Rufus said, "Nothin'! I would just want him to be wealthy so he would be able to do what he wanted and live easier."

Rufus describes his mother as "beautiful people." "She is a very affectionate, outgoing person, understanding and strong. My mother is a very rational woman; she made us sort things out in our heads. She went to college for two years, but dropped out when I was born. She is fifty-five now. She worked as a clerk in a department store when I was ten to fifteen years old. My father didn't like for her to have to work; he said if we had stayed in Houston, she wouldn't have had to work. I wanted to be a doctor; my father told me that if we had stayed in Texas maybe I could have been one."

Rufus says his mother was very protective of her children. "Hell, she'd get out and fuss and cuss the neighbor women if someone was bothering us. We'd get in a fight with some other kids, and my father would have to tell my mother, 'Let them fight. My boys will do OK. There is nothin' sissy about my boys!'"

His mother was an awesome disciplinarian. "Shit, she would spank us harder than my father! I would rather my father spank me any time than my mother. As I got older, though, the more she would whip me, the less I would cry."

Rufus says he would do nothing to change his mother. "I'd just want to make her happy every day of her life." He indicates that while he loves both parents, he was closer to his mother. "I can talk about things with her. She's con-proof!"

Rufus describes his younger brother with affection, but said he is a hothead. "He always lived in the shadow of me. For example, I was a good athlete and he was jealous of me. He got into a fight with an older dude; he wouldn't ask me for help. The dude beat the hell out of my brother. My brother told me to stay out of it so I did. He did nine flat years for two murder raps. But doin' time in prison made him worse. He has withdrawn from people — from everyone except my mother."

Although Rufus cares for his younger sister, they were not close. "There was too much age difference between us. She is a nice gal, quiet and reserved. She is married and left home; she lives in California with her husband."

One other "family member" plays a significant role in Rufus's life. "That's my Uncle James. He lives in Texas, has a big painting company. He can do or buy anything he wants. He's done well. I always wanted to be wealthy like my Uncle James."

While his family had the necessities, they were not well off financially. "We were poor, man. My father worked his ass off, and we were still poor. I didn't want to have to live like that, always scrapin' along and just gettin' by. I wanted to have things, have money like my Uncle James, and have nice things, big cars, live good, and dress nice; and I did. The most important lesson I learned as a kid was that you can do most anything if you've got enough money behind you."

Rufus made average grades in school. "I didn't like studyin' much, but my mother and father pushed me hard. They wanted me to excel! I didn't excel too much in the classes, but I did as an athlete. Man, I was good in baseball, basketball, and football! My father was really proud of me when I made the all-star baseball team as a kid. I was a good athlete till I was sixteen; I got kicked off the football team for drinking. I wasn't really drinkin', I was with guys who were, though. My father was disappointed. I started gettin' disinterested in school and just quit during the eleventh grade."

Even before he dropped out of school, Rufus began his history of altercations with the law. "I was arrested for car theft when I was fifteen; my people came and got me out of the detention home. The police picked me up again when I was sixteen, for joy-ridin' in some guy's car. My mother was upset as hell when she came to get me. She gave me a tongue-lashing! The whole thing with the law turned me against work; I couldn't find a job because of my record.

"I was arrested for second-degree burglary when I was seventeen. They sent me to the reform school. I spent most of the time in the hole for fighting; they tried to break me, but they couldn't. I ended up in the penitentiary. People didn't give me any shit, 'cause they knew I would fight and I pasted several dudes too. It meant more time, but I wasn't gonna take no shit off no one! I finished high school in the penitentiary and got my diploma. That made my mother proud.

"I paid my dues with the atrocities the whites done against me. I know violence, and I know violence begets violence. I am talking about things like having to go to the joint when I was just a kid. They beat me, but they couldn't *beat* me because I wouldn't knuckle under to them! I know that if my parents had had some money, I wouldn't have gone to the joint for all those years. The dudes who actually perpetrated the burglaries had money; they didn't have to go to the joint, but a poor kid like me with no bucks behind him had to go. I vowed when I was there that I would have the money I needed one way or another!

"I came back when I was nineteen. I tried to get work, but I couldn't find any because I had a record. Then the police picked me up on two armed robbery charges; I had to stay in jail six months because I couldn't make bond. All of my people's money was tied up with the lawyer, but shit, I took their lie detector test and I beat them!"

At age nineteen, Rufus met the woman who became his first wife. "She was just a nice kid when I went to the joint, but when I came back she was a woman, a helluva woman! I was tryin' to catch her, but shit, man, she caught me! She is a very intelligent woman. She is a strong and amorative woman. We had a son. Her parents didn't want her to marry me at all, because I was doing a little hustling in those days. Her father completed college and is a professional man."

Rufus married Rosella when he was twenty-one. After his marriage, Rufus found employment. "I worked as a maintenance man in a hospital. Then I worked as an apprentice pressman for a while. Then I worked in construction. I wasn't making any real money; They were union jobs and you have to be there ten to fifteen years before you make any real money. I didn't want to wait ten years, so when I was about twenty-six I just kind of drifted into pimping. I had a couple of hustling broads working for me on the side since I was about twenty-two. My lady didn't like it, but they made money for us. Finally I just decided to go into it all the way."

It did not take Rufus long to discover he had special talent. "I was a very successful pimp, very successful! I know how to 'stir' a woman and turn her on to me. Shit, within a year I had two Cadillacs, fine clothes — all tailor-made — custom jewelry, and more money than I knew what to do with. Within two years, I had five good-looking whores out working for me every night. Kansas City pimps are strong dudes, and I was the *best* in Kansas City! It takes initiative, man. I wanted money and the things it could provide and I got it! My wife didn't like it. Her parents didn't like it either, but hell, man, I was doing my thing and doing it *good!*

"A lot of people think pimping is a physical thing, but it's not. It's a mental thing. You put a mental thing on a broad that makes her dig you and makes her want to do anything you want. You may think the pimp chooses his whores; that's only partly right. It's the broad who chooses who she will work for. The pimp's job is to put himself into a position where the broad he is tryin' to get in his stable wants to choose him.

"I built my thing around peace and harmony with my broads. There was no nagging or bitching. Occasionally I'd have to knock one of them down 'cause she was getting out of line, but that didn't happen too often. Basically, I treated them all good and all equal. I took good care of their needs, and they literally worked their asses off for me.

"Sometimes I'd give my working broads some coke to snort after they had taken care of business. Sometimes we would just all pile in bed and have a coke party after work. The girls would get all giggly and high. I never would let a working broad use a needle; you let a whore get to using the needle and, sure as hell, she'll start 'chipping' on you. You would have to kick her ass out on the street. I did that a couple of times. It always upset the other broads, but it has to be done. That's why coke is about all I would let them have; it's not habit-forming and it keeps their drive up for work."

Rufus had another advantage over some pimps. "I had a good 'bottom woman,' my main woman. She was five years older than me. She was a seasoned whore, who was a killer herself. She taught me the business, how to be an exquisite pimp, and how to control females. She would keep the other broads in line; as long as I kept her in line, she kept the others in line. We were a good team. She bought all the clothes for my broads and took good care of them, and I took good care of her. In fact, I divorced my first wife and married my bottom woman, to tighten her up to me. It was strictly a business thing. I gave her one of the Cadillacs, too. Of course, it was easier for her to work across state lines, being married and all. Shit, after that she pushed my working broads! We did well.

"My bottom woman and I were always on the lookout for better broads to upgrade our stable. We'd spot a broad in some town we wanted with us, and I'd get her, turn her on to me, even if I had to take her away from another pimp.

That created problems occasionally, but if the other pimp raised too much hell, I'd beat the shit out of him. I got shot once doing that.

"I did well pimping for about six or seven years. I had a new El Dorado Cadillac every year, I had all the money I could spend. Shit, I lived like a king!" But Rufus's occupation was not all sweetness and light: "Shit, man, it is dangerous. A pimp lives in such luxury, man, that everyone envies him. People want to kill you, take your women, shit like that. You have to be flamboyant and flashy to keep your broads; they expect their man to look good for them. The hell of it is, man, all that flashy shit makes ghetto dudes want to do you in! I was shot twice because of the envy shit. The police are always after your ass; I must have been arrested a hundred times. Of course, you can't roll into a town dressed fit to kill with a Cadillac full of good-looking broads and not attract attention. Again, you don't sleep good nights because you're always afraid some motherfucker will bust your door down and try to kill you. After we were around a town a while, people wouldn't mess with us much; they were afraid of me and my bottom woman. I would beat the shit out of dudes who crossed me, and she would simply shoot them. She shot one man three times in Nebraska; he shot me first, and she filled him full of holes. Word like that gets around. Nobody wants to mess with a killer broad."

Despite these occupational hazards Rufus continued pimping for several years. "Shit, man, it was good despite all of that. That stuff was just part of that business and there was no way I could avoid it.

"We must have moved, aw, shit, over a hundred times. We'd go with the conventions, where there would be big crowds of dudes on the make. Then my bottom woman got hit with a boostin' (shoplifting) and assault charge in Denver. Besides that, the police started trying' to frame me, like I am sendin' my bottom lady across state lines and all of that shit. I was heavy into 'boy' and 'girl' then and couldn't concentrate on my business. The whole thing started to cave in.

"They busted my bottom woman and put $25,000 bond on her. My lawyer said they had a case against her and were determined to put her away. I told my bottom woman about it, and she said she wanted to run as long as she could, so we jumped bond and took off. We ran all over the country for two years. I got picked up in California for having needle marks and paraphernalia; then I was picked up in New York on a robbery charge. I guess I have done three to four years in jails and the penitentiary all told. Anyway, after two years she was picked up on a boostin' charge in Philadelphia. They found out about her jumpin' bond in Colorado. Now she's doing time for murder in another state.

"I tried to make it alone, but I wasn't successful after I lost my bottom woman. Finally, I just came on back to Kansas City to my wife. She always loved me and was glad to have me home again. I found out how lucky I am. I discovered I needed peace of mind, being able to live without havin' to always look over my shoulder. My wife was still in love with me, despite the broads.

"I have been home with my wife for over a year now, and it's the best thing that ever happened to me. It is a good feelin' to know that you are loved despite large faults. Sometimes I tell her I ain't good enough for her, and she cries. She says she was born for me; it makes me feel good. I love bein' with my woman. I want things to be good for her, I don't want nothin' too strenuous for her. She's the greatest! I am happy I got her, man!"

Rufus found when he returned that his seventeen-year-old son was incarcerated for armed robbery. "I guess he did it. He ultimately got two five-year sentences running concurrently. It took every dime I had for his lawyer. Shit, I am broke now, but if I hadn't gotten him a good lawyer, he would have gotten twenty years! I even lost my Cadillac. It worries me what the joint will do to his head, do to him mentally. Making money as a pimp isn't fast enough for him — Shit, he wants quick stuff like from robberies and all. He just wanted nice things, I guess. I guess all blacks go through that kind of thing, like, 'I want the things other people have even if I have to take them!'"

Rufus stated with obvious pride that his son was "a chip off the old block." "He likes sports and likes to dress well. He is a kind of an introvert, he doesn't like to talk and rap like I do. He's cool, but he is kind of mean; I am not mean. He is not street-wise like I am. I wanted him to be an athlete, but he wanted to be like me, I guess. He gets into violence. I don't like violence. It creates too much disturbance and puts the Man on your ass.

"When I did that kind of thing, I was smooth. They couldn't pin anything heavy on me except that first burglary charge, and I was just a green-ass kid. When he does that kind of thing, he does it rough, and got caught. He is in school in the joint and is doin' all right, I guess. We are closer now than before. I love the boy because he is cool and relaxed all the time; he dresses sharp like me. He loves his father and digs him as a man. I would really like to stop him from robbin' before he hurts someone or someone hurts him."

His financial situation since he left home has sharply varied. "When we were first married, it was all financial; first I couldn't get a job, but then when I got one it didn't pay much. When I was pimpin', I had more money than I could even spend. Since I came back to my wife, it is all financial problems again. Here I am thirty-five and I am scratching out a living. I have been doin' some construction work, but hell, you get laid off in bad weather and use up all the money you saved in the summer. It's no way to live."

Despite the problems with their son, Rufus feels his family now is very stable and very affectionate. "Overall things aren't as bad as they always seem. I've had my bad luck, but I got a whole lot of things to be happy for. I am in good health and I've got a woman who loves me, man, in spite of my faults. I don't have to worry about people busting in my house and tryin' to kill me or my wife now. I guess you could say I am a rich man in a lot of ways."

Rufus states he has two goals in life: (1) to own his own business, "like a clothing store. I like to dress, and I like to see everyone dressed and have the best of everything at prices people could afford," and (2) to "just live in peace. I am tired of hassles, man. I would just like to live in peace and be in a position where I could look after my family and help my friends. One thing I learned is not to put my family in danger. I want to protect my family and keep them from all harm."

Rufus has no political interests, though he describes himself as a liberal. "I'd make room in the world for everyone, man."

He states that he would like his epitaph to read, "Here is a man who was well-respected and helped his fellow man."

Interpretive Integration

Eight themes define the framework for the evolution of Rufus's life style:

- Relative poverty during childhood — but with sufficient resources to meet basic survival needs
- Open and enduring expressions of affection and acceptance by both parents
- A father who encouraged Rufus to be a fighter, and a college-trained mother who inculcated expectations that Rufus excel and achieve
- No great emphasis, apparently, on religious or ethical training
- Early recognition of the importance of money and what it could provide in the ghetto culture
- A "rich" uncle who became a symbol to Rufus of how he wanted to live
- Failure of Rufus's efforts to achieve in high school athletics
- Initial failure as an adolescent thief, but an education in the rules of how to beat "John Law" in the reformatory and prison

Reared in this type of environment, Rufus developed an adult life style characterized by the following:

- A masculine self-image emphasizing fearlessness and willingness to fight for goals
- Lack of regard for social rules and a poorly developed sense of responsibility to other people
- A high level of self-confidence and self-assurance in a man who is not easily discouraged
- Relative absence of long-range goals and preoccupation with short-range opportunities
- Limited marketable occupational skills in a man nonetheless determined to be on top and have money
- Anger at a world which would allow a poor boy to go to prison while equally guilty persons with money do not, and a vow that he would find ways to have money but not be caught

• A driving need to excel, to be noticed and attended to by others, recreating the status he enjoyed with his parents

Rufus is a charming, manipulative man who desires money and the things and status it can provide. He has limited skills that are marketable in lawful work. It is not surprising then that this sensuous and energetic man chose a career as a pimp. When asked what kind of animal he might be if he had the choice, Rufus stated, "Shit, I'd be a lion, the King of the Jungle! I'd be a male lion. He's a lazy dude. The females do all the work. Hell, that's what I've been, man!" When asked what kind of car he might be, Rufus stated without hesitation, "I'd be a Rolls-Royce, 'cause they are the ultimate in luxury!"

Although Rufus may not have marketable work skills, he knows how to survive. Apparently, he learned his lessons well in the penitentiary, because he has only done occasional jail time since he was a youth. Rufus has learned not to push the law enforcement system in a direct fashion, because, as he says, "It puts the Man on your ass!" Rufus has learned another important rule of survival, namely, never to put himself out front where he would have to take the fall. Thus, although Rufus admits he was arrested on numerous occasions, it was his "hustling broads" and "bottom woman" who were charged.

During the last two years Rufus has suffered reversals. He lost his "bottom woman," and has been unable to make it as a pimp on his own. Although he expended all his financial reserves, he was unable to prevent his son from going to the penitentiary. He is unemployed and must rely upon his wife for financial support. Also, he has lost his "cool status ride" — his Cadillac. In a ghetto street culture such reversals signal considerable status loss.

There are indications that Rufus may have become involved in difficulties with important figures in the drug community. Normally, Rufus is a restless, energetic, and action-oriented "street man." However, for the last six months he has been holed up in his house. He has made no efforts to seek employment, has rarely gone out, and has all but vanished from the street. Friends and acquaintances have been keeping their distance, apparently providing him little, if any, encouragement or support. Rufus has stayed home and banked upon his "brothers" to keep him informed of events and happenings on the street. When Rufus made his first cautious trip back on the street, he did so only because they told him it was safe.

Rufus appears to be waiting it out in the hope that the situation will pass and he can return to his customary life without threat of harm. He toys with the idea of attempting to again become "the best pimp that ever came out of Kansas City." At the same time, he recognizes that the money, the Cadillac, and the jewelry did not make him happy. Perhaps even more important, Rufus has been shot twice in the last few years — he may have become cognizant of his own mortality.

FORMAL PSYCHOLOGICAL ASSESSMENT

Dimensional Test Findings

Intelligence Tests

Tests show that Rufus functions in the Normal range of intelligence, a fact which may help account for his failure to do exceptionally well in school and meet his parent's expectations that he excel there. It may also account for his ability to succeed on the street only when he has the support of a brighter, more capable person such as his "bottom woman."

MMPI

Rufus's MMPI profile presents an almost classic picture of a hypomanic pattern of adjustment. That is, the MMPI depicts Rufus as hyperactive, aggressive, and manipulative (figure 11.1).

Despite some elevation of the F Scale, the relatively low Validity Scale scores indicate the test is valid and that, by and large, Rufus attempted to answer questions honestly. However, he is not reflective or introspective; and he has little self-insight. Though he has lived much of his life in dangerous circumstances, he will actively deny emotional distress.

In general, the MMPI pattern is that of a colorful, expressive, and ebullient man — alert, restless, and ambitious. Rufus lives in a world of constant action. His activity serves essentially to minimize and hold in check feelings of depression, self-doubt, and worry; it is a flight from depression. This is a stubborn and willful man who ordinarily seems peaceful but flares up and becomes belligerent if crossed in trying to get what he wants.

Rufus is also somewhat disorganized and distractible; he lives in a narrow time-life perspective bounded by preoccupation with immediate needs and events. Rufus is ambitious, but he has difficulty in completing tasks because of his impatience and distractibility; he has poor control and is prone to act without deliberation. And he sometimes becomes so expansive — even grandiose — that he takes on more activities than he can complete.

Rufus is, however, a shrewd judge of others. He is socially perceptive and persuasive; he communicates ideas clearly and effectively and is able to win others to his point of view. He is an effective manipulator who shows no hesitance in using charm, guile, deceit, or even physical force to achieve his goals. Rufus would be noticed in any crowd; however, while he can be charming and engaging, few people know him well — there is only a limited number of people to whom he will make any personal commitment.

Rufus views the world as a hostile place. To him others are selfish and preoccupied with personal gain; they will take quick advantage if he shows the slightest hesitance or weakness. The world to him is composed of two types:

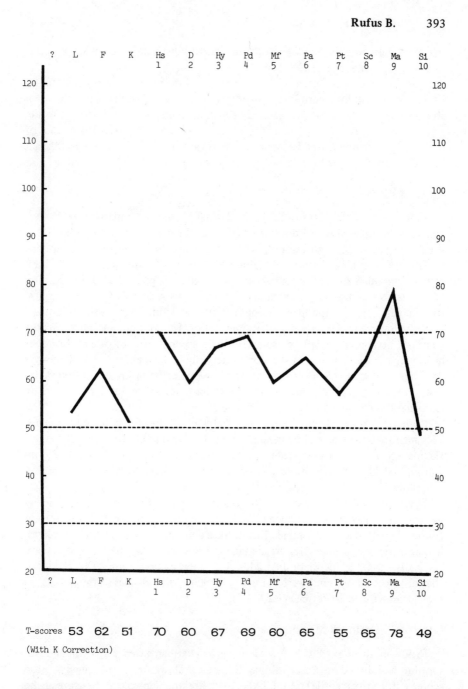

?	L	F	K	Hs 1	D 2	Hy 3	Pd 4	Mf 5	Pa 6	Pt 7	Sc 8	Ma 9	Si 10
T-scores 53	62	51		70	60	67	69	60	65	55	65	78	49

(With K Correction)

FIGURE 11.1.   MMPI Profile: Rufus B. *Reproduced from the Minnesota Multiphasic Personality Inventory Profile and Case Summary form, by permission. Copyright 1948 by the Psychological Corporation, New York, N.Y. All rights reserved.*

the exploiters and the exploited. Rufus will not hesitate to do what is necessary to avoid being one of the latter.

Although action is Rufus's primary method of maintaining personal stability, he has an alternative method for handling tension. He is sensuous, and when stresses become too great, he withdraws into a dependent role: He will hole up, let his wife — or some other woman — nurture and care for him, perform a lot of sex, and get high on drugs. He continues these activities until he feels good again — or until his anxieties become so intense that he is forced back into action.

Sixteen PF

Table 11.1 reveals Rufus to be a charming but manipulative, exploitive, and ruthless man who will do whatever is expedient to achieve his goals. He is tough, resilient, and self-assured, with little need for approval from others.

The most striking feature of Rufus's Sixteen PF Profile is his lack of inhibition. This man lives in a "now" world; he has no plan for his life. Rather, he focuses on immediate, momentary events. Rufus is socially alert and aggressive; he can quickly capitalize on opportunities and turn them to his advantage.

Rufus does not feel a sense of responsibility. He does not moralize. On the contrary, he is a narcissistic person with little commitment to others. Nor does he experience guilt, apprehension, or anxiety about his behavior; he will always do what he thinks will meet his immediate needs or be in his own interest. He does not accept social conventions. Laws have relevance for him only if he feels that there is some danger of being caught.

Rufus is concerned only about what helps him achieve his immediate goals. This man maintains a cool demeanor under stress and adjusts quickly to change. He may seek out danger because of the excitement and tests of courage involved, and he may feel more completely alive in these situations than at any other time.

There are two major flaws in Rufus's functioning. First, he has a tendency to leap into action before giving sufficient consideration to consequences or considering alternatives. Second, Rufus takes a piecemeal approach to problems; he has difficulty in planning, organizing, and implementing methods to achieve his goals, and his distractibility adds a further complication. The boldness, charm, street savvy, and verbal fluency which Rufus displays compensate to some degree for these deficiencies.

Other Dimensional Measures

Rufus obtained extremely low scores on Zuckerman's General, Thrill and Adventure, and Boredom Susceptibility Subscales. However, he obtained average scores (fiftieth percentile) on the Experience-Seeking Subscale and a score at the sixty-ninth percentile on the Disinhibition Scale. Taken together, these scores are not remarkable, but the relatively high Disinhibition score may reflect Rufus's unconventional style, active sexual life, and narcissistic life orientation.

The mean scores obtained by Rufus on the Novelty Experiencing Scales are, by and large, comparable to those obtained by airmen and college males. None of his scores was more than one standard deviation from the mean of either group. These findings suggest that Rufus is not remarkably different from the two comparison groups on these dimensions.

Rufus earned a score of 38 on Garlington and Shimota's (1964) Change Seeker Index. In comparison with mean scores obtained by college males (49.06; $N = 187$) and army males (43.30; $N = 60$), Rufus exhibits lower needs for sensory input and change.

Rufus obtained scores of 12, 15, and 5 on the Eysenck Personality Inventory Extroversion, Neuroticism, and Lie Scales. These correspond to percentile levels of sixty-eight, eighty-seven, and eighty-nine, respectively, when compared with industrial norms. The high Lie Scores suggest that these results are invalid and Rufus was dissimulating. However, he earned a standard score of 7.3 on the Extroversion Index of the Sixteen PF, a result which, independent of the Eysenck Inventory, suggests Rufus is highly extroverted.

Integration

The picture of Rufus that emerges on dimensional tests is consistent with the life style described above under "Evolution of Life Style" and, by and large, substantiates other findings. The MMPI and Cattell Sixteen PF document why Rufus had so little difficulty controlling prostitutes. This is a strong, socially aggressive, and bold man with obvious charm. His narcissism, poise, and willingness to resort to physical violence would undoubtedly make Rufus attractive to certain kinds of women.

The dimensional measures also suggest why Rufus failed in his efforts to continue as a pimp after he lost his "main woman." Rufus has difficulties with managerial functions, i.e., the development and organization of effort and the implementation of plans. Also, his distractibility, lack of self-discipline, and willingness to leap into action without deliberation limit his managerial effectiveness. Thus, some of the same personal characteristics which have made him attractive to women have handicapped him in his efforts to succeed in his chosen occupation.

Findings From Morphogenic Measures

Overview

Throughout the morphogenic data, Rufus shows a few persistent characteristics. Most obvious is his tendency to find his own identity only through the reactions he provokes from other people. Rufus's self-concept is apparently not stable enough to stand up on its own. Instead, he gains his sense of selfhood by

TABLE 11.1. Cattell 16F Profile: Rufus B.

Standard Score	Low Score Description	Standard Ten Score (Sten) 1 2 3 4 5 6 7 8 9 10	High Score Description
6	Reserved, detached, critical, cool, aloof, stiff, precise, objective	A (5)	Outgoing, warm-hearted, easygoing, trustful, good-natured, participating
3	Less intelligent, concretistic thinking, less well-organized, poor judgment	B (3)	More intelligent, abstract-thinking, bright, insightful, fast-learning, better judgment
5	Affected by feelings, emotionally less stable, worrying, easily upset, changeable	C (5)	Emotionally stable, mature, unruffled, faces reality, calm (higher ego strength)
6	Humble, mild, easily led, docile, accommodating, submissive, conforming	E (6)	Assertive, aggressive, stubborn, headstrong, competitive, dominant, rebellious
6	Sober, taciturn, serious, introspective, reflective, slow, cautious	F (6)	Happy-go-lucky, enthusiastic, talkative, cheerful, frank, quick, alert
3	Expedient, disregards rules, social conventions and obligations to people (weaker superego strength)	G (3)	Conscientious, persistent, moralistic, persevering, well-disciplined (stronger superego strength)
10	Shy, timid, withdrawn, threat-sensitive	H (10)	Venturesome, uninhibited, socially bold, active, impulsive
4	Tough-minded, self-reliant, cynical, realistic	I (4)	Tender-minded, sensitive, dependent, seeking help and sympathy
6	Trusting, accepting conditions, understanding, tolerant, permissive	L (6)	Suspicious, hard to fool, dogmatic

Factor	Low pole			High pole
L	Practical, "down-to-earth" concerns, guided by objective reality	4		Imaginative, bohemian, absent-minded, unconventional, easily seduced from practical judgment
M	Forthright, unpretentious, genuine, spontaneous, natural, artless, socially clumsy	6		Astute, polished, socially aware, shrewd, smart, "cuts corners"
N	Self-assured, placid, secure, self-confident, complacent, serene	6		Apprehensive, self-reproaching, insecure, worrying, troubled, guilt-prone
O	Conservative, respectful of established traditional ideas	7		Experimenting, liberal, free-thinking, non-moralistic, experiments with problem-solutions
Q_1	Group-dependent, depends on social approval, a "joiner" and sound follower	4		Self-sufficient, resourceful, prefers to make own decisions
Q_2	Undisciplined self-conflict, lax, follows own urges, careless of social rules	5		Controlled, exacting willpower, socially precise, compulsive, persistent, foresighted
Q_3	Relaxed, tranquil, torpid, unfrustrated, composed, low ergic tension	5		Tense, frustrated, driven, overwrought, high ergic tension

Average

putting up an impressive front. This serves two purposes: First, it conceals the real Rufus. Second, the admiration and attention it draws gives him the personal identity he otherwise lacks. In the theoretical language of Carl Jung, Rufus presents a classic case of *inflation of the persona:* overdevelopment of a social mask at the expense of inner differentiation.

Beneath the happy and competent surface appearance, Rufus knows that his actions are not always exemplary. And he is becoming tired of fighting feelings of being worthless and rejected, and weary of forever trying to be someone he is not. Besides, doubts about his ability to maintain appearances are beginning to trouble him.

The Q-Sort data show the favorable picture of himself that Rufus has been trying to sustain. Hints of his inability to evaluate himself except in relation to others appear, as does the suggestion that he feels a need to be more in touch with his inner self. It seems that he uses cocaine to buttress his esteem and generate feelings that he can believe are truly his own.

The Rep Test data were particularly revealing because this test enabled Rufus to talk about himself indirectly by describing his impressions of other people. Here he identified with his own worst self and indicated his dissatisfaction with this identification. Rufus showed that he does not entirely enjoy being a hustler, a liar, and a wrongdoer. Indeed, he dislikes the self he finds when he looks behind his own facade. The problem is that without constant support from others it is the only self he has.

Q-Sorts

Standard Items

Rufus's descriptions of his usual self are consistent, both within testing sessions (median $r = .660$) and between them (median $r = .675$). His other sortings are moderately consistent, varying little from an overall median of $r = .576$. At first glance these values suggest that he was following instructions conscientiously. Subsequent analyses showed that this statement is not entirely accurate.

All of Rufus's descriptive sortings of the standard items tend to correlate positively with each other. For example, the median correlation between his description of his usual self and that of his ideal self is .639. The median correlations between his descriptions of the typical cocaine user, on the one hand, and those of his usual and ideal selves, on the other, are .631 and .645, respectively. These findings are subject to at least two interpretations: One possibility is that Rufus is remarkably well integrated; The second is that he was not so much following testing instructions as presenting a single picture of himself that may conceal more than it discloses. Qualitative analyses suggest that the latter possibility is correct.

Factor analysis.   From all fifteen of Rufus's descriptive sortings of the standard Q-Sort items only one factor emerged. Consequently, it is safe to conclude that, with minor variations, Rufus placed the items into the same over-all configuration, regardless of instructions, at all assessment sessions.

Rufus's self-presentation is hardly credible: According to him he is: happy, pleasant, strong, deep, humble, wise, and easygoing. Traits he rejects are: crying, being sad, violent, explosive, hostile, cruel, smug, or foolish. He also described himself as a person who is not often ignored or snubbed. Possibly, Rufus really believes himself to be like this. More reasonable, however, is the proposition that he presented himself to the investigators in a carefully guarded way. Such a conclusion should come as no surprise; his whole life is built around putting up a good front.

Another possibility is that while Rufus is competent in psyching out others he is so unpracticed in self-examination that he is unable to respond accurately to a procedure like the Q-Sort. Perhaps he in fact did the best he could on these testings, but, because he does not know his inner life, his best is not satisfactory. Evidence from the Rep Test (cited below) is consistent with this possibility. Nevertheless, the likelihood that Rufus consciously attempted self-concealment on the Q-Sortings cannot be discounted, for his self-revelation on the more indirect Rep Test could have been unintentional.

Individualized Items

In general, the picture is the same here as it was for the standard Q-Sort items. Nearly all reliabilities are at least moderately high. (There are no data for Rufus as he is during an amphetamine high because he claimed to be unfamiliar with the effects of amphetamine.)

Only one shift in reliability values occurred, but it had profound effects on subsequent analyses: Rufus's description of his bad self changed completely at the time of the second reassessment session. As is shown later, the change was such that Rufus became even less revealing of his true feelings.

For the most part, correlations among descriptions that Rufus provided with his own individualized items are positive and fairly high, showing also a general trend to increase from one assessment period to the next. Thus, for example, the median correlation between Rufus's descriptions of his usual self and those of his ideal self increased from .505 to .790 and then to .801. When describing himself as he is when he wants cocaine and as he is during a cocaine high, the correlation between sortings was at first .385; at the first reassessment this value increased to .657, and by the second reassessment it was .828 (a remarkably high value). The implication is clear: Rufus's sortings became more homogeneous as time went by; he hid his real self more and more completely.

The median correlation between his description of his usual self and what he thinks most nonusers of drugs are like also went from .480 to .691 and then to .721. This finding is hard to take at face value, because a high correlation between these descriptive sortings is inconsistent with Rufus's life style; he tries to be as unique and as different from others as possible.

Finally, there was a remarkable shift in the correlation between Rufus's

TABLE 11.1. Individualized Q-Sort Items: Rufus B.

Achievement
Positive
1. Getting ahead
2. Success
Negative
3. Playing on a person for personal gain
4. Cheating to win

Affect
Positive
5. Laughter
*6. Happiness
Negative
*7. Sad
8. Crying

Anxiety
Positive
*9. Mellow
10. Relaxed
Negative
11. Irrational
*28. Impulsive

Chastity
Positive
13. Not doing adultery
*14. Faithful to your wife
Negative
15. Not fertile
16. Sexless

Dependence
Positive
17. Need someone
18. Have to have someone
Negative
19. Relying on somebody else
20. "Manless"

Dominance
Positive
*21. Strong
22. Fearless
Negative
23. Weak
24. Punk

Excitement
Positive
25. Thrilled
26. Joyous
Negative
27. Anxious
*28. Impulsive

Humility
Positive
29. Doesn't have to put on a floor show
30. Self-assured
Negative
*31. Ignored
32. Put down

Independence
Positive
33. Independent
34. Stand on your own two feet
Negative
35. Egotist
36. Snob

Knowledge
Positive
37. Intelligent
38. Hip
Negative
39. Dummy
40. Stupid

Restraint
Positive
41. Having a level head
42. Beling relaxed, calm
Negative
*43. Slow
44. Late freight

Self-satisfaction (Stasis)
Positive
45. Feel proud
46. Someone who digs what he's doing
Negative
47. Bum
48. Good-for-nothing

Sexuality
Positive
49. Pretty
50. Freak
Negative
51. Garbage can
52. Vulture

Interpersonal Relations
Positive
53. Good
*54. Friendly
Negative
55. Bully
56. Overbearing

Social Recognition
Positive
57. Popular
58. Getting over
Negative
59. Jive dude
60. A fool

Note: Items marked with an asterisk (*) are not significantly altered from their original, standard wording.

400

descriptions of his bad self and those of his usual and ideal selves. As is expected in normal cases, the correlations were negative at the first assessment and first reassessment periods (median $r = -.488$ and $-.660$). At the second reassessment, however, they shifted to the median value of .752, reflecting a complete reversal of the relationship. Other data show that the change took place in the bad-self sorting, which suddenly became like the usual self and the ideal self. If one were to take Rufus at his word, one would be forced to believe that even his bad self became good with time!

Factor analysis. When applied to the twenty-seven sortings Rufus provided with the individualized Q-Sort items, the factor-analytic procedure yields three factors, one quite strong, the other two rather weak. The first factor shows progressively heavier loadings from one assessment session to the next; it therefore represents the uniform self-presentation that Rufus was developing throughout the research. The second factor is identified only with the description of his bad self provided by Rufus in the first assessment session. The loading of this description is negative, so the factor seems to represent a kind of backhanded presentation of a set of ideals or moral values. Only one descriptive sorting loads heavily on the third factor. It is Rufus's description, provided at the first assessment session, of himself as he is during a cocaine high.

Factor I — self-presentation — portrays Rufus as: a person who is getting ahead, a success, someone who is popular and "getting over," and a hip, intelligent person. The traits he rejected as part of his self-presentation were: being sexually unattractive (a vulture, a garbage can), being a dummy or being stupid, and being a fool or "jive dude" — someone who is socially recognized, but in a negative or undesirable way. Again, Rufus described himself in entirely desirable terms.

Factor II is more difficult to describe. Here Rufus seemed to be expressing dissatisfaction with people he classifies as bums, snobs, good-for-nothings, and egotists. Such people display a host of undesirable traits: Among other things, they are irrational, uncool, weak, punk; they are overbearing bullies who are dummies and are stupid. At the other end of this scale, Rufus seems to admire people who can laugh and are happy, are self-assured, and don't have to put on a floor show. These people are mellow, relaxed, faithful to their wives, good, and friendly.

Apparently, Rufus feels many good things while under the influence of cocaine (Factor III). He is strong and fearless, thrilled and joyous, good, friendly, and self-assured. Of special interest is his inclusion in this factor of the item "doesn't have to put on a floor show." Since Rufus's life *is* a floor show, it may be that cocaine gives him some relief from the need to impress others. Items describing the negative end of this factor confirm this suggestion, for Rufus says that when he is taking cocaine he is not a bully or overbearing, nor does he worry about being a fool or "jive dude."

A word is in order about Rufus's colorful language in his individualized items. In part, Rufus's vocabulary is merely the jargon of the culture in which he lives; in part, however, it is also a device for gaining attention and for obscuring, rather than clarifying, meanings. These uses of language serve adaptive purposes. In Rufus's world self-preservation depends on his cleverness and ability to conceal his intentions, while success depends on his ability to attract attention and gain recognition. Colorful language is like colorful clothing or a diamond in an ear; it attracts attention and distracts the observer from what is underneath the surface.

Rep Test

Role Groups

Rufus's descriptions of people in his life range in reliability from those that are remarkably stable to those that display contradictory tendencies over time. Some people whom he described consistently were his wife — who does, in fact, occupy a central position in his life — his mother, his father, and associates connected with cocaine use. These are probably the people he cares about most and knows best.

Rufus's interpersonal constructs are as follows:

Interpersonal Constructs

1. Treats other people good
2. Lovable
3. Lies to gain advantage
4. Rational
5. Plays on people
6. Wrongdoer
7. Hustler
8. Square
9. Hardworker
10. Can take care of themselves
11. Got a lot of class
12. Strong
13. Selfish, uses people
14. Easy to talk to
15. Talks, acts violent

Descriptions low in reliability include: a person who drinks a lot of alcohol, a person you feel sorry for, a person who dislikes you, a person who behaves strangely, and an employer you dislike. A reasonable guess is that Rufus did not describe these people reliably because he has never cared to get to know them. He is not the type to study or try to understand people who do not "turn him on" or to whom he otherwise reacts negatively.

Also included in the low-reliability sortings are Rufus's descriptions of his usual self, his ideal self, and his self while on cocaine. The only description of himself that is reliable is his description of his worst self. Apparently, Rufus only knows what he is like when he is bad.

In general the Rep Test is more revealing of Rufus's self-concept than are the Q-Sorts. Perhaps that is because Rufus is not naturally inclined toward introspection — which is, after all, required for performance of the Q-Sort. He lives his life wholly in relation to other people; this is the source of information that the Rep Test taps directly. And when describing others, Rufus indirectly describes himself.

Factor analysis. Three role groups appear in the outcome of the factor analysis. The first and third groups are the most important, involving as they do all of Rufus's self-descriptions. The second grouping, Factor II, contains the people for whom Rufus seems to feel genuine affection, or who he believes feel genuine affection for him: wife, mother, father, and liked employer. All these are described as square (probably not used in a derogatory way in these instances), hardworking, and rational; they are kind and helpful and treat others well.

Factor I — the major factor — provides as complete a self-picture of Rufus as is available anywhere. Contained in this factor with high positive loadings are: usual self, worst self, people associated with cocaine, and successful person. All of these persons play on people, are hustlers and wrongdoers, can take care of themselves, will lie to take advantage, use people, and are selfish. In contrast to what he said of himself on the Q-Sorts, here Rufus seemed to believe that he is not a good person.

Factor III shows that Rufus has an ideal for himself which does not include lying, hustling, or wrongdoing. In this ideal he is easy to talk to, has a lot of class, and treats other people well but can still take care of himself. Though his ideal self is kind and helpful, it is also strong, does not play on people or lie to take advantage, and is not mean or selfish.

The integration of these findings is straightforward. Rufus feels that the bad behavior which he engages in but disapproves of is essential to his survival. Cocaine makes him temporarily into the person he would like to be, and helps him escape from admitting the possibility that he dislikes himself. The data provide little evidence that anxiety or guilt play any part in this process. Rufus identifies so closely with his own facade that whatever potentially distressing impulses he has are deeply hidden from personal awareness.

Construct Groups

Factor analysis produced four groups from among Rufus's list of constructs. Of these, the first group is the strongest and clearest. It is bipolar, containing at one end most of the bad characteristics Rufus identified with himself — a hustler, a wrongdoer, plays on people, and selfish. The other end contains nearly all the descriptors of the people he likes — treats other people well, kind, rational, hardworking, and square. It therefore seems that the most important dimension for Rufus is the extent to which a person belongs to the group of those similar to him or to the group of those similar to the people he likes, such as his wife and parents. Someone in the first group is merely to be used, and is not taken seriously. Anyone in the second group is to be loved and cared for.

The second factor is also bipolar and reveals a fascinating twist to Rufus's personality. One end of the factor is the trait: having a lot of class. The other has the traits: being mean, talking and acting violent. Rufus is capable of violence, but it is not his preference; he prefers class, and would rather live by his wits. These data suggest that he regards violence not as an occasion for guilt or shame, but as a matter of bad taste.

The last two factors are each associated with a single construct. The third factor underscores the importance to Rufus of being able to take care of oneself. The fourth contains only the construct "strong," the importance of which is obvious.

Setting Survey

In Rufus's case all data values relating to settings are misleading, because his report of his activities given at the second reassessment session was much more sparse than those at previous sessions. For example, at this session he accounted for a total of only nine hours, as compared to twenty-eight hours at the first assessment session and more than sixty hours at the first reassessment session. These data are therefore consistent with the hypotheses, noted elsewhere, that Rufus generally tended to conceal his activities and that this tendency increased, becoming quite strong by the time of the second reassessment session.

Integration

The most dominant themes in Rufus's morphogenic data are the importance of being noticed and the lack of a self-structure capable of existing without constant support and sustenance from input by others. Rufus was sharply conscious that he might reveal his true feelings on the tests. He therefore did what he always does in life: He set up a screen by describing himself in colorful language and in only favorable ways. However Rufus's strategy was not entirely the product of deliberate intent; he has lived for so long in the light cast upon him by others that he may have become incapable of understanding himself in any other terms. This explains in part his intense ambition and need to be on top, admired, respected, feared, or even hated. Without these responses from people, Rufus would have no intrinsic identity. Consequently, achievement of dominance over others is essential to his personal psychological survival.

More so than other forms of data, the morphogenic tests give hints about Rufus's underlying fears. In view of his past and of the attitudes and general values of the middle class, it is easy to see why Rufus would resist attempts to convince him that he is an evil person. His early family experiences gave him the strength to attain personality integration, but in a unique though peculiarly effective way. He learned to build his life around the proposition that he must use his talents to their best advantage and should be as ruthless as necessary to become the most successful person in his profession. Of course, what seems bad to others may not seem so to Rufus. On the surface, he is, at best, indifferent to such considerations and, at worst, proud of his ability to be anti-social, to be violent if the occasion demands it, and to use others for his own self-enhancement.

Underneath, however, he realizes that because his existence depends on his ability and willingness to do bad things better than anyone else, any diminution of his powers constitutes the gravest personal threat. His current setbacks have aroused doubts and fears that he may have lost his ability to live as he has in the past. He wonders whether a calmer, more peaceful life is possible; yet, despite his wonderings he has realized that for him the answer must be no. Rufus is incapable of compromise. If he cannot be the King of Beasts he is vulnerable to feeling worthless — and he will never allow himself to feel that way. Consequently, the only fate one can see for him, in light of the data currently available, is eventual defeat at the hands of a younger man who feels the same about himself and life as does Rufus.

STYLES OF DRUG USE

General Pattern

Rufus's pattern of drug use (table 11.3) is rather narrow. He reported that he has never tried five of the thirteen classes of substances listed and that his drug-usage pattern as an adult has been limited primarily to cocaine, heroin, and marijuana.

The first drug he used was marijuana, at age sixteen. He used it only on an intermittent basis till age thirty-one, when it intensified — he had entered a methadone maintenance program for two years. "When I got on methadone, weed tasted better. I just stayed with it."

At age seventeen, Rufus began experimenting with a variety of drugs, most of which he dropped within a year. "I really never got into alcohol much. I like beer pretty well, but I am not much for hard stuff. Besides, alcohol is a depressant; who the hell wants to be depressed? Most dudes who do much heroin don't drink much; it's a good way to get yourself killed. My thing is boy and girl." Rufus also has tried barbiturates — "I did T-Birds off and on for awhile, but I got strung out and crazy on barbs and said to hell with them"; morphine in tablet form — "I shot them for awhile but didn't like them as well as heroin"; and tranquilizers — "I tried them awhile but they are downers like barbs. I don't want to be down, man. Forget that shit."

From age twenty-one to twenty-five he experimented with snorting cocaine, intravenous heroin use, and for a short period, paregoric use. "Shit, man, I

TABLE 11.3. Genealogy and Pattern of Drug Use and Abuse: Rufus B.

Drug Substances	Age (13–36)	Frequency of Drug Usage	Comments
1. Marijuana	(dashed line, ~14–36)	Regular	I just like weed.
2. Alcohol	(dashed line, ~17–36)	Intermittent	I don't like to drink much now except at parties, maybe.
3. Barbiturates	(dashed arrow, ~16–18)	Intermittent	They depress you, man. Who wants to be depressed?
4. Psychotropics (Librium, Valium, etc.)	(dashed arrow, ~16–18)	Intermittent	I don't use them but I tried them a while.
5. Other opiates Morphine Paregoric	(arrow ~16–18; dashed arrow ~24–25)	Intermittent	I tried the tablet form a while. I shot some when heroin was not available.
6. Cocaine	(dashed line, ~20–26)	Daily	I nod on heroin, but on coke I function together. You would never know I was high.
7. Heroin	(solid line, ~23–26)	Daily	I like the high. It keeps you relaxed.

Drug	Frequency	Comment
8. Polydrug (cocaine/heroin)	Daily	Boy and girl are beautiful together. They make me mellow.
9. Illegal methadone	Never	It's available, but I never tried it.
10. Amphetamine	Never	I don't mess with them. They make you crazy.
11. Hallucinogens (psychedelics)	Never	I never did it. I saw a couple of dudes get their heads screwed up on it.
12. Inhalants	Never	I never tried them at all.
13. Non-prescription, over-the-counter drug	Never	That's not for me.
14. Other		

Legend

——— Denotes regular usage

- - - Denotes intermittent usage

just like the high I got from heroin. You don't hurt at all, you just feel good. It is just a mellow, nice high, particularly if you speedball with girl. Boy keeps you relaxed. You feel good! I did boy off and on until I was twenty-five. Then I got hooked the first time. I have been hooked maybe three to four times since then, but I have always been able to get off. I only had to go into metha-done maintenance once. I was on methadone for a couple of years, but I worked it down till I could get off."

Rufus reported he has never used illegal methadone or amphetamine. "I don't mess with those amphetamines. Everyone I know says they make you crazy. I have never wanted to mess with that crazy shit. I don't want my head screwed around. I want to be on top of my thing." He said he has never tried a hallucinogen (and doesn't intend to — "I have known several guys who got their heads all screwed up on that stuff. I don't want any part of it"), inhalants, or non-prescription, over-the-counter drugs.

At age twenty-five he began regular use of speedball mixtures of cocaine and heroin which has continued to the present. "Boy and girl are beautiful together! They make me mellow. You never get strung out on girl. I have used girl to drive boy out of my system; you have to have a lot, though. I nod off on boy, but with girl I am all together. I like to do both because it makes me feel good."

Rufus indicated that he has taken cocaine and heroin daily (when available) since he was twenty-five years old. On the average, his usage cost approximately $80–100 per day. The longest time he has not used drugs was for thirty days, but he was incarcerated at the time. Rufus indicated he has overdosed only once. "I was doing boy. I started getting dizzy and things started getting dark. I could feel it, so I went out and walked in the rain until I was OK."

Preference Rankings

Table 11.4 presents Rufus's preference rankings for nine drug substances. His rankings are quite consistent and slow clearly his preference for speedballs of heroin and cocaine. They also show clearly his distaste for LSD, barbiturates and amphetamine.

Ratings

Analysis of Rufus's ratings of various drugs yields two factors: The first factor is bipolar; the substances at the positive pole of this factor are mari-juana, cocaine, and speedball. He described all of these as being safe, strong, positive, secure, creative, protected, sheltered, and healthy. Substances at the negative pole are amphetamine, barbiturates, and LSD; these he regards as bad, ugly, unpleasant, wrong, dirty, and worthless. The loading of the concept of drugs in general was only moderate on this factor, indicating that Rufus does not regard these substances as drugs.

TABLE 11.4.   Drug Preference Rankings: Rufus B.

Substance	First Assessment	First Reassessment	Second Reassessment	Mean	Composite Rank
Amphetamine	7	7	8	7.3	8
Barbiturates	8	8	7	7.7	9
Beer	4	4	4	4.0	4
Cocaine	2	2	2	2.0	2
Hard liquor	6	6	6	6.0	6
Heroin	3	3	3	3.0	3
LSD	9	9	9	9.0	9
Marijuana	5	5	5	5.0	5
Speedball	1	1	1	1.0	1

Factor II suggests that the term "drug" for Rufus means heroin, for both heroin and drugs in general have substantial positive loadings on this factor. They are described as good, beautiful, pleasant, right, valuable, and clean. At the negative pole of this factor is hard liquor, which Rufus evidently regards as the opposite of a drug. He describes hard liquor as unsafe, weak, negative, insecure, trite, exposed, hazardous, and sick.

Beer had low loadings on both factors, indicating that Rufus does not think it belongs in the same ball-park with the rest of the substances. His rejection of beer on the rating scales does not contradict his moderately strong preference for it expressed in his rankings; ratings of water might have produced the same result.

Pattern of Use

Social Context

Rufus reported his first use of cocaine was at age twenty-one, first as a snorter and then as a shooter. He found snorting a pleasant but not remarkable experience. "You feel good, warm inside. It gives you a lift, but it is not as good as shooting. I still snort some when I am with a broad and we are into sex." He continued to take cocaine intermittently (both snorting and shooting) until age twenty-five, when he began regular, daily intravenous usage of cocaine. "I snorted off and on, then graduated to banging coke when I was twenty-five. I have been banging girl and girl-and-boy ever since."

Rufus made the following observations about his first intravenous use of cocaine: "This friend of mine came by and asked me if I wanted to try cocaine with the needle. He said it gave you a nice, mellow high and kept you relaxed. Shit — we mixed some speed, heroin, and coke — it gave me one *helluva* feeling!

There was this helluva rush! Wow! I have never had anything like that again in my life. I get hot thinking about it even today. It was like having a climax with a woman, only intensified a hundred times. It was so good I thought I would die."

As indicated, Rufus prefers speedball. "Some people use girl to give them drive. I use it to get high, to feel good. I don't like to speed, I like to relax, that's why I use them both. It makes me very mellow, and that's good. You can stay all night with a woman. You never get strung out with girl, because girl keeps you all together. Hell, I could come in here loaded with girl and you would never know it — girl keeps you all together and you feel *good!*"

Rufus estimates that he has done 10 percent of his cocaine alone, 25 percent with one other person — "usually when I am with a broad" — and the remaining 65 percent with four or five close male friends. "Hell, man, shooting girl makes me high. I don't want to be alone when I am high, I want to share it. I want people around me that are having a good time, too."

Rufus indicates he uses one gram of cocaine per day. "It is always available, because the same man who sells you boy will always have girl, too, so if you've got the money he's got the stuff." The largest amount of cocaine he has used is two grams: "That's pretty typical for a run. I would shoot two grams of girl, then use boy to speed by and bring me down. I would use boy behind girl because if you OD on girl it is hard to bring you back."

Rufus enjoys doing cocaine runs for a couple of days with a few close friends. He indicates that he has done perhaps thirty or forty such runs using two grams per day. "We'd fire up on girl, relax, visit, sleep a little, fire some more and get high." There are only two circumstances needed to trigger a cocaine run: having money and the availability of good coke. He indicates no daily pattern in his use of cocaine: "I would do it morning or night or any other time I can get it." He does admit, however, that reversals or setbacks in life would cause him to turn to cocaine: "If I got discouraged or depressed, I would want some girl."

Rufus estimates that 25 percent of the cocaine he has used has been street cocaine — "Street stuff can be bad news" — 25 percent pharmaceutical or liquid cocaine — "liquid cocaine blinded me once, but boy brought me back" — and the remaining 50 percent rock crystal. He says he can determine the difference between street and high-quality cocaine by the rush or "drive" he gets with the first (free) shot and the bitterness in the taste. The third criterion is brilliance. "Rock crystal coke has high drive, a bitter taste, and a high brillance!"

In Rufus's opinion one develops temporary tolerance for cocaine. He states that on a run he would have to increase the size of the hits after taking a total of about one-half gram of cocaine. By the end of a run he might be shooting as much as one-half gram in each hit. "Then I'd have to start thinking about how to get down. I used boy to come down on. It's the best; I have heard guys say methadone brings you down better and faster, but I don't know about that. When I was on methadone you could speed by the methadone with girl and still get a good high."

Rufus concludes that the body's tolerance for cocaine lasts about a day. "In twenty-four hours you're clear and can start all over again and get that good rush with the first hit." He does not consider withdrawal from cocaine to be discomforting: "You're tired as hell, worn out, and kind of depressed that it's all gone, but I would always fire boy behind girl and go to bed and go right to sleep; after a good night's rest I felt OK."

Reactions to Cocaine

Physiological Reactions
The physiological reactions which occur every time Rufus uses cocaine include sweaty palms, dryness in the mouth and throat, increased heart rate, increased mental activity, and loss of sensations of fatigue (table 11.5). A second group of reactions occurring with high frequency — up to 90 percent of the time — include vomiting, clogging of the nasal airways — perhaps an allergic reaction in an intravenous cocaine user — ringing of the ears — "They ring like bells" — dizziness, and local anesthesia.

Surprisingly, while Rufus reported an increased heart rate — "It pounds like hell" — every time he has used cocaine, he says that an increase in pulse and respiration rate occurs only half the time. It may be that he misunderstood these questions, or he may simply have been insensitive to these bodily reactions. It seems that both reactions should be regular sequelae to stimulation of the central nervous system. Rufus did note that cocaine would trigger a dumping evacuation of the bowels about half the time. He also reported that he occasionally experiences tremors, gooseflesh, and headache (which he attributed to the cut).

Rufus never experiences a running nose, tears, nosebleed, inflammation, infection, hepatitis — "You don't get that if you use new spikes" — allergic reactions, yawning, weight loss, or loss of sensations of hunger and pain.

Psychological Reactions
The psychological reactions Rufus reported fall into four clusters (table 11.6). First, cocaine causes increased thinking power and imagination, acclerated mental activity, and garrulousness. Further, he finds cocaine to be an aphrodisiac — "It stimulates the sex drive for both men and women" — prolonging sexual intercourse and providing a more spectacular orgasm. Most of the time, cocaine makes Rufus feel he is "more together" and has better self-control.

Rufus described a second cluster of psychological reactions that occur about half the time (40-60 percent) in his cocaine use. These reactions include increased restlessness, excitement, sense of well-being, euphoria, insomnia, and feelings of increased strength and ability to work.

Rufus reported increased feelings of tension and anxiety about 30 percent

TABLE 11.5. Physiological Reactions to Cocaine Use and Abuse: Rufus B.

Commonly Reported Reactions to Cocaine Use/Abuse	Reactions Observed Yes	Reactions Observed No	Percent/Time Observed	Qualifying Comments and Observations
Dizziness – feeling of light-headedness	Yes		70	If it is a good grade of cocaine. You get real "light-headed" with the rush on high grade coke.
Sweating – perspiration or increases in temperature	Yes		100	I always sweat a lot on coke. My hands would sweat a lot.
Rhinorrhea – running nose		No		Not shooting. Your nose runs, snorting.
Tremors – muscle spasms	Yes		25	If you do too much. I would be twitching or "trembly" in my arms and legs in the last stages with girl.
Lacrimation – tears to eyes		No		I never did, snorting or shooting.
Mydriasis – dilation of pupils, light sensitivity		No		Not that I ever noticed.
Gooseflesh	Yes		35	If it's good, high-grade coke it will make me have goosebumps with the rush.
Emesis – vomiting	Yes		90	I would vomit about 80–90 percent of the time with high grade coke (40–50 percent pure). You feel nauseous most of the time.
Reactive hyperemia – clogging of nasal air passages	Yes		80	With good girl my nose would be clogged with snorting or shooting.
Anorexia – loss of appetite, sensation for hunger		No		I never noticed it. I could always eat on girl.
Dryness of mouth and throat, lack of salivation	Yes		100	It always happened with me.
Increased heart rate	Yes		100	Your heart pumps faster, you can feel it.
Tightness in chest or chest pains		No		I never noticed it with girl.
Local anesthesia, numbness	Yes		70	I would get numb after a gram or so, particularly my face and throat.
Nosebleed		No		It didn't happen either snorting or shooting.
Elevation of pulse rate	Yes		50	You could feel your pulse pounding just like your heart.
Increased respiration rate	Yes		50	Your body is stimulated.

412

Cellulitis – inflammation following administration	No		It happened to me snorting girl though.
Infection of nasal mucous membrane	No		No, I got a couple of "burns," that's all.
Yawning	No		Not for me.
Hyperphrenia – excessive mental activity	Yes	100	Your mind and imagination go like crazy.
Weight loss	No		I never did enough at one time. I guess if you did a lot you might.
Fainting	No		I never fainted on girl. I did on boy a time or two.
Increased sensitivity to allergies	No		I was never allergic to anything.
Diarrhea or explosive bowel movements	Yes		Sometimes you have to go to the john right after a hit.
Hepatitis or liver infections	No		I have never had hepatitis with girl.
Headaches	Yes	5	You can get a hell of a headache if the coke is not up to par or if it has been cut with garbage. Sometimes they use strychnine in the cut.
Loss of fatigue	Yes	100	You don't feel tired at all.
Ringing in the ears	Yes	80	They ring like bells with high-grade girl.
Convulsions	No		I get sick and vomit. I never had convulsions.
Visual flashes with the rush	No		I never had anything like that with girl.

TABLE 11.6. Psychological Reactions to Cocaine Use and Abuse: Rufus B.

Commonly Reported Reactions to Cocaine Use/Abuse	Reactions Observed Yes	No	Percent/ Time Observed	Qualifying Comments and Observations
Increased feelings of self-control	Yes		90	You feel you're on top of it all.
Increased optimism, courage		No		Shit, I never had problems about courage or self-confidence, man!
Increased activity, restlessness, excitement	Yes		40	It always makes me feel restless and excited.
Feeling of increased physical strength or ability to do physical work	Yes		50	It depends on the quality. Good girl makes you feel like you could do anything!
Intensified feelings of well-being, euphoria, "floating," etc.	Yes		50	You feel good but you only get that floating feeling with boy.
Feeling that everything is perfect		No		Shit, man, I never believed any garbage like that!
An exquisite "don't care about the world" attitude		No		You get that feeling with boy.
A physical orgasm with the "rush"	Yes			I literally came on myself with high-grade girl. My ears were ringing like bells then, too.
Increased thinking power and imagination	Yes		100	Every time, man, your mind moves fast. It's quicker.
Feeling that the mind is quicker than normal, the feeling that one is smarter than everyone else	Yes		100	Every time, man, your mind moves fast. It's quicker.
More talkative than usual, a stream of talk	Yes		100	You talk like a goose. You just babble on and on.
Indifference to pain		No		I never felt that.
Decreased interest in work, failure of ambition, loss of ambition for useful work.		No		Hell no, it makes me want to work!
Insomnia	Yes		30	It's hard to go to sleep if you do too much girl.
Depression, anxiety	Yes		30	I have never been depressed on girl, but I have been anxious as hell. Heroin makes some guys violent. It puts some dudes in a depression, a depressed mood and they react with violence. Hell, people use coke to be happy-go-lucky.
Prolonged sexual intercourse	Yes		100	You last longer.

An aphrodisiac or sexual stimulant	Yes	100	Yeah, it turns you on, women in particular.
Better orgasm on coke	Yes	100	It's great!
Irrational fears	No		Never.
Terror or panic	No		Never.
Tactile hallucinations — the feeling that insects are crawling on or under the skin (particularly fingertips, palms of hands, etc.)	No		Never.
Changes in reality or the way a room or objects look — the wall waving or in motion, etc.	No		No, girl keeps you right in reality. It doesn't take you away.
Paranoid ideas — the feeling that people are after you. You believe you are being watched, talked about or threatened, a wife or girlfriend is unfaithful, untrustworthy, etc.	No		Never.
Causes one to carry a gun or run from imaginary enemies	No		Never. I've carried a gun, but not on girl.
Visual hallucinations	No		Not for me.
Auditory hallucinations — hearing voices talking about you, threatening, etc.	No		Not girl.
Olfactory hallucinations — new odors, smells, etc.	Yes	40	Girl makes your sense of smell keener, so you notice odors you wouldn't normally pay attention to.
A trigger for violence.	No		Hell no, man, girl makes me passive. Anything that makes me want to have sex with a woman is not violent. I have had my share of violence. I should know.

of the time he used cocaine. He was the only participant to report an orgasm with the cocaine rush. He stated, "It was so good I actually came on myself. This only happened four times, though."

Rufus's psychological reactions are more uniquely defined by reactions he has not experienced than by those he did report. Cocaine does not make him feel more optimistic or courageous — "I never had trouble with courage" — make him feel every thing is perfect — "I never believed any shit like that" — create a don't-give-a-damn attitude towards the world — "Boy does that, not girl!" — or decrease interest in work. Rufus has not experienced paranoid ideas, visual, auditory, tactile, or olfactory hallucinations, changes in perceived reality, irrational fears, or panic reactions causing him to carry a gun or run from imaginary enemies. He does not feel that cocaine is a trigger for violence: "It isn't for me. Girl makes me mellow, puts me in a happy-go-lucky mood; it makes me passive. Anything that makes me want to have sex with a woman is not violent. I have had my share of violence; I should know."

Integration

Rufus does not take cocaine to maintain his energy level or drive. He does not need to; in fact, he has more energy than he is able to manage. His problem is finding some way to relax. Use of cocaine — and more particularly speed-ball — represents one way this man can rest, yet temporarily drop the cloak of worry that seems to follow wherever he goes. When Rufus pauses in life, he must wrestle with the feelings of dysphoria and perhaps remorse that constitute the shadow side of his personality. He wonders what life is all about, what he is all about, what success is, why he failed as a pimp, what he did wrong, how he failed his son, what he could have done differently, what will ultimately become of him, and what he should do with the remainder of his life. Rufus feels trapped because the problems appear unsolvable. However, with cocaine or speedball Rufus can stop, pause, relax, feel mellow, and be passive and at ease with himself, a woman, or a few close associates without having to deal with these concerns.

Rufus is almost as skillful in manipulating his emotional states with drugs as he is in manipulating other people. In fact, Rufus shows better judgment in his use of cocaine than in other areas of living. His usage of one or even two grams per day (buffered with heroin) permits him to relax, feel mellow, perform sex, visit with his friends, and listen to his records, all the while avoiding adverse reactions. Using cocaine and heroin together Rufus gets the cocaine high but never experiences the paranoia, hallucinations, anxiety reactions, or urge to take excessive amounts of cocaine that are typical sequelae to heavy usage.

Although Rufus has never discussed it directly, there is at least one other reason he uses cocaine. Among all of the substances in current usage in the ghetto, cocaine is the prestige drug, the Cadillac of substances. Rufus is a status-conscious man. It is important for him that others know he uses "only the best stuff," just as it is important for him to communicate his status by his exquisite dress and his "cool status ride."

LIFE ACTIVITIES AND EXPERIENCES:
IN RUFUS'S OWN WORDS

Overview

This section provides accounts of two days in Rufus's life. These days occurred in early February and late May 1975.

The previous year was one of the most difficult in Rufus's life. He suffered reversals that might have devastated less resilient men: He lost his "bottom woman" who played a significant role in his success as a pimp; his stable of "hustling broads" is gone; he came home to find his son in the penitentiary for armed robbery; and he himself is broke and unemployed. To make matters worse, Rufus has apparently antagonized some powerful figures in the drug community. It was rumored that there was an open-ended contract on his life payable to whoever could claim it. Though Rufus has never admitted it, he makes an allusion to this matter below, at the end of the second day. For four to six months Rufus had rarely left his home. For all practical purposes, this impatient, restless man withdrew from the world. He avoided going onto the street and disappeared from his regular haunts. His friends of long standing had withdrawn and were standing clear of whatever might occur. During this period, Rufus was isolated and alone. The only people he saw regularly were his wife and two "brothers" who live with him.

It is clear that Rufus was frustrated by all that had happened — he may even have feared for his life. Apparently he decided that if he would "lay low" long enough it would pass. It was only on the second day that Rufus made his first cautious foray back on the street — and only then because his "brothers" told him the word was out that it was all over.

During his self-enforced exile Rufus has been thrown back upon himself. On the first day he shares his reflections on his life as a pimp, his concern about his son in the penitentiary and his fear that he must have let the boy down, his daily routine (which includes polishing his diamond and listening to his "sides" — his jazz records), and his frustration. At the same time, he tells of his love for his wife and his buoyant optimism and hope for the future. He tries to tell himself all is well, but he is nervous, restless, and edgy.

As indicated, on the second day Rufus straps on a "piece" and makes his first tentative trip back into the "street." The lion is leaving his den. He is constantly moving, watchful, alert, and ready. The tension of the first few hours on the street underscores the intensity with which the game is played. Rufus has been told it is all over, but he knows full well this could be a trick. Two stories are going on, one revealed by what Rufus describes and the other by the things that remain unsaid. He is not sure what will "come down," but he is trying to find out where he stands. Everyone he meets feigns a pleasant camaraderie; at the same time, they are almost as nervous, cautious, and edgy as Rufus. From these experiences Rufus concludes he still has a few friends. He gets home safely, but there is a flurry of concern resulting from a garbled phone message; he is relieved when his "brothers" arrive home safely. During the evening Rufus shares more of what he was thinking and feeling during the day. Since he made it home safely he concludes it was a good day, and that "it" was perhaps all over.

Activity and Experience Audits

First Day: A Monday in February

12:00 p.m.–2:45 a.m.
I was laying in bed at home; my wife was asleep. I generally watch TV till it goes off. I'm into the movie, man. TV relaxes me; I'm a TV addict. My son is on my mind, though. Some friends have been down to see him over the weekend. They told us he was in good spirits. He's big, I don't worry about him being able to protect himself, but it's hard on him mentally. I'll be glad when he gets home. I was feeling kind of gloomy about him, sad 'cause I miss him. His mother worries about him, too, I know. She don't say much, but she worries about him like mothers do.

Melvin and Joe, my brothers, are in and asleep.

2:45–5:30 a.m.
The TV programs go off. I go check the house, lock up, and turn the tube off.

Then I went to bed, but couldn't sleep. I tossed and turned, just laying there thinking. I feel bad. I'm thinking that somewhere I failed the boy; I didn't want him to be like me, I wanted him to be better. He didn't do it for pleasure, but did it because he wanted better things. Having more things doesn't make him happier, though.

As I get older, things don't mean what they did when I was younger. I appreciate the simple things in life more now. I got a woman who loves me and I love her. As much as I love drugs, I don't enjoy them the way I used to; I want to stop. It doesn't bother her as long as I do it at home. I've learned to conserve; I don't take bill money now to spend on it. Extra money I get, that's OK to get high with, but I enjoy being with her.

I finally went to sleep.

5:30–6:30 a.m.
The phone rings, my sister-in-law makes her wake-up call.

I wake my wife. She gets out of bed, cleans up, gets dressed, and starts getting ready for work. She is not feeling too well, she was thinking about her son, too. We made plans to go see him again in a couple of weeks.

I told her, soon as she left I was sure gonna sleep good. She said she envied me. She kissed me goodbye and told me that if I got lonesome to call her. I told her to take the phone out of the room because I wasn't going to answer it; I didn't want to be woke up — most of the calls are for Melvin and Joe, my brothers, anyway. She did.

6:30 a.m.–12:30 p.m.
I slept.

12:30–4:00 p.m.
I got up, went to the bathroom, cleaned up, and polished my diamond. You use a special paste kinda like Brasso. Let it dry, then you buff it down, and that diamond will really shine!

I was still feeling kinda gloomy. I decided I had better eat. (I don't eat breakfast too much, but I decided it might make me feel better.)

I let my German shepherd out of the basement and fed him. Then I let him out in the back yard. It's all fenced in and he's safe there. I had two, a boy and a girl, but the girl was hit by a car and killed during the winter; that's when I put the fence up.

I fixed some breakfast. I ate three eggs and a beef hot dog that I stuck over the raw fire, some toast, and a glass of milk. I took it all in the front room to eat. I ate and listened to some jazz on the box while I ate. I was alone; Melvin and Joe were out somewhere. It was quiet and I was by myself, listening to John Coltrane, digging the instruments; I was feeling better now.

I took the dishes in the kitchen, came back, and put some old Miles Davis tunes on. It made me think about when I was younger and had a tiger by the tail — I had broads, sure enough, clothes, and money to burn! I was also thinking about when I first met my woman. I dug her then and I dig her now! It's hard to believe, but I love her more now than I did then; I wouldn't think it would be possible. I am thinking I'll sure be glad when she comes home.

I heard the dog barking outside, and it's getting close to time for her to come home. The dog is barking at some kids in the back; some little kids back there are throwing rocks at him. I have had him since he was a pup, I bought him for my son. However, I overprotect him now. I don't want him run over like the female. When she died, he stopped barking for a long time; he just moped after she died. When my son was incarcerated, we — my wife and I — took up with the dogs, maybe to fill the emptiness.

I went out back and told the kids to stop throwing rocks.

4:00–6:30 p.m.

My lady comes home and the sun starts to shine again. She always greets me and asks how my day was. I tell her how terrible it was till now. She smiles, we embrace, and she asks me what I want to eat, what she should fix, and stuff like that. I'm feeling good with her there.

I walked up to the corner to get some cigarettes, milk, and stuff. I kept my eyes open. I'm thinking how nice it is, and how the walk will do me good. I would like to have a ride, but I lost my Cadillac trying to help my boy. I start tripping on the fact that I don't need Cadillacs anymore, and thinking on how I lost it on legal fees for my son. Hell, it kept him from getting twenty to thirty years! I don't need a Cadillac, any kind of car will do, I'm thinking.

I ran into some friends at the store and got a ride back home. We just chatted about jive, where the good stuff is at, and things like that. I thanked the dudes. I went in the house and unloaded the groceries and just relaxed. My brother Melvin was there. He had two friends over; they were smoking weed.

If I am not high, weed will intensify my pain. If I am already high, I can smoke weed. If I am sick though, weed will hurt a thousand times worse! I felt pretty good, so I smoked a joint. I turned the box on and ate in the front room. I was still doing some sides.

I had missed most of "Star Trek," so I didn't watch it, but had gotten into playing some old Lou Rawls records for my wife. We were chatting about the music and feeling pretty good. It reminded me of old times, when I had a lot of money.

6:30 p.m.–2:30 a.m.

Melvin and the dudes left.

I went in the bedroom, took my clothes off, and just stretched out and relaxed. My wife is cleaning up the dishes and everything. I am watching the tube and relaxing.

She finishes and sits down with me, waiting on "The Rookies" to come on. Then she usually watches "S.W.A.T."! Shit, man, they're just nothing but professional killers!

Her "Rookie" program comes on.

We got this big queen-sized bed and big pillows and all. She just cuddles up right behind me, puts her arm over my shoulders, and watches the tube. I feel the warmth of her behind me; she holds my hand. About 9:00 she falls off to sleep. I covered her up.

I turn over and tell her I love her while she sleeps. She smiles.

I check her occasionally to see if she is all right, if she is resting cool. If she has a bad dream, I put my hand on her face and tell her it's all right. She smiles and sleeps like a log; she gets to snoring, but hell, man, that's cool! It's all right. I am thinking about TV; it ain't too bad. I am laying there thinking life could be better, but it ain't too bad. It's a good feeling knowing, man, that you're loved genuinely. It's a good feeling that somebody loves you despite large faults. It makes you want to be better and do better! As long as I got her, I will be better.

Sometimes I tell her I ain't good enough for her, and she cries. She says she was born for me. It makes me feel good. I know; I haven't always felt like that! I love being with the woman, but I enjoy helping her. I don't want nothing too strenuous for her.

I was laying there watching TV and thinking about stuff like that.

2:30 a.m.

The programs went off TV. I get up, turn the tube off, and lock the house. My brothers are in and asleep. I got to bed and right to sleep.

The Day: A *good* day! I am happy I got her, man!

Second Day: A Monday in May

12:00 p.m.–2:30 a.m.

I was home in bed, watching TV till it went off. I was into the tube and feeling pretty good. I really get into those movies! When the program went off, I got up, turned the tube off, and went to bed.

5:30 a.m.

My wife got up and was getting ready to go to work. I woke up and chatted with her a few minutes, then went back to sleep.

10:30 a.m.–12:00 n.

I got up, went to the bathroom, shaved, took a bath, and cleaned up. I felt good! I felt like getting high.

I fed the dog and let him out in the back yard.

I didn't eat any breakfast because I wasn't hungry, so I went in the front room and sat down. I put some sides on the box, and sat down and smoked a joint, just trying to get myself together. I was wondering what I was going to do.

I decided, fuck it! I am going up on the street! I have been *through* the street a lot this winter, but with the mess I had I had not stayed there. I was trying to make up my mind whether I was going to walk or try to catch a ride. Also, I was wondering why the hell I was doing all of this staying in. I knew from what I had heard it was over!

When those dudes put me in the mess, I didn't want to be around people; I was disgusted with them. They didn't want me around and I didn't want any part of them. They had all believed a lot of shit which wasn't true, and just let me hang! But it is over now, so I went and got dressed. I strapped on my piece, just in case.

I went out on the porch and checked the mail.

A friend was driving by. He slowed down as he went by the house, and I hollered at him; he stopped and backed up. I asked if he would give me a lift up to the street. He said yeah, so I went back and put my dog in the house.

12:00 n.–4:00 p.m.

Nathan — my friend — was drinking a can of beer and asked me if I wanted one. I told him, sure, I would like a cold beer, but I didn't have any money. He said OK, and drove down to a place where he could get some beer. Instead, he came back with some alcohol, some screwdrivers. Nathan is a good-natured dude. He used to mess around, but has squared up and cleaned up his act; he's a beer drinker now. I told him, "Man, you know I am no drinker." He said one wouldn't hurt me, so I took it.

We drove up to the street; we're chatting about old times, but I'm watching. I felt pretty good. Told him I had been trying to get my head together from the mess I had gotten into. He said he understood.

We drove up and down, checking the streets out. The weather was real nice and I was feeling good, drinking my screwdriver. I was wondering if I was going to turn out to see ex-partners or sure-enough partners. I was gonna try to figure out, after this long time, who liked me and who don't. I wanted to see who was faking. I was gonna tell those dudes who were faking to stay out of my face!

We stopped and I got out of the car. Nathan and I chatted with two–three guys. I had seen two of my friends; I wanted to find out where I was with them and see if everything was alright. I saw John; he's a good-natured fellow. I have known him ten to fifteen years. He was glad to see me, he wasn't faking.

I told Nathan I would check with him later. He wanted to know when he could come by and beat my ass at chess. He drove off.

John and two or three other dudes were standing there on the street bull-shitting. John and I started to rap. I am trying to feel the dude out and see where he was at. He asked if I knew where he could get some Freon for his air conditioner; I told him I didn't know. He said he needed some, and wanted to know if I wanted to ride with him to find it. I said OK.

I felt OK after he told me he had heard what had come down on me. He said it was a pretty screwy deal to lay on a man. He said he had been told I was trying to stop, and that's why he didn't come by — out of consideration for me. That's probably not why. He simply didn't want to be caught in some kind of crossfire, but I let it go.

We drove to three or four stores trying to find a quart of Freon. As it turned out, we didn't get it. They only had it in gallons.

John asked if I had had any breakfast yet. I told him no, so we drove out to a restaurant.

I am feeling a little more relaxed, a little better. I told him I didn't have no money, but he said that was OK. We go in this place, sit down, and give the waitress our order. He's treating me. The place is crowded; there are fifteen-twenty people in there. John's talking about waffles, of all the damn things! He's a waffle nut, and is talking about where you get good waffles, and the prices and all. I just sat and listened and watched; I had a sandwich. We ate and just chatted. He paid and we left.

John was supposed to meet some people on the street, but he stopped and took his glasses into an optical place; he said they had been bothering his eyes. He came back in a minute. They told him they couldn't do nothing with them (they only cost him $1.59). He asked me if I wanted them. I didn't care, but I said OK, and put them in my pocket.

He got tickled about the glasses. They had told him in the optical place that they were dime-store glasses, and no damn wonder his eyes had been bothering him! He thought it was funny as hell! I got amused by it, too. I didn't know what the hell to do with the dime-store glasses he gave me, though.

We parked the car, and he walked down the street a ways to see his friends. Two old partners of mine came up and we chatted awhile, feeling each other out. I was getting a little more relaxed, but was keeping my eyes open.

Everyone comes up and greets me (three-four guys I knew). I am thinking this one is a sure-enough partner, that one is faking! That's what is going on in my mind. I am chatting, looking, and watching. The dudes are talking about how good I am looking now. I am listening to all that shit, but that is the only thing some of them are telling the truth about, how good I look — and I do look good, man!

My sure-enough partner, Ed, is a good-natured guy. He's big and strong. We have done a lot of shit together. I had only seen him two–three times in the last six–eight months, and had never had time to rap with him like I wanted to. We were just standing there on the street visiting, so he just said, "Let's ride!" So we got in his car and left.

4:00–5:30 p.m.

Ed had his lady in the car. I have known her a long time; she's a working gal, a booster. I felt real good that he asked me to join him.

We go to my place. He's a Coltrane fan, and we went by my place to listen to some sides. We smoked a joint and chatted. He said he had heard about the mess I had been in; he said that if someone did that to him, he would be tempted to kill them. I didn't say much, just listened. We chatted about the sides. Ed's lady left to go take care of some business for him. We just chatted and dug some sides after that.

Momma came home and I helped her carry the groceries in. I was glad to see her.

Ed and I went for a walk and came back. I felt good after that walk, *real good!*

Ed's lady came back with another broad; Ed has two working broads, they're both boosters, but they're nice.

5:30–6:30 p.m.

The broads dropped Ed and I up on the street, and then they go on to work. We ran into another old partner of mine, Fred, on the street. He was glad to see me out, I could tell. We wanted to see Fred because he, Ed, and I were all raised together; we had done a lot of things together. Ed hasn't been out of the penitentiary too long, and we wanted to chat about old times.

I felt good. I wasn't high, just a little mellow, but still watching and very much alert. You don't get high and go up on the street, shit! I want to know what is going on. Particularly right now, I want to be on top of my action! I hadn't been out among a lot of people in a long time, and I don't want some crazy s.o.b. who doesn't know it's over starting something.

We just drive up and down the streets checking things out. Fred was glad to see me back; he had heard about the shit, too. We would drive along in Fred's car, and if we would see someone we knew, we would pull over and visit a few minutes. I am feeling I've got some sure-enough partners with me. The dudes just come up to the car and visit, then we would pull off down the street until we saw some more. One of the dudes was a working guy, but most of them are still chasing that jive and everything. I don't have to get out there and chase that jive.

6:30–8:30 p.m.

Fred drives Ed home and drops him off. He has to stay home by the phone in case his women need him. If they get into any trouble with their stuff, he will be there.

Fred then drops me off at my place. We just chat in a general conversation; I am still checking him out. I told him I would see with him later. He said if he heard anything or anything came up, he would give me a ring.

Momma is glad to see me. Supper is ready. I felt real good! I decided I wasn't going to be staying in no more! As best I could tell, the thing is over. I had been checking it all day and trying to figure it out. People had been putting out lies on me, but that shit don't work now. It's over.

My wife fixed our dinner, and we watched TV and ate supper.

After my wife had finished eating, Joe's woman — Joe's one of my brothers — came in and fixed her hair. I ate by myself. Apparently Joe is kind of getting the little hustling broad straightened up. He had her on punishment this week; she couldn't go out of the house for two days.

I told my wife what all had happened during my day, and she was pleased. While I was gone, she had gotten a call from her sister about some emergency; the connection was mixed up, so she had been worried about me. She relaxed some when I came home, but Melvin was still out and she was worrying about him. It was kind of crazy, because we couldn't get her sister back on the phone to find out just what the hell it was.

Melvin came in, so he was OK. We never did find out what the hell the call was all about. However, we were both relieved he was home in one piece.

8:30 p.m.—3:00 a.m.

We went upstairs. I felt *super;* real, real good! I felt like my old self again. I had decided that shit was not for me; I had to get my head and heart together and stay low awhile. I will try to take care of my business and hope that others take care of theirs. I don't really know exactly how I got into such a mess, but, man, I felt very relieved! I will do my business, but if I go with a dude I'll go with him all the way no matter what comes down! I give that kind of loyalty and expect my friends to do the same. However, man, I am not putting my life out there for just anybody! Those dudes had tried to use me, then bad-mouthed me and get my ass into a lot of risky trouble. It was tearing my head apart. I had no one to talk to. I talked with my wife about it some, but with that kind of thing a man needs a man to talk with.

We got ready for bed. I was feeling real comfortable rapping with my wife about the day, where I had been, who I thought was OK, who I thought was faking. I was really feeling good it was over!

We got off into the tube. She fell out to sleep about 9:30.

I woke her up about 10:15 and made her go get us something to eat. She did, but was kind of pissed at me about it. She went back to sleep a little pissed.

I am into the tube. I felt good. I fell off to sleep myself about 11:00. I didn't know how tired I really was.

I woke up about 3:00 a.m. and the tube was still on. I got up, turned it off, and went back to sleep.

The Day: A *good day!* A *super day!* It was just like the rest of them are going to be! It all seems kind of silly now, but it was damn serious then. The way it was, there was no way I could win. I've got to learn how to strengthen my mind to deal with that kind of thing if it ever comes down again. I hope it doesn't! They had me thinking I was gonna perish and all that shit!

_____ Part 3

Interpretation

12

Interpersonal Comparisons

Chapters 3-11 emphasized the uniquenesses of nine men. This chapter will focus upon the participants as a group. The task is approached in three ways: by examining social-demographic data, examining information from the formal psychological assessments, and examining information concerning drug use and its effects.

SOCIAL–DEMOGRAPHIC COMPARISONS

As indicated in chapter 2, these men vary widely in socio-demographic characteristics. They come from two racial groups (Negro and Caucasian) and range from twenty-one to forty-four years of age (mean age = 30.11 years). They come from families ranging from four to ten members per household (mean = 5.56 persons per household). Five are the youngest in their family, two are the eldest, and two occupy intermediate positions.

Arky, Tom, George, John, and Fred have had defective relationships with their fathers or stepfathers, who are deceased, absent, or rejecting. Seven participants — Arky, Bill, Tom, George, Al, John, and Willie — feel closer to their mothers than their fathers. Rufus is proud of his father, while Fred has difficulty determining which parent he dislikes more. In seven families the mother has been dominant — those of Arky, George, Al, John, Willie, Rufus, and Fred.

The number of years of formal education ranges from ten to thirteen. The mean of 12.1 years corresponds to the average of 12.3 years for the six-county

Kansas City Standard Metropolitan Statistical Area (SMSA) in the 1970 Census. Although three participants — Bill, Tom, and George — enrolled in college full-time for one or more semesters, none has a college degree. The average IQ of the group, as measured by the Revised Beta, is 105.8; the standard deviation of this value is 11.21; the range is from 93 to 119.

Specifying the marital status of these nine men is difficult because three — Arky, George and John — married during the project, while Willie obtained a divorce during the same period. Arky, George, Al, John, Willie, and Rufus were married at some time during the project. Five men had obtained divorces from a prior marriage. Only three — Arky, Willie, and Rufus — have children.

Six participants live in rental housing (apartments or homes) while the remainder are home owners. Two — Al and Rufus — live in the inner city, five — Arky, Bill, Tom, Willie, and Fred — live elsewhere in the city proper, and two — George and John — lived in the suburbs.

Eight of the nine men are healthy. Only Tom had a serious medical problem, a defective heart valve.

Bill, George, John, and Willie maintained full-time legal employment during the project, while Arky and Fred maintained irregular or intermittent employment. The remainder — Tom, Al, and Rufus — were unemployed or engaged in illegal occupations. Only Bill, George, John, and Willie have work skills that are marketable in the larger society.

All the men — except Bill and Tom — had one or more arrests for drug-related criminal activity. The total number of arrests per man ranges from one (Bill) to more than a hundred (Rufus), averaging 21 per man. Excluding Rufus, the arrest rate averaged almost 9 per man. However, the conviction rate was low, averaging only about 1.4.

Four men — Bill, George, John, and Willie — are achievement-oriented and upwardly mobile. Tom was also ambitious, but he was only able to succeed in an illegal occupation. Rufus is ambitious, but, like Tom, his talents are illegal. Although Fred comes from an exceptionally wealthy family his aspirations are lower than those of his parents. Arky's life goal is simply to stay out of the penitentiary, if he can. Al G. has limited resources, knows it, and has come to terms with this fact.

As a group, the nine men show normal sexual activity. John has intercourse with his wife almost every day; Arky, Tom, Willie, and Rufus reported having sexual intercourse with theirs two or three times per week. George had once been very active sexually, but reported little sexual involvement during the project; he was temporarily too depressed to be interested in sex. Bill's and Fred's sexual activity has been irregular. Al is probably the least sexually active man.

These men rarely attend church and show little interest in religious activities. They also have a low regard for politics. Only Willie takes a lively interest in political activities. He knows many local politicians and has been involved in events involving black affairs.

These participants are not like the man who lives next door. Nevertheless, were it not for their often unusual occupations and high arrest rates, they would be difficult to identify as heavy cocaine users from social-demographic characteristics alone.

Formal Psychological Assessment

In general, factor-analytic and cluster-analytic techniques show that what seems a good way of grouping persons on one instrument is not necessarily good on another. The men we interviewed may be sorted into types according to per- formances of one kind; they may also be sorted into types on the basis of performance of another kind. Yet, for the most part these typings resist being merged into a single scheme. The nine men are individuals and behave as such in every thing they do.

Dimensional Data

MMPI Profiles

Cluster analysis suggests that a uniform profile could be said to characterize the MMPI scores of seven of the men (Cluster I in table 12.1).

TABLE 12.1. Mean MMPI T-Scores for Participants

	Cluster I	Cluster II (Fred)	Cluster III (Tom)
L	49.0	63	43
F	57.7	104	68
K	49.1	46	40
Hs	57.4	72	47
D	58.6	94	66
Hy	57.6	73	58
Pd	68.1	81	96
Mf	65.7	72	51
Pa	53.9	95	73
Pt	60.4	87	74
Sc	56.0	96	90
Ma	70.1	63	83
Si	55.3	65	55

The data look like that for the classic picture of a sociopathic individual; note the high values on the *Ma* and *Pd* Scales. Fred (Cluster II) differs from the main cluster by virtue of his high *F* Scale score and his elevations on at least nine other scales. Tom's *Pd* and *Ma* scores (Cluster III) are especially high; in addition, his profile shows high values on *Sc, Pa,* and *Pt* Scales. Signs of tension, anxiety, and introspective concern are less prominent in Tom's record than in that of Fred.

Sixteen PF Scales

Cluster analysis of the Sixteen PF data shows such wide individual differences that conceptualization of any group or subgroup by scale means is not justified. The averages reported in table 12.2 are presented here for informational purposes only, not as a group profile of personality traits.

TABLE 12.2. Group Mean Sten Scores on the Sixteen PF Scale

Factor	Mean	Standard Deviation
A	5.6	1.9
B	5.0	2.3
C	4.7	2.3
E	6.1	2.5
F	5.3	2.1
G	4.3	2.4
H	5.7	2.3
I	6.6	1.7
L	5.7	2.1
M	6.6	1.9
N	4.9	1.8
O	5.3	1.1
Q_1	7.3	1.3
Q_2	6.9	2.2
Q_3	4.3	1.4
Q_4	6.2	2.1

Morphogenic Data

Q-Sorts

Because the Q-Sort method was originally designed as a way of discovering similarities among people, it lends itself readily to the problem at hand. At least fourteen separate typologies could be constructed: one for each instructional condition with the standard items (five in all) and with the individual items (nine in all). Taking assessment sessions into account, a total of forty-two cluster analyses are technically possible.

Three instructional conditions have been selected for scrutiny; these are the conditions of greatest importance to the investigation — usual self, ideal self, self during a cocaine high. Because sortings for these three instructional conditions were obtained with both standard and individualized items, a total of six sortings has been used for analytical purposes.

Procedures

Item-placement values were added together so that each man was represented by composite sortings (sixty sums each) for the six conditions described above. Each composite was factor-analyzed separately. The question was whether persons grouped together on one summed sorting tend to be similar on the other five as well. The analysis indicates that Arky, Rufus, George, Al, John, and Bill form a coherent group while Fred, Tom, and Willie are isolates. Of possible importance is the confirmation of the MMPI finding that Fred and Tom differ from the rest of the men.

Rep Test

Data from the Rep Test are so individualized that only limited interperson comparisons are possible. The best opportunity for this lies in the fact that all participants described all twenty roles with six *standard* constructs: kind-helpful, mean, selfish, strong, wise, and sexy. The data for this analysis are, therefore, counts of the number of times each person used a given standard construct to describe each role. Correlation coefficients represent the similarity between one person's use of the construct and that of another. The matrix of correlations was factor analyzed; the table of factor loadings shows which persons used the construct similarly. The same procedures were performed on the other five constructs; resulting groupings were then compared for similarities. The comparison shows that Willie, Tom, and John make up one group while George, Bill, Al, and Rufus make up a second. Fred is a loner. The meanings of these findings are not obvious. Except for the isolation of Fred, this grouping could not have been anticipated. Possibly the ambiguity results from applying quantitative procedures that are too sophisticated for the data.

Other Morphogenic Measures

Ratings

Each person rated ten drugs on twenty-six scales. In chapters 3-11, factor analyses show how each groups the ten drugs in his own mind. It has also been possible to factor persons as well as of drugs. For example, all persons' ratings of cocaine have been intercorrelated and factor-analyzed. The result is that persons rating the drug similarly have high loadings on the same factors. Similar procedures have been followed for the other concepts rated.

The complex structure that has emerged does not lend itself to interpretation. These men are far from uniform in their ratings, and any attempt to represent their opinions by averaging scale values would be misleading. The true state of affairs virtually requires that each person be treated separately.

Setting Survey

For each of eleven environmental settings every participant described his penetration into the setting (i.e., the type of activity he engaged in), his satisfaction with what occurred, the number of times he entered the setting in the previous week, and the number of hours spent there during the previous week. Each of these measures was summed for each person, and four factor analyses among persons were performed.

Three groups of persons emerged. The first consists of Willie, John, George, and Bill; the second of Arky, Rufus, and Fred; and the third of Al and Tom. The first group displays conventional patterns of activity, especially with respect to work. The second group is less conventional. The third describes unconventional patterns of activities — they reported not working at all.

Drug Preferences

The existence of a large single factor on drug preference rankings would indicate that the men share a common set of values about drugs. Actually, two preference factors and one isolate appear. The first factor contains six persons. Arky and George — who like amphetamine more than most others — form a second factor. Bill — the lone snorter — is unique; except for cocaine use, his pattern is so different that he does not belong in the same analysis with the others (table 12.3).

TABLE 12.3. Ranked Preference for Drugs

Substance	Members of Factor I	Members of Factor II	Bill
Amphetamine	8	3	5
Barbiturates	7	5	6
Beer	5	7	3
Cocaine	2	1	1
Hard liquor	6	8	4
Heroin	3	4	9
LSD	9	9	7
Marijuana	4	6	2
Speedball	1	2	8

Note: Factor I contains Rufus, Willie, Fred, Al, John, and Tom. Factor II contains Arky and George. The main difference between the two factors is in the preference for amphetamine. Low rank indicates high preference.

DRUG USE PATTERNS

Years of Experience with Drugs

Overall, black participants were older (mean = 38.67 years of age) than the whites (mean = 25.93 years). Black participants ranged from twenty-one to twenty-three years of age when they first tried cocaine, and ranged from seventeen to nineteen years old when they first tried other hard drugs (mean = 18 years). White participants were somewhat younger (sixteen to twenty-three years old), when they first tried cocaine (mean = 17.83 years) as well as other hard drugs (fourteen to twenty-two years of age; mean = 17.50 years).

However, due to age differences, black participants appeared in our project to have more years of experience with hard drugs than whites. The blacks had used cocaine for an average of 9.67 years and other hard drugs for an average of 15.67 years. White participants had used cocaine for an average of 5.17 years and other hard drugs for an average of 7.50 years.

The genealogies of drug use reveal that all participants initiated drug use with either alcohol or marijuana; both black and white participants used an average of five drug substances prior to their initial use of cocaine, which drugs included an average of two other hard drugs — primarily heroin and other opiates among blacks and amphetamine, barbiturates, or opiates among whites; and white participants experimented with a somewhat wider variety of substances (mean = 10.83 drugs) than blacks (mean = 8.33), who avoided hallucinogens and had only limited experience with barbiturates or amphetamine.

Introduction to Cocaine and Reactions to First-Time Use

All but one man was introduced to cocaine by friends or acquaintances. The exception was Bill, who sought out a dealer himself and purchased a small quantity.

Six men — Arky, Rufus, Fred, George,Tom, and Willie — were surprised by the intense sense of well-being that accompanied their first intravenous use of cocaine. John, however, reported a neutral, if not negative, reaction. He may have injected low-grade cocaine at this time, because when he later tried pharmaceutical cocaine his reaction mirrored that reported by others. Bill was disappointed by his experience, while Al was frightened. Though seven men had had previous experience snorting it, the effects accompanying injection were so unique that some said it was as if they were using a different drug.

Social Context

Low-level use of cocaine (see "Level of Use" below) often took place in gatherings of from four to a dozen or more users. Among moderate users — Arky, Rufus, and John — from two to four other persons might participate. However, among heavy users — Fred, George, Tom, and Willie — the drug was typically taken either alone or with no more than one or two trusted friends.

Daily Patterns

Most of the men took cocaine at night. Five definitely preferred to use cocaine in the evening hours, except during a run. Many reasons were offered for this, including the facts that some participants worked during daytime hours; others used cocaine to stay alert on evening jobs; it is safer to transact drug sales after dark, and it is also safer to use cocaine at night in the privacy of one's home.

Two men began daily cocaine use in the morning hours. George practiced intravenous use after breakfast to "fire him up" for a day's work. John had no legal employment while practicing his heavy cocaine use; while eating, he started his day with the elevation of mood the drug provided. He admitted, however, that he did not always adhere to this pattern. Bill and Rufus would use the drug whenever it was available.

Procedures for Determining Drug Quality

A wide variety of procedures were reported for determining the quality of cocaine. These include looking for brilliance in flakes or crystals, determining quality by cost or reputation of the dealer, using Clorox; testing its solubility in water, knowing where the drug was obtained (if obtained in a drugstore burglary, the participant was certain it was pharmaceutical cocaine), assessing the rush and alcoholic fume or taste accompanying injection, and assaying the drug in a professional laboratory. This last method was used only by Tom when purchasing in kilo amounts.

Bill and Al relied on the dealer. Most intravenous cocaine users were very pragmatic about how to determine quality; they preferred to shoot a sample and felt that they could determine the quality by the accompanying rush and the fume. Both Tom and Willie indicated that most cocaine users were unable to discriminate between cocaine and procaine; Tom ridiculed the idea that anyone would be able to determine quality by visual inspection.

EXTENT OF COCAINE USE

The effects of cocaine result from a complex interaction of several factors, including method of administration, amount used, quality or purity, frequency of use, whether an antagonistic agent is used in conjunction with the cocaine (for example, as in speedballing), and idiosyncratic reactions to the drug. Given these considerations, we have ranked our nine men in terms of their habitual level of cocaine usage from low to intermediate to high ("heavy"). We have taken into account the use of opiates in conjunction with cocaine, our reasoning being that cocaine buffered with heroin would produce more moderate reactions than the same amount of cocaine without buffering. By contrast, the use of opiates only at the end of a cocaine high constitutes an effort to eliminate unpleasant after effects of the cocaine experience, not to moderate the experience itself.

One additional consideration was taken into account, that of access to the drug. Even people with a great deal of money may not use all the cocaine they would like to, because it is hard to have access to a large supply. Ready availability of high-grade cocaine was therefore regarded as a condition for a high level of usage.

Level of Use

At the lowest level of use is Bill, an intranasal user who consumes at most about a quarter gram of street cocaine in two or three days. Next is Al, who uses about one-third gram of street cocaine a day. Al takes cocaine intravenously and probably could get more of the substance than Bill, because he has better access to it.

The next two (intermediate) positions are occupied by Arky and Rufus. Arky reported intermittent use of about a gram a day of pharmaceutical cocaine, while Rufus reported a daily use of one gram of cocaine, primarily "rock crystal." John used a gram or more of pharmaceutical cocaine per day. He was better situated to regulate his supply — for example, by living with a woman dealer — than Arky. Consequently, John is placed slightly higher than Arky or Rufus on the continuum.

Fred, Tom, Willie, and George all reported taking three grams or more per day. Thus they form a group whose use is distinctly higher than those below them. Fred uses primarily street cocaine, Tom used rock crystal, and George used pharmaceutical cocaine. Fred was therefore placed lowest on our scale, with Tom next. Willie reported having used about four grams of rock crystal daily. However, he estimated that his cocaine was only 50-60 percent pure; George was therefore identified as the highest user in the group because of the greater purity of the substance he used.

Usage Level and Psychological Test Scores

Rank-order correlation coefficients (Kendall's τ) have been calculated to compare usage level with data from dimensional and morphogenic tests. On the MMPI, usage level correlates positively and significantly ($\tau = .500$) with scores on the F Scale and Scales 4 (Pd) and 7 (Pt). Another positive, though not quite significant, correlation ($\tau = .444$) appears between usage level and scores on Scales 2 (D), 6 (Pa), and 8 (Sc). These findings suggest that heavier usage of cocaine is associated with unconventionality, antisocial attitudes, self-assertiveness, tension, anxiety, depression, suspiciousness, and tendencies to withdraw.

Scores on the Novelty Experiencing Scale tend to correlate negatively with usage level, indicating that heavier usage is associated with lowered interest in novel or unusual experiences. The trend was very strong on the Internal Cognitive Subscale (τ = $-.889$), a finding consistent with the observation that heavier users take cocaine not to activate thought but to deaden it.

On the Q-Sorts, reliabilities of sortings relate negatively and significantly to use level (τ = $-.556$ for standard items; τ = $-.500$ for individualized items). Thus, heavy use is associated here with relative instability — or else with inconsistency of descriptions. Self-satisfaction, as measured by correlations between the usual self and the ideal self, relates negatively and significantly to dosage level on the individualized items (τ = $-.500$). The relationship of dosage level to self-dissatisfaction, as measured by correlations between usual-self and worst-self sortings, is positive and significant (τ = $.611$).

Usage Level and Drug Reactions

An examination has been conducted of participants' estimates of the frequency with which cocaine produces specific physiological and psychological reactions. Five patterns appear in the relationships between usage level and frequency of occurrence of specific reactions to the drug. In the following discussion, each pattern is first described; then the physiological and psychological reactions that apply to each pattern of relationship are identified.

These findings must be interpreted in light of the fact that participants' responses to direct questions about specific reactions (phrased in quantitative terms) were sometimes not consistent with spontaneous comments they made in less structured interviews. Such discrepancies appear primarily in Pattern N, a pattern that implies no relationship between dosage and effect. For example, mydriasis (pupilary dilation) was reported as infrequent by some men who nonetheless commented spontaneously about visual disturbances (misty vision, etc.) that implied its occurrence. Also, sexuality does not seem to be dosage-related when examined in a purely quantitative manner. Nevertheless, as is shown in chapter 13, interview data reveal a clear inverse relationship between sexual interest and level of usage.

Discrepancies like these are not frequent in the data. However, when findings were affected by this methodological problem, the difficulty usually arose from poor wording of specific items or from failure to follow up leads, rather than from inherent defects in the general approach to measurement.

Pattern C (Common Reactions at All Usage Levels)

This pattern consists of reactions said by seven or more participants to occur at least 50 percent of the time they use cocaine. These reactions are therefore frequent, regardless of habitual level of usage of the drug.

Physiological Reactions
One reaction was virtually universal; all nine men said it occurs 100 percent of the time cocaine is used. It is loss of fatigue. The other reactions in this

category are: intensely accelerated mental activity, dryness of mouth, increased heart rate, sweating, loss of appetite, increased pulse rate, and increased respiration rate.

Because higher levels of usage are more frequent than lower ones among these nine men, the data are not conclusive; but they do suggest that inclusion of more cases at the low-usage level might show all reactions — except loss of fatigue — to diminish at these lower levels of use. To illustrate this, figure 12.1 shows the relationship between usage level and reports of the frequency of occurrence of increased pulse rate. Data for this figure were obtained by averaging within each group the percentages reported by the four highest-level users, the three intermediate-level users, and the two lowest-level users. The figure shows that, although the reaction is common at all levels, there is a tendency for frequency of occurrence to diminish at lower levels of cocaine usage.

Psychological Reactions

Although no psychological reaction is universal, six meet the criteria for inclusion as common responses to cocaine. These are: increased activity and restlessness, increased thinking power, more talkative, insomnia, euphoria, and mind quicker than normal.

FIGURE 12.1. Relationship between Dosage Level and Increased Pulse Rate (Pattern C).

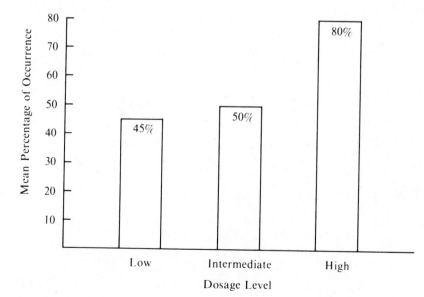

Pattern HI (Heavy and Intermediate Users Only)

This pattern consists of reactions reported by from three to six men as occurring for at least 50 percent of their cocaine use and that are more prominent among heavy and intermediate-level users than among low-level users. Figure 12.2 illustrates pattern HI for the reaction tinnitus (ringing in the ears). It also shows the tendency, common in these data, for frequency of occurrence to drop off slightly at the highest usage level; in many instances, however, this tendency is due to the exceptionally low reports of deviant responses by Willie.

Physiological Reactions

Pattern HI appears in reports of the occurrence of tinnitus, diarrhea, weight loss, vomiting, dizziness, and tightness in the chest.

Psychological Reactions

The three psychological reactions displaying Pattern HI are indifference to pain, increased feelings of self-control, and depression and anxiety.

Pattern H (Heavy Users Only)

This pattern consists of reactions reported by from three to six men as occurring at least 50 percent of their cocaine use and that are prominent only among heavy users. Figure 12.3 illustrates Pattern H for the reaction of paranoid ideas.

FIGURE 12.2. Relationship between Dosage Level and Tinnitus (Pattern HI).

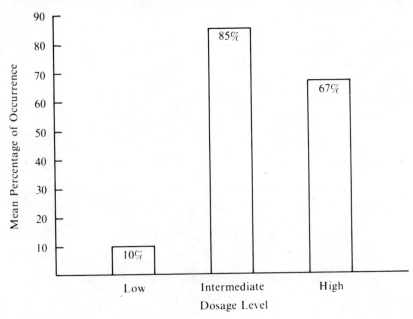

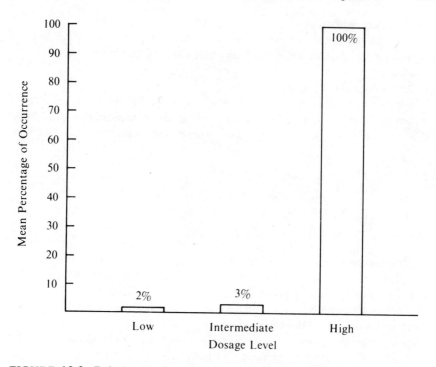

FIGURE 12.3. Relationship between Dosage Level and Paranoid Ideas (Pattern H).

Physiological Reactions

No physiological reactions display Pattern H.

Psychological Reactions

A large number of psychological reactions (seven) are characterized Pattern H. One such reaction is a pleasant one — feeling everything is perfect. Another is neutral or ambiguous — decreased interest in work. The rest reflect distortions of reality — changes in perception of reality and auditory hallucinations — and frightening mental conditions — paranoid ideas, irrational fears, and terror and panic. Along with the depression and anxiety reported as part of Pattern HI, these reactions can only be construed as indicating that a high price in mental anguish is paid for a few moments of ecstasy.

Pattern N (No Relation of Reactions to Usage Level)

This pattern consists of reactions reported by from three to six men as occuring at least 50 percent of the time but that are not clearly related to habitual level of drug use.

Physiological Reactions
Four physiological reactions appear to be unrelated to habitual level of cocaine use: gooseflesh, mydriasis, headache, and local numbness.

Psychological Reactions
Five psychological reactions appear to display Pattern N. Three involve sexual behavior — prolonged sexual intercourse, better orgasm, and aphrodisiac; the other two are: increased physical strength and olfactory hallucinations.

Pattern U (Uncommon at All Levels)

This pattern contains reactions reported by only one or two men to occur at least 50 percent of the time they used cocaine. They are therefore uncommon at any level of habitual use.

Physiological Reactions
A large group of the uncommon physiological reactions reflects the fact that only one participant administered cocaine intranasally. The occurrence of many of these reactions would have been higher in a group predominantly of lower-level intranasal users: rhinorrhea, hyperemia, nosebleed, nasal infection, lacrimation, cellulitis, yawning, and increased sensitivity to allergenic substances.

Three other reactions represent disturbances or pathological effects that were not reported at all by any of the men: fainting, convulsions, and hepatitis (attributed to poor care of injection apparatus). Although convulsions were denied, several men admitted to tremors or muscle spasms: Four said these occurred less than 50 percent of the time; however, one high-level user (Tom) and one intermediate level user (John) said they occurred 100 percent of the time cocaine was used.

Psychological Reactions
Three uncommon psychological reactions deserve special note because, although they occurred infrequently, when they did occur it was *only* at the highest level of usage: visual hallucinations, cause you to carry a gun, don't care about the world. Other reactions displaying Pattern U were: physical orgasm with rush, increased optimism and courage, and tactile hallucinations.

Integration

The findings reported above are summarized in Table 12.4. On the one hand, the data clearly display the stimulating effects of cocaine at all rates of use. Physiologically, the drug is associated with arousal of the central nervous system and the sympathetic nervous system. Psychologically, it is associated with pleasurable feelings, wakefulness, and a more rapid general pace of behavior.

On the other hand, at the high and intermediate levels of usage the number of unpleasant — not to say pathological — responses is also great. On the physiological side these perhaps are not so serious, consisting of such reactions as dizziness, vomiting, tinnitus, and diarrhea. Psychologically, however, they can be quite serious, involving intense fear or anxiety, paranoid ideation, and severe depression. Paradoxically, at high levels of use cocaine produces some of the same problems — especially depression and anxiety — that low-level users may be taking cocaine to alleviate.

There seems to be a threshold effect, in that certain reactions almost never reported at intermediate or low levels of usage appear suddenly, and fairly frequently, at the highest usage level. This threshold effect is especially noticeable for paranoid ideas (see figure 12.3), but it occurs for nearly all psychological reactions listed under Pattern H. Even the three psychological reactions described under Pattern HI show a sudden increase from no occurrence at low-level usage to common occurrence at intermediate and high levels of habitual use.

Possibly the reason for this rests on the dependence of psychological reactions on cognitive processes. A physical symptom such as diarrhea or emesis can be recognized, accepted, and reported relatively easily. However, terror, panic, paranoia, and depression may be less easy to admit. Perhaps the natural tendency is to deny unpleasant feelings, such as fear, unless they reach such intensity that they cannot be ignored.

LIFE STYLE AND COCAINE USE

The preceding discussion has not considered molar or inclusive relationships that are difficult to quantify. This section describes correlates of usage level that become apparent only upon examination of the more subtle, qualitative, and integrative features of each participant's life.

Pleasure as a Reason for Taking Cocaine

Participants at the low end of the usage continuum (especially Bill) tend to take cocaine mainly for pleasure: to enhance sensory experience and sociability or open up a joyful world of fantasy and wish-fulfillment. Bill seems to be seeking a kind of Disneyland existence in which all is sweetness, light, and good clean fun. Neither Al nor Arky ever express much wish to use cocaine for any purpose other than sensuous enjoyment.

John and Rufus are transitional cases. In John one occasionally sees the same adolescent desire to use cocaine for sheer pleasure found with Bill; but he also uses the drug for more serious purposes. Cocaine certainly produces enjoyable states for Rufus — the only participant who reported having had an orgasm

TABLE 12.4. Summary of Relationships between Usage Level and Reported Reactions to Cocaine.

Pattern	Physiological Reactions	Psychological Reactions
C Common at All Levels	Loss of fatigue (universal) Hyperphrenia Dryness of mouth and throat Increased Heart rate Sweating Anorexia Increased Pulse Rate Increased Respiration Rate	Increased activity, restlessness Increased thinking power More talkative Insomnia Euphoria
HI Heavy and Intermediate Users Only	Ringing in Ears Diarrhea Weight loss Emesis Dizziness Tightness in chest	Indifference to pain Increased feelings of self-control Depression, anxiety
H Heavy Users Only	(None)	Paranoid ideas Irrational fears Terror, panic Feeling everything is perfect Decreased interest in work Changes in perception of reality Auditory hallucinations

N

No Relation to Usage Level

Gooseflesh
Mydriasis
Headache
Local numbness

Increased physical strength
Prolonged sexual intercourse
Aphrodisiac
Better orgasm
Olfactory hallucinations

Visual hallucinations
Cause me to carry a gun
Don't care about world
Tactile hallucinations
Trigger for violence
Physical orgasm with rush
Increased optimism, courage

U

Uncommon at all levels

Hyperemia (stuffy nose)
Tremors, spasms
Increased allergic sensitivity
Rhinorrhea
Lacrimation
Cellulitis
Hepatitis
Fainting
Yawning
Nasal infection
Nosebleed
Convulsions

445

with the rush — but cocaine is also the "pimp's drug," and taking it is necessary for Rufus to retain the prestige he needs in order to stay in operation. Above Rufus's level of usage, cocaine seems to be taken for reasons more central to life style.

Sustaining the Self-Concept

Except for Rufus, persons mentioned so far do not take cocaine to prop up their personality integration. However, Fred needs drugs to support his self-concept. Taking cocaine identifies him as an important person. More significant, cocaine provides the ideal weapon in the running battle with his father around which Fred's life is built. Finally, cocaine provides him with a necessary release for the tensions of his lonely, self-defeating existence.

The relationship of cocaine to self-concept is obvious with both George and Tom. George used the drug to keep himself in a sufficiently high state of drive to maintain a competitive edge in his profession. Cocaine helped keep Tom on his toes and helped sustain the continuous level of tension he seemed to need to preserve his identity — and perhaps his life.

Finally, Willie is in a class by himself. In Willie's life cocaine makes a hopeless existence endurable. Willie built a successful career in a dangerous, violent, and demanding profession, but now he doubts the value of his accomplishments. Willie takes cocaine to escape, not into paradise but into forgetfulness.

Emotional Intensity (Anger)

The correspondence between usage level and emotional intensity is close, especially where anger is concerned. Bill will run from situations in which strong feelings are aroused. Al floats along on the surface of his emotional life; though he is often frightened, his fears are realistic.

Arky would like to be emotionally low-toned, but there are rumblings that speak of angry impulses ready to break through. In John's case the expression of hostile feelings takes on a cyclical character; it makes him sometimes intensely emotional, sometimes depressed and miserable.

Rufus's feelings seldom get out of hand. They often influence his behavior, but they are rarely inappropriate. Rufus knows what he wants and is not afraid to feel strongly about getting it.

Fred, Tom, Willie, and George are all highly emotional people. They are keyed up, vibrant, alert, on edge, and capable of acting passionately. Fred seems nearly psychotic when his emotions threaten to take over his personality. Tom was in many ways like a caged beast likely to leap out at anyone carelessly opening the door. Willie is so full of anger — transformed into despair — that he is ready to burst. George channels his strength into his effort to become a machine or fortress. Compared to these men low-dosage users seem to be made of cardboard, at least with respect to this characteristic of depth and intensity of feelings.

Escape

All nine participants may be using cocaine for escape, but not all are escaping from the same thing or into the same state. Willie is fighting a losing battle with a seemingly pointless, degrading life, but he will not give up the struggle. Something similar applied to Tom and George. They used cocaine to escape the vulnerability of their true selves; it became an ally in their battles against harsh, unvanquishable consciences.

Toward the center of the usage continuum, Fred uses cocaine both as a weapon and as an escape from his own personality. For Fred cocaine provides an escape from tension, but it is also an integral part of his life.

Rufus, too, is characterized by tendencies to escape. Rufus is escaping from the internal self that he has tried to eliminate. Cocaine is only part of a total life style directed toward avoidance of inner experiences.

John represents a transitional state. On the one hand, John wants middle-class respectability; On the other, he has such low tolerance for middle-class life that he takes drugs to make life endurable. It is as if he were using the drug to escape from being well-adjusted. At the same time, John also uses cocaine for the fantasy-like existence it supports.

Engagement

Most of what has been said regarding the integration of cocaine into life styles can be related to the complex but important variable of level of engagement with life. At low levels of usage engagement is not intense; in fact, it is often avoided. Cocaine provides a ticket to an ecstatic reality where life is pleasant and troubles are few. Several men give the impression that if they had to face the stern realities of life unaided they would cave in or give up. That is certainly true of Bill, who runs from conflicts. It is also true of Al, who knew he would never be a success; he would have loved to take cocaine all the time, though he had learned to accept the likelihood that that was impossible. Arky gets by as a thief, but his basic wish is to live an easy, carefree life away from the complexities of what he described as a "fucked up" world.

John tries to engage life, but cannot do so for long; he slips back to using cocaine whenever ordinary responsibilities become too heavy to bear. Rufus engages the external world effectively, but he cannot face his inner self. He invariably returns to active encounter with his environment; indeed, without such encounters, Rufus could not exist.

Fred, Tom, Willie, and George take life very seriously. They are totally immersed in their problems. Furthermore, they are all in their own ways strong, competent, and, in at least one case, dangerous individuals. They pay a price for their immersion and engagement. Without a miracle — which George has sought from God — each of these men seems fated to disaster or despair. Cocaine offers a respite, but no disentanglement, from life. One might suppose that the contrast with life that it provides only makes their suffering worse.

Additional Psychosocial Considerations

Nearly all participants have had serious problems in their relationships with their fathers. In most cases, these problems have led to identifications with the father that were weak, faulty, or conflictual. Tom and Fred provide two clear examples of antagonistic identifications. Arky exemplifies the problems that arise from having in effect no father at all, psychologically speaking.

Several men also reported having tough, resilient, firm, and domineering mothers. As a result, intimate relations with persons of the other sex are lacking in many participants. For some, the impossibility of intimacy spreads to all persons.

All participants are products of American culture, perhaps to an extreme. All want to escape from the world unless they can achieve what they regard as the ultimate in success — acquiring wealth and admiration through aggressive self-assertion, winning the war of life by competing harder than anyone else.

Of course, the characteristics noted above might well be found in people who use other drugs or no drugs at all. More data are needed if these possibilities are to be fairly and objectively evaluated.

Conclusions

13

SPECIFIC EFFECTS OF COCAINE

Introduction

Petersen and Stillman (1977) state that a "bewildering array" of physical and psychological effects have been said to be associated with use of cocaine. They are unquestionably correct, for in preparing this report we found more than 200 different — and often contradictory — cocaine-related reactions reported in the literature. Our research was designed to test many beliefs about the effects of cocaine. It has examined both intranasal and intravenous methods of drug administration (though only one man practiced snorting exclusively, seven others had snorted and were familiar with its effects). Also, our studies measured the effects of cocaine at differing usage levels, ranging from intranasal use of from fifty to a hundred milligrams of cocaine on weekends to intravenous use of three or more grams per day for several years. Many factors can modify subjective drug effects; therefore we selected users who had sufficient experience with the drug to speak with authority about it, questioned all participants extensively using the same interview items, and concentrated interview questions on typical rather than unusual or idiosyncratic reactions.

This chapter evaluates several categories of belief about cocaine's effects. First it considers a variety of physiological reactions said to be associated with use of cocaine. It then discusses a large group of psychological reactions reportedly associated with use of the drug. Within each category of effects, find-

449

ings and conclusions that have been reported by other investigators are summarized first. These are then evaluated in the light of our data.

The physiological and psychological effects of cocaine discussed in this section are as follows:

Physiological Effects
    Cardiovascular Effects
    Sensory-Motor Effects (General Sensory-Motor Effects; Visual-Motor Effects; Stereotypy)
    Vegetative-Metabolic Effects
    (General Vegetative-Metabolic Effects; The Issue of Addiction; Dosage; Method of Administration; and Lethality)
Psychological Effects
    Affective-Psychosocial States
    Affective-Psychophysical States: Sexuality
    Affective-Psychophysical States: Other
    Cognitive Effects
    Characterological Effects
The Toxic Cocaine Reaction

The sections that follow present some methodological notes and our assessment of the value of the Representative Case Method in this type of research. A preliminary theory describing cocaine's effects upon human behavior is presented and its effects are compared with those of another stimulant, amphetamine. Finally, we summarize our conclusions concerning the relationships between life styles and cocaine use and present some preliminary ideas for a theory of psychological structure that has emerged in this research.

Physiological Effects

Cardiovascular Effects

Previous reports. Some of the most firmly established responses to cocaine involve sympathomimetic stimulation of the cardiovascular system. These effects include increased heart and respiration rates (Fischman et al., 1976; Post et al., 1974; Resnick et al., 1977) as well as increases in systolic or diastolic blood pressure (Byck and Van Dyke, 1977; Fischman et al.; Post et al.; Resnick et al.). Evidence as to whether cocaine produces cardiac abnormalities is mixed, with some investigators reporting cardiac arrhythmia, including bigeminal rhythms and multiple ectopic ventricular contractions, and angina pectoris (Orr and Jones, 1968; Young and Glauber, 1947), and others reporting no evidence of such effects (Post et al.; Resnick et al.).

Our findings. Our studies, by and large, confirm the findings reported by other investigators. All participants agreed that cocaine increases heart and pulse rate, and every one, with the exception of Willie M., reported increases in respiration rate. (Even Willie M. said that intravenous administration would "take [his] breath away.") Most of our men reported tightness in the chest immediately after injection, which then eased within a few minutes. Three high-dose users (Tom P., Fred S., and Willie M.) described incidents of severe precordial chest pains.

Sensory-Motor Effects

The sensory-motor effects of cocaine can be divided into three types: *general sensory-motor effects, visual-motor effects,* and *stereotypy.*

General Sensory-Motor Effects

Previous reports. Research findings indicate that increased restlessness and heightened activity and locomotor responses in animals — the mouse, rat, dog, and rhesus monkey — and man, accompany use of cocaine (Deneau, Yanagita, and Seevers, 1969; Fog, 1969; Ho, Taylor, Estevez, Englert, and McKenna, 1977; Johanson, Balster and Bonese, 1976; Tatum and Seevers, 1929). Other sensory-motor effects include increased muscle tone (Grinspoon and Bakalar, 1976), increased energy and alertness (Ashley, 1975; Reinarman, 1977; Siegel, 1977), chills, gooseflesh and piloerection or erection of the hair (Ritchie et al., 1970; Woods, 1977), hypersensitivity to noise (Chopra and Chopra, 1930/1931), *tinnitus* or a ringing or buzzing sensation in the ears (Grinspoon and Bakalar), dizziness and vertigo (Chopra and Chopra), tremors and *dyskinesia,* an inhibition or impairment of voluntary movement producing fragmentary or incompleted responses (Post, Kopanda, and Black, 1976), *dysmetria,* or the improper measurement of distances in muscular acts (Deneau et al., 1969; Johanson et al., 1976), deafness (Chopra and Chopra), convulsions, particularly with overdose (Eddy, Halbach, Isbell, and Seevers, 1965; Post, 1977; Woods), and numbness or anesthesia at the site of drug application (Barash, 1977; Goldberg, 1967; Waldorf et al., 1977).

Our findings. This research supports the contention that cocaine produces increased restlessness, excitement, and need for activity. Although the effects upon muscle tone could not be determined, there was a consensus among the men that they felt more alert and energetic when using the drug. While all experienced increased restlessness, excitement, energy, and need for activity, only a few could use these capabilities constructively. The following comments are typical: "You feel strong and powerful, but you're not interested in work"; "You feel like you could do anything you wanted but the only thing that you're interested in is the next hit."

Reports of chills and gooseflesh were not uncommon, but were interpreted differently by different users. Arky L. described it as electricity going through his body, while Fred S. described the chills and gooseflesh as anticipatory responses. There was only one report of piloerection (Arky L.), but the absence of other reports of this effect is probably due to the fact that the investigators failed to ask about it directly.

None of the low- or intermediate-dose users reported hypersensitivity to noise in conjunction with their use of cocaine. However, some high-dosage users, particularly Tom P., Fred S., and George B., reported intense auditory hypersensitivity and strong startle reactions. They often misinterpreted normal sounds − "A guy turned on the water in the bathroom. I thought it was a snake and jumped up with my gun to kill the son of a bitch!" "When I was shooting, I would hear a noise and almost jump out of my skin."

Tinnitus or ringing in the ears was a common reaction, and most men reported that dizziness or light-headedness accompanied the rush. Occasional tremors in extremities occurred, but no one reported dyskinesia, dysmetria, deafness, or convulsions. All experienced anesthesia at the site of drug application and some heavy users reported generalized body numbness after injection of two or three grams of cocaine.

Visual-Motor Effects

Previous reports.   A variety of visual-motor effects are reportedly associated with the use of cocaine. One of the most firmly documented ocular effects is *mydriasis* or extreme pupillary dilation (Byck and Van Dyke, 1977; Johanson et al., 1976; P. Schultz, 1898). Kuroda (1915) attributed mydriasis to paralysis of the smooth muscle fibers of the iris. Woods and Downs (1973) contend, however, that it is caused by enhancement of norepinephrine released tonically from sympathetic fibers that normally innervate the radial muscles of the iris. Among users this effect is described as increased light sensitivity, visual haziness, "fuzziness" of objects, halos around lights, and difficulties in binocular vision. Siegel (1977) says that *exophthalmos,* or protrusion of the eyeball, and *cycloplegia,* or paralysis of the ciliary muscles of the eye, are associated with use of the drug.

Siegel's 1977 study of intranasal use of cocaine cites a variety of other visual disturbances. These effects, which Siegel labels "pseudohallucinations," include sensations of movement in the peripheral visual field similar to that reported by amphetamine abusers (Ellinwood, 1972) and flashes or spots of light ("snow lights") in the visual field. During the later stages of use, Siegel's subjects saw geometric patterns − straight lines, points, curves, stars, stripes, zigzags, herringbones, checkerboards, and lattices − in peripheral visual fields. Other visual effects include double vision or *polyopia, micropsia,* and *macropsia,* disturbances in which objects and people appear smaller or larger than actual size, and *dysmorphopsia,* or distortions in the shapes of perceived objects.

Our findings.   Most of the men in our study would agree with the user who said, "Cocaine really screws up your vision." All but one (Rufus B.) reported that mydriasis or related visual anomalies were common sequelae to the use of cocaine. Most reported increased sensitivity to light —"Bright lights hurt your eyes" — difficulties with binocular vision — "You can't see things so well on coke" — visual haziness — "Everything looks fuzzy." "Everything got so hazy that sometimes I'd miss a vein" — and the classic "snow" effects — "After two grams everything gets misty, milky, and hazy." "After two grams the room looks like a fog or a snowstorm." Two men reported that colors appeared richer, warmer, and brighter, and two reported that occasionally the room would darken as if someone had turned down the lights. Several reported "squiggles" in the visual field and visual floaters, but none reported apparent movement in peripheral visual fields or perceptions of geometric patterns. Given the difficulties in binocular vision some of these men described, some may have experienced double vision, though they did not specifically report it. There were no reports of exophthalmos, cyloplegia or any marked distortions in the apparent size or shape of persons or objects (micropsia, macropsia, or dysmorphopsia). With heavy intravenous use of cocaine, visually perceived reality became fuzzy, hazy, and misty, but apparently retained its objective characteristics.

Stereotypy

Previous reports. A major response reported as resulting from heavy or chronic cocaine use is *stereotypy,* a compulsion to rigidly repeat certain acts. In animal studies, stereotypy is the tendency to perform a single activity or sets of activities — sniffing, licking, biting, gnawing, circling, head-rearing, and other motor behavior — continuously after drug administration.

Amphetamine and some of its derivatives can produce marked stereotyped or compulsive behavior in humans. Ellinwood (1972) aptly described such stereotypy in amphetamine psychosis: "Watches, doorknobs, television sets, radios and phonographs, tape recorders, typewriters, and children's toys were among the common items of curiosity and repetitious analysis. . . . One man dismantled a $1,200 hi-fi set. Another sorted, filed, and put on display repainted electronic parts, both new and worthless ones. . . . Many of the prepsychotic patients reported a sense of satisfaction just from repetitious performance of an act. Some would literally spend days cleaning a room or polishing a car. One man polished and painted everything around. He tiled his apartment, including the walls, in Armstrong vinyl pebble tiling, then painted the individual pebbles red, yellow, gold, and black" (p. 151).

Stereotypy has been demonstrated following administration of large (100–600 mg./kg.) doses of cocaine in the rat (Fog, 1969; Randrup and Munkvad, 1970), the cat (Wallace and Gershon, 1971), the dog (Tatum and Seevers, 1929), and in some studies with rhesus monkeys (Tatum and Seevers, 1929; Wilson, Bedford, Buelke, and Kibbe, 1976). Stripling and Ellinwood (1977) have demonstrated that chronic administration of cocaine (20–40 mg./kg.) produces stereotyped behavior in rats. Scheel-Kruger, Braestrup, Nielson, Golembiowska, and Mogilnicka (1977) note, however, that while cocaine can induce stereotyped behavior in laboratory animals it never produces the characteristic compulsive, continuous, and restricted performance so easily demonstrated with amphetamine, its phenethylamine derivatives, or apomorphine.

Post (1977) obtained contradictory findings with rats and rhesus monkeys. Chronic administration of 10 mg./kg. i.p. of cocaine increased hyperactivity and stereotyped behaviors in rats; however, chronic administration of 10-17 mg./kg. i.p. of cocaine in rhesus monkeys produced some initial stereotypy but was more predominantly associated with motor inhibition. The animals became cataleptic, engaged in staring and visual tracking of nonexistent objects, and evidenced oral-buccal-lingual dyskinesias.

A number of investigators (Fischman, Schuster, and Krasnegor, 1977; Jaffe, 1970; Kramer et al., 1967) have postulated that stereotyped behavior can be a symptom of heavy or prolonged cocaine use in humans. Post (1975) reports stereotyped behavior can be one of the symptoms of cocaine-induced paranoid psychosis, while Grinspoon and Bakalar (1976) state that stereotypy may be evidenced in the chronic cocaine users' "exaggerated sense of meaningfulness" and their compelling desire to put things in order.

Our findings. Our studies provide no support for the hypothesis that heavy cocaine use produces stereotyped behavior in humans, nor do the data support a hypothesis that users undergo dyskinesic or cataleptic reactions. The absence of stereotyped behavior among these chronic, high-dose cocaine users contrasts sharply with the easily recognized stereotypes — taking a motorcycle apart in a living room and polishing all the parts, playing a guitar for two days, washing a car fifteen or twenty times, cleaning an already immaculate apartment again and again — found in our subsequent research with amphetamine abusers. The cocaine users in this study experience intense excitement, restlessness, and anxiety, feel alert and energetic, experience euphoria and acceleration of ideational activity, but, typically, they do not go anywhere or do anything; instead, they sit in a locked room experiencing the "rush" or readying themselves for the next injection.

The absence of stereotypy in the behavior of chronic cocaine users injecting from one to eleven grams (George B.) of cocaine per day brings into question reported similarities in effect of cocaine and amphetamine, and suggests that insufficient attention has been given to the differences between these drugs (Ashley, 1975). Our findings, plus observations from animal research, suggest there may be important phylogenetic differences in response to cocaine. Stereotypy occurs in rats and dogs in response to both cocaine and amphetamine. However, in primates, such as rhesus monkeys and man, stereotypy occurs consistently only in response to amphetamine. Human responses to heavy use of cocaine seem to involve cognitive and affective processes more than motoric activities.

Vegetative-Metabolic Effects

There is a group of central effects triggered by cocaine which, for lack of a better term, we call vegetative-metabolic responses. These effects may be divided into four categories: a large group of diverse reactions which we have labeled *general vegetative-metabolic effects,* a cluster of drug-induced reactions having to do with whether cocaine produces *addiction or physical dependence* and *tolerance,* the effects of varying *dosage* and *methods of administration,* including consideration of the drug's *lethality,* and, finally, the *medical complications* associated with use of cocaine.

General Vegetative-Metabolic Effects

Previous reports. The general vegetative-metabolic effects of cocaine include *anorexia* or loss of apetite (Balster and Schuster, 1973; Eddy et al., 1965; Isbell and White, 1953; Kolb, 1962), weight loss (Dale, 1903; Grinspoon and Bakalar, 1976), insomnia and other sleep disturbances such as the reduction of REM and total sleep (Eddy et al.; Post et al., 1974; Wesson and Smith, 1977), reduction or abolition of fatigue (Ashley, 1975; Dale; Freud, 1884, in Byck, 1974; Hanna, 1974; Siegel, 1977), *hyperthermia* or elevation of body temperature (Clark, 1973; Van Dyke and Byck, 1977), dry mouth and throat (Grinspoon and Bakalar, 1976), nausea or vomiting (Byck and Van Dyke; Eddy et al.), pallor (Ashley, 1975), increased metabolic rate, *hyperglycemia* or abnormally increased blood sugar, reduction or decrease in stomach and intestinal activity, and constipation (Chopra and Chopra, 1930/1931; Grinspoon and Bakalar).

Our findings. All participants except the two who buffered cocaine with heroin (Al G. and Rufus B.), said that cocaine is a powerful anorectic. As a consequence, most reported that weight loss (frequently undesired) regularly accompanied prolonged use of cocaine. The general physiognomy of the men supported their comments. While none showed evidence of the emaciation, malnutrition, feebleness, or general debility described by early writers (Dale; Kolb, 1925b; Lewin, 1931), our men, as a group, were physically trim and displayed little extra body fat. Most reported that they could eat while on cocaine, but they had no appetite. They reported none of the physical distress, nausea, or pain associated with attempting to eat that was reported in subsequent research by a comparable group of amphetamine users.

All the men concurred that the insomnia and inability to rest, relax, or slow down mental activity after prolonged use of cocaine was one of its most troublesome side effects. The effect was sufficiently intense that they used opiates, tranquilizers, or even alcohol to terminate the drug's effects. While some investigators (Gay et al., 1973b; Waldorf et al., 1977) report that barbiturates are used to terminate the cocaine high, no one in these studies took barbiturates for this purpose; most disliked the unpleasant synergistic effects of the two drugs. High-grade heroin or Dilaudid were preferred because of their potency, "smoothness," and lack of adverse side effects.

At least three men (Tom P., George B., and Fred S.) became addicted to opiates in their efforts to control the adverse effects of cocaine. These results are consistent with the early findings of Mills (1905) and Gordon (1908) and the more recent observations of Kolb (1962) and Gay et al. (1973b). Paradoxically, two persons in these studies broke their opiate addiction with heavy use of cocaine; a third (George B.) underwent a "cold turkey" withdrawal from Dilaudid.

Although all our intravenous users reported insomnia and related symptoms to be a serious adverse effect of prolonged cocaine use, this effect is ignored in some studies. For example, none of the subjects in Siegel's research (1977) — some of whom reported effects suggestive of the toxic cocaine reaction — even mentioned insomnia. Our research indicates that cocaine is a powerful anti-fatigue agent; all users agreed that it not only reduced physical sensations of fatigue, it obliterated them. These findings are consistent with those reported by other investigators.

Most of our men said that heavy or profuse sweating regularly accompanied their cocaine use. If heavy or profuse sweating is symptomatic of hyperthermia or elevation of core body temperature, then our studies may be interpreted as confirming this effect.

Most of the men agreed that a dry mouth and throat ("cotton mouth") was a regular sequel to their use of cocaine. Vomiting was a frequent toxic reaction after prolonged or compulsive use, but nausea was even more common. Most of them felt nauseous whenever they used cocaine.

Increased pallor — which could result from peripheral vasoconstriction — is frequently mentioned in the literature as a symptom of cocaine toxicity. No one in these studies noticed paleness, lack of coloration in their skin, or *cyanosis* while using cocaine. This is not to say that such reactions did not occur. When one considers the intensity of the intravenous cocaine effect, its brevity, and the men's preoccupation with readying themselves for the next injection, it would hardly be surprising if they paid little attention to changes in skin coloration.

Clark (1973) reported that cocaine acts directly upon the CNS thermostat, setting it at a higher level. Thus, it would be logical to expect that cocaine might alter the body's metabolism. However, there was no way to test this hypothesis in our study. Similarly, the question of whether cocaine produces hyperglycemia could be best answered in the laboratory.

Grinspoon and Bakalar (1976) report that reduction in stomach or intestinal activity is a common reaction to heavy or prolonged use of cocaine, but Ashley (1975) reports that cocaine is a natural laxative that stimulates bowel movements and the bladder. Chopra and Chopra (1930/1931) reported that the stimulating effects of cocaine on the ganglia of Auerbach's plexus will often produce evacuation of the bowel as soon as it is taken. They noted, however, that this reaction is followed immediately by "obstinate" constipation. The men in our studies said that cocaine acted as a laxative and triggered complete bowel evacuation shortly after injection; they also reported increased urination. Our findings support Ashley's observations but seem contrary to those reported by Grinspoon and Bakalar. The apparent contradictions could be resolved if the bowel evacuation, increased urination, and subsequent reduction of intestinal activity are merely steps in physiological mobilization. A powerful CNS stimulant could produce these effects in mobilizing the organism for the emergency "fight or flight" reaction.

One might be inclined to attribute laxative effects to the cocaine "cut," for a variety of substances, including epsom salts, are used as cutting agents. However, given the consistency in response reported by people using varying qualities of cocaine obtained from diverse sources, the "cut" itself seems an unlikely causal agent.

The Issue of Addiction

Previous reports. According to Grinspoon and Bakalar (1976), the World Health Organization has concluded that cocaine produces neither *physical dependence* nor *tolerance,* but can produce an intense psychic dependence. Dependence of the cocaine type is "a state arising from repeated administration of cocaine or an agent with cocaine-like properties on a periodic or continuous basis. Its characteristics include: (1) an overpowering desire or need to continue taking the drug and to obtain it by any means; (2) absence of tolerance to the effects of the drug during continued administration; in the more frequent periodic use, the drug may be taken in short intervals, resulting in the build-up of an intense toxic reaction; (3) a psychic dependence on the effects of the drug related to a subjective and individual appreciation of these effects; and (4) absence of physical dependence and hence absence of an abstinence syndrome on abrupt withdrawal; withdrawal is attended by a psychic disturbance manifested by a craving for the drug" (p. 186).

Most investigators agree that since there is no physical dependence on cocaine there is no characteristic withdrawal or abstinence syndrome (Ashley, 1975; Burroughs, 1959; Isbell and White, 1953; Tatum and Seevers, 1929; Woods and Downs, 1973).

Evidence from animal studies suggests that with chronic use a *reverse tolerance* develops, so less cocaine is required to produce measurable effects. In animals, increased sensitivity is evidenced in hyperactivity, stereotypy, hyperthermia, and lowered thresholds for seizures and lethal doses. Recovery from drug-induced sensitivity may require from thirty to forty days of abstinence (Downs and Eddy, 1932a, 1932b; Matsuzaki et al., 1976; Post and Kopanda, 1975; Post and Rose, 1976; Stripling and Ellinwood, 1977).

Some investigators differ with the majority on these matters. Eiswirth et al. (1972) have claimed that with heavy use tolerance to cocaine develops rapidly, much as it does with amphetamine. They postulate that increased tolerance explains why heavy intravenous users can inject as much as ten grams of cocaine a day without lethal effects. However, Hatch and Fischer (1972) and Gunne and Johnsson (1964) were unable to demonstrate either tolerance or supersensitivity with repeated administrations of cocaine to animals. Wesson and Smith (1977) feel that, while psychological dependence definitely does occur, whether cocaine produces true physical dependence remains a question. They contend, however, that the depression that follows cocaine use may be viewed as a withdrawal state.

Our findings. The men in these studies agreed that cocaine is not physically addicting like the opiates. It was the opinion of most, though not all, heavy users that they developed *temporary tolerance* to the drug. They cited as evidence the fact that on "runs" they would have to increase the dosage to obtain a potent "rush": "When I first fire up I'm using a tenth of a gram and get a fantastic rush. . . . Before the night's out I'll be shooting a quarter gram a whack, but I never get back to that first rush." "After a gram I had to start increasing the hit to get the rush I wanted." In contrast, Willie M. stated that he never developed tolerance to cocaine and could inject the same amount all night and get the same effects, if the quality of the drug was good.

The development of "temporary tolerance" substantiates similar findings reported by Waldorf et al. (1977) with intranasal cocaine users. They noted that after regular use ("snorting" every twenty or thirty minutes) for a ten- or twelve-hour period, the user no longer experiences positive effects and may for that reason stop taking the drug. However, the next day he can take the original dose and experience the same effects. Most participants in these studies would agree with Arky L., who reported, "After approximately seventy-two hours, two good nights' sleep, and lots of water you can go back, start all over at the bottom, and get off good."

No heavy chronic cocaine users reported reverse tolerance. (Given their compulsive cocaine use and the relatively high cost of the drug, most would have been delighted had this occurred.)

The withdrawal or abstinence reactions that these men reported — physical and mental exhaustion, insomnia, an intense "wired" feeling, and inability to relax, along with depression and anxiety, and, in one case, suicidal ideas — do not resemble the abstinence syndrome accompanying opiate or barbiturate abuse but are similar to the overstimulation and post-reactive symptoms frequently described with amphetamine abuse (Ellinwood, 1972; D. E. Smith, 1969).

The participants in this research were clear about the strength of their attachment to cocaine. For them it is a powerful attachment, but not one of absolute necessity. Most know from experience what it is like to be addicted to a drug such as heroin. Although they might spend every cent they can get on cocaine, their need for it is of a different sort. For one thing, cocaine produces no long-term withdrawal or addictive symptoms. Some adverse effects were attributed to fatigue or to substances used to cut the drug. Other unavoidable ill effects are regarded as unimportant in comparison to benefits. The participants would undoubtedly say that their need for cocaine does not arise from any fear of withdrawal, but from an inability to give up the intense pleasure they feel the drug bestows.

Dosage, Method of Administration, and Lethality

Previous reports. Dosage is a critical variable because many of cocaine's effects are dosage-dependent. Woods (1977) contends that the magnitude and quality of every effect of cocaine depends on dose and route of administration.

However, aside from our studies, there has been very little research with humans designed to measure cocaine's effects at differing dosage levels.

Most recent research on humans involves relatively low dosages — ranging from 4 mg. to 105 mg. at one administration — or else street usage — ranging from 1 g. to 4 g. per week or month, with daily dose unspecified (Ashley, 1975; Byck et al., 1977; Fischman et al., 1977; Post et al., 1974; Siegel, 1977). In contrast, early research tended to focus upon clinical studies of heavy, chronic cocaine users (Gordon, 1908; Kolb, 1925a; Mills, 1905). Not surprisingly, this divergence in dosages studies has produced considerable variability, and even contradictions, in the conclusions drawn about cocaine's effects.

The most popular methods of cocaine administration today are *intranasal insufflation* or "snorting" and *intravenous injection*, with the former being far more popular than the latter.

These two methods of administration produce qualitatively different effects. With intranasal administration, cocaine reportedly produces a subtle, gradual sense of mild exhilaration and well-being that the experienced user becomes aware of within two or three minutes (Sabbag, 1976; Waldorf et al., 1977). Typically, the user becomes talkative and feels energetic and self-confident. Wesson and Smith (1977) report that the effects of a single dose diminish after twenty to forty minutes, generally with no discernible aftereffects. Ashley (1975) reports, however, that the effects can be felt in subdued form by a sensitive observer for some two hours after inhaling only 20–30 mg.

Intravenous administration involves larger doses, and produces almost instantaneous effects which endure in a pronounced way for approximately ten minutes (Ashley). Intravenous users experience an intense "rush" and dramatic "high." "This rush is almost universally described by sexual analogies, namely the orgasm. Unlike snorting, the effects are far from subtle and gradual, but take hold of the user immediately. Some users are startled by the immediacy of the effects" (Waldorf et al., 1977, p. 35). Burroughs (1959) described the intravenous experience somewhat differently: "The euphoria centers in the head. Perhaps the drug activates pleasure connections directly in the brain. I suspect that an electric current in the right place would produce the same effect. The full exhilaration of cocaine can only be realized by an intravenous injection. The pleasurable effects do not last more than five or ten minutes. If the drug is injected into the skin, rapid elimination vitiates the effects. This goes doubly for sniffing" (p. 249). Both the peak experience and "come down" arrive much more quickly with intravenous use than when snorting.

It is difficult to speak unambiguously about the lethal effects of cocaine, since reports vary greatly. A large number of cases of cocaine poisoning and death were reported in the early medical literature (Mattison, 1891; Mayer, 1924). Some of these were associated with substantial doses of cocaine. However, in some cases, death was associated with urethral administration of very small amounts of the drug — one to four grains, and in one case a third of a grain (Scheppegrell, 1898). It has been long known that a dose that might produce euphoria in one man could produce acute poisoning or even death in another; Such idiosyncratic responses may account for some of the deaths reported in the early literature.

A variety of other factors affect the lethality of cocaine. For example, Woods (1977) describes marked species differences in response. Doses that produce only a modest increase in locomotor behavior in a mouse will kill a rhesus monkey. Crowding or grouping mice increases lethality. Similarly, electrically shocking animals after administering cocaine will kill more of them, even though the shock alone is not strong enough to be lethal. Heat and exercise decrease the dose necessary to produce death, as does pretreatment with phenobarbital (Evans, Dwivedi, and Harbison, 1977).

In 1905, Mills estimated that the lethal dose of cocaine for humans under normal conditions lies between .5 g. and 1.25 g. More recently, the fatal dose has been estimated to be 1.2 g. or 1200 mg. after oral ingestion, and the LD_{50} (a dose which is lethal for 50 percent of test subjects) is estimated to be approximately 500 mg. after oral ingestion in a 150-pound man (Gay et al., 1973b). However, the fatal dose after application to mucous membrane may be as low as 20–30 mg. (Eiswirth, et al., 1972).

The incidence of deaths due to cocaine seems to be small, however. Finkle and McClosky (1977) conducted a retrospective survey involving twenty-seven medical examiners' and coroners' offices in the United States and Canada in a geographic area that contained 30 percent of the U. S. population. They found a total of 111 sudden deaths in which cocaine was involved, but only 26 in which cocaine was the only drug detected. When compared with deaths due to opiates and sedative-hypnotic drugs, this incidence appears to be small. However, Grinspoon and Bakalar (1976) urge caution in interpreting such statistics. They note that deaths from cocaine may have not been recognized or reported, that the drug is metabolized quickly and is therefore difficult to detect in the blood or urine, and that statements about the causes of drug-related deaths are often influenced by socially accepted myths.

Our findings. Systematic efforts were made in these studies to sample the dose continuum. Although our coverage was skewed towards heavy use, the strategy employed does provide a clear picture of some of the effects produced by cocaine at differing dosage levels. As previous discussions have shown (see chapter 12), some common effects persist across the whole dose continuum, other effects are only observed with low doses, others make their appearance only after sustained, regular use of more than one gram per day, and some reported but uncommon effects are not related to any variance of dosage.

No findings are more unambiguous than the difference between intranasal and intravenous use of cocaine. Most of our men were introduced to cocaine through "snorting," and most described this as a pleasant but unremarkable experience – "You feel a warm glow inside." "You feel good." "It's a good party high." "It gives you a lift, that's about all." Their descriptions of the intravenous experience were of an entirely different phenomenon – "Wow! I never had anything like that. It was like having a big bolt of electricity running through your body, but I was relaxed at the same time." "I thought, shit, this is how Superman must feel." "It was a total surprise. I couldn't believe it." The intensity of the intravenous reaction is underscored by the statement made by several men that once they had experienced it they never snorted cocaine again; it was like using two different drugs.

There was general agreement among the men that the intravenous cocaine reaction is also more transitory — "It's a quick up and a quick down for me." "You have to fire up in ten or fifteen minutes to get it again." Such findings support the distinctions between intranasal and intravenous use of cocaine reported by other investigators.

The findings also leave little question that some individuals can practice intravenous injection of exceptionally large doses of cocaine daily for extended periods without lethal effect. Thus, George B. reported daily intravenous use of three grams of pharmaceutical cocaine for two years; Fred S. injected three grams of street cocaine (estimated at nearly 50 percent purity) for a year and a half; and Willie M. practiced intravenous use of four grams of cocaine (estimated at 50 percent purity) per day for five years. These unquestionably qualify as massive amounts. It should be noted however, that in 1923 Dixon cited cases involving the use of 100 grains of cocaine (6.49 g.) per day. No one in our studies reported intravenous use of a gram of cocaine in a single dose. However, single doses of 250–500 mg. at the end of a long "run" were not uncommon.

We believe our participants' reports are unexaggerated, but we have no explanation for how people can inject these amounts of cocaine and survive. Whether it is a matter of temporary tolerance or of a healthy liver working overtime to detoxify the drug can be resolved only by the drug toxicologist. Our data simply indicate that in the period of a day some of these men injected massive amounts of cocaine and did not die.

Despite these findings, it is our opinion that efforts to "decriminalize" cocaine are inappropriate at this time. First, cocaine is not benign; when used in excess it can produce paranoia, hallucinations, and psychosis. Second, while the current practice of "snorting" small amounts may seem safe enough, even "snorting" can kill (Finkle and McClosky, 1977; Wetli and Wright, 1979). Thus, in some individuals cocaine can produce acute adverse reactions, including death, at doses that might produce only pleasurable reactions in others. Efforts should be made to better define the parameters of risk with cocaine prior to efforts to alter its legal status.

Medical Complications
Previous reports. The major adverse medical effects associated with intranasal use of cocaine are said to be *inflammation of the nasal mucosa,* accompanied by *nasal irritation, sores,* and *bleeding.* These effects are due to particles of cocaine that become lodged in the small hair follicles of the nasal membrane

(Ashley; Waldorf et al., 1977). Such particles may also lodge in the sinus cavities, producing *headaches* and *congestion*. These symptoms may resemble a common cold, with congestion and a "runny nose" (Petersen and Stillman, 1977). To avoid these effects, experienced users chop up their cocaine with a razor blade to keep it finely grained and "snort" a little water or use nose drops and nasal sprays to dissolve any bits of the drug in hair follicles. Although *perforation of the nasal septum* (the membrane dividing the halves of the nose) can occur with nasal administration of cocaine, this reaction is more rare than was earlier believed.

People who practice intravenous use of cocaine are vulnerable to all the medical complications that can arise from non-sterile intravenous drug use: *overdose, hepatitis, pneumonia, multiple embolic thrombosis, embolic pneumonia, lung abscess, endocarditis, tetanus, local sepsis at injection sites,* and *generalized septicemia* (Ellinwood, 1974).

Our findings. The eight men in these studies who had practiced intranasal use of cocaine reported few serious adverse effects. All reported rhinorrhea, numbness, and nasal congestion as common reactions — "You get the sniffles." "It numbs my nose, throat, sinuses, and gums." "My nose gets congested for a couple of hours." Several reported that their eyes would water with a "big snort," most reported occasional inflammation of the nasal membrane, one reported an occasional nosebleed, but none reported infections. None reported perforation of the nasal septum, though one man said that he knew individuals with this condition.

Most men reported no severe medical complications associated with intravenous use. Four — Tom P., John B., Fred S., and Willie M. — did say that on a few occasions they felt they had experienced symptoms of overdose. None contracted hepatitis, and none had ever received emergency medical treatment for drug-related medical conditions. One intravenous user (Tom P.) apparently caused irreparable damage to a heart valve through what may have been use of unsanitary paraphernalia. He and one other high-dose intravenous user required hospitalization for pneumothorax or collapsed lung, which they thought was related to their use of cocaine. George B. and Willie M. both reported incidents in which they had produced severe external "burns" or abscesses with intravenous use of cocaine. Others, notably Tom P. and Fred S., reported that failure to hit the vein would occasionally produce a large bump, which was absorbed within a few days.

The absence of hepatitis in this research contrasts sharply with the reported incidence of hepatitis among amphetamine abusers (D. E. Smith, 1969; Smith and Fischer, 1969). Beyond that, the relative freedom of these men from medical complications associated with non-sterile injection appears to be due not only to their more sanitary practices but also to the social isolation in which they used cocaine, a situation reducing the likelihood of sharing needles and syringes with other users.

None of the participants reported allergic reactions. One (Arky L.) reported itching of the hands, which he interpreted as an allergic response; this was more likely an instance of the tactile hallucinations associated with high-dose cocaine use. Allergic responses to cocaine are apparently quite rare; in their review of the literature, Van Dyke and Byck (1977) were unable to find a single case of anaphylactic reaction to cocaine.

Psychological Effects

Affective-Psychosocial States

Previous reports. Several affective states are reportedly associated with cocaine use. There is a general consensus that the most distinctive of them are *euphoria* and a *sense of well-being.* These states have been variously described in terms such as a subtle exhilaration, a pleasant feeling of well-being and mastery (Waldorf et al., 1977), an illusion of supreme well-being (Grinspoon and Bakalar, 1976), a thrill throughout the body (Kolb, 1925b), a high and pleasant feeling (Resnick et al., 1977), an exhilaration and lasting euphoria, which does not differ from the euphoria of the normal person (Freud, 1884, in R. Byck, 1974), illusory satisfaction of desires (Gutierrez-Noriega, 1944, cited in Grinspoon and Bakalar, 1976), an elevation of mood that can reach proportions of euphoric excitement (Gay et al., 1973b), and an ecstatic sensation of extreme mental and physical power (Isbell and White, 1953).

A second cluster of affective states concerns the drug's impact upon sociability. Cocaine is said to increase self-confidence, (Eiswirth et al., 1972; Kolb, 1925a; Waldorf et al., 1977), make the user more garrulous and talkative (Gordon, 1908; Reinarman, 1977; Waldorf et al., 1977), and increase friendliness and enhance sociability (Fischman, et al., 1977; Siegel, 1977). For example, Waldorf and his co-workers (1977) state that snorting cocaine is a highly social activity. People tend to give up their reserve and become more open, personal, talkative, and outgoing after "doing" cocaine. They listen better and feel more rapport with others. They report that this sense of heightened friendliness can create a bond between cocaine users.

Some investigators report that with heavy or prolonged use, the psychological state of pleasant sociability is replaced by withdrawal from social contacts and a desire for social isolation (Joël and Fränkel, 1924, and Mendizabal, 1944; both cited in Grinspoon and Bakalar, 1976; Waldorf et al., 1977), impatience and irritability with other people, hypersensitivity, increased agressiveness, drug-related crime and the emergence of a potential for violence due to the paranoia, anxiety, and delusions of persecution that accompany the cocaine psychosis (Cohen, 1975; Isbell and White, 1953; Kolb, 1925a; Lewin, 1931; Louria, 1966; Mills, 1905; Siegel, 1977; Wesson and Smith, 1977). Woods (1977), summarizing a number of animal studies, notes that cocaine does not by itself induce aggression. However, the drug may increase or decrease aggression that has been elicited by environmental events.

Another psychosocial factor that is associated with the use of cocaine is a sense of status. Cocaine, the "Champagne" or "Cadillac of the drug market," is commonly considered a status drug. Sabbag (1976) states, "And, like high-quality caviar, it [cocaine] most frequently embellishes the diet of the avant-garde and the aristocratic, a leisure class — in New York, a *Who's Who* among actors, models, athletes, artists, musicians, and modern businessmen, professionals, politicians, and diplomats, as well as that sourceless supply of socialites and celebrities of no certifiable occupation. The common denominator is money. And it is fashionable in the high-profit purlieus of Harlem — with pimps, prostitutes, and drug dealers, any neighborhood heavy-weight with influence on the street. Coke is status" (p. 68).

Some of the accoutrements of modern cocaine users further mark it as a status drug. A recent article in *Newsweek* magazine (Steele et al., 1977) states, "Some coke buffs wear neck chains with a razor blade and a tiny spoon dangling like amulets. Maxfred's, a San Francisco jewelry store, provides diamond en-crusted razor blades for $500 and custom-designed spoons that sell for as much as $5,000.... A Los Angeles store called Propinquity stocks vials of glass and 14-karat gold at $4,000 as well as bargain-basement coke kits (mirror, razor blade, spoon, and cocaine container) at $10. At an L.A. boutique, a $150 sterling fountain pen has a chamber to hold cocaine — and, just in case the buyer actually wants a pen, a cartridge that holds ink" (p. 21).

Our findings. The findings of this research indicate unequivocally that cocaine produces euphoric effects, a sense of enhanced well-being, and, for some individuals, increased self-confidence. With the exception of Al G., all our participants agreed on this. One described the euphoric effects as a "flash of life"; another stated, "You feel nine feet tall"; a third added, "You feel like a million dollars and have this fantastic self-confidence." Three men described the cocaine "high" in sexual terms: "It's like having a climax with a woman, only intensified a hundred times." "The flash is like coming in intercourse, only far better." "It's an orgasmic feeling like you get in sex, but far better — but it only lasts a few minutes."

All agreed that cocaine made them talkative, but two different patterns, depending on degree of use, were reported regarding the drug's effects on friendliness and sociability. Relatively low-dose cocaine users (Arky L., Bill F., and Rufus B.) often used the drug in groups of four, six, or more persons to enhance social relationships. These findings provide some support for the report of Waldorf et al. (1977). At low-dosage levels, cocaine loosens people up, reduces inhibitions, and produces mild euphoria. If one wants to enjoy being with others, these effects are helpful; but they are just as helpful when one wishes to be alone, to escape from others whose behavior or constant presence has become aggravating. Arky L. captured these dual effects when he stated, "It's not like amphetamine. You can't relax on amphetamine, but you can on coke. It will go with you wherever you want to go; whatever mood you are in, it will carry it."

While most low-dose users felt that the drug enhanced social relationships, heavy users reported that the drug produced the opposite effect. When taking cocaine they found it necessary to restrict social contacts, withdraw, and isolate themselves, because of the intense paranoia the drug produced. These men tended to use the drug with no more than one other person. As Tom P. said, "The more people there are, there are just that many more plotting against me." With the exception of one participant (Al G.), the degree of social participation seemed to be inversely related to dosage and chronicity of use.

Heavy cocaine users not only reduced social contact sharply, but to further ensure their isolation took such steps as locking or barricading their doors, closing the window blinds, and turning off all the lights. Additionally, contacts with members of the opposite sex tended to be sharply limited during periods of heavy cocaine use. The user is apparently preoccupied with the ecstatic rush and euphoriant reaction accompanying intravenous use of the drug, and the presence of others of either sex seems to be not only unnecessary in this situation but may actually be undesirable. The withdrawal and isolation reported by high-dosage users in these studies are the opposite of the social effects of cocaine reported with intranasal users; this is consistent with earlier observations of heavy intravenous users.

There is no question that violence and drug-related crimes occurred in the lives of some of the cocaine users in these studies. Several were engaged in illegal activities such as pimping, dealing drugs, and burglarizing drugstores, and two participants were shot and killed during the course of this research or shortly thereafter. However, there was little evidence that cocaine itself makes users violent. With the possible exception of Tom P., none of our men considered themselves violent individuals. Low- and moderate-dose cocaine users stoutly denied that they had ever experienced a proneness to violence while using cocaine. Some did say that alcohol or barbiturates made them violent, but not cocaine. Several had seen men become violent while using the drug, but pointed out that these individuals exhibited the same pattern of uninhibited, antisocial behavior at all times.

The responses of heavy cocaine users regarding violence differed somewhat from those of low- and moderate-dose users. George B. and Willie M. were of the opinion that, while they had never acted violently, the potential for violence was always present. Tom P., a normally volatile person, reported that he felt less violent while using cocaine. He did note, however, that he might attack an individual who he felt was blocking his efforts to purchase more cocaine and continue a run. Fred S. was the only participant who admitted an act of violence while under the influence of cocaine; though this mild-mannered man was probably surprised at himself, he stated that he had attempted to assault a police officer who had apprehended him during an extended cocaine run.

The conclusion of some of our heavy cocaine users was that there is loss of inhibition and an emergence of hostile impulses into consciousness which the user has to control carefully. Add to this the visual and auditory hallucinations, fears of discovery at any moment by the police, and generally paranoid thoughts, and one can readily agree with George B. that "the potential for violence is always there."

There was no evidence that cocaine makes people into antisocial fiends. At least one person (George B.) used very high doses to achieve a perfectly acceptable, even admirable social end, that is, gaining success in sales work. Several participants have engaged in antisocial acts, some of them violent. But, with one exception, none of these men could be said to be violent by nature, and most would go out of their way to avoid doing anything "fiendish." Those who live in a subculture in which crime and violence are regarded by many of its members as necessary engage in crime or violence when they feel they must. Several participants do it in a matter-of-fact way; none does it because of the direct effects of cocaine, and all seem to regard their acts as rational responses to the conditions under which they live.

That cocaine is a high-status drug is certainly true. At $80–120 a gram (approximately one twenty-eighth of an ounce) and $1,800–2,300 an ounce it is hard to get, always expensive, and usually in short supply. Therefore, being able to use it regularly makes one special.

If money, as Sabbag (1976) asserts, is the factor that determines status among cocaine users, the heavy users in these studies (Tom P., George B., Willie M., and Fred S.) had unquestionable status. Their personal annual consumption of the drug (regardless of cut) ranged from 26 ounces to almost one-and-one-half kilos, amounts that might make many cocaine users cry with envy. George B. and Fred S. admitted spending from $35,000 to $40,000 a year for the drug. Tom P. and Willie M., both dealers, reported spending considerably less for their personal use. However, even at a low dollar cost of $80 per gram, the current street value of Willie M.'s annual cocaine consumption would be almost $117,000.

While access to money is an obvious factor in regular cocaine use, other factors are also important. One is having powerful connections who can assure continuing access to the drug; another is dealing the drug to reduce the cost of personal use. For obvious reasons, the investigators did not attempt to pursue the matter of how these men maintained regular supplies of cocaine. However, all the heavy users apparently had good connections, good enough so that George B., for example, could use pharmaceutical cocaine almost exclusively.

One reason none of the heavy cocaine users seemed particularly disturbed by costs may be that all were, to some degree, dealing, and were thereby able to reduce the cost of their personal use. Dealing in substantial amounts of cocaine can involve such large sums that money takes on a certain unreality, and the dealer may become insensitive to its value. Tom P. described the effect this way: "It's weird. When you deal in large amounts of coke you can make

$60,000 to $70,000 in a week. Have you ever seen $70,000 in small bills? It's damn near a suitcase full! What are you going to do with it all? You can't put it in a bank. I can buy a car with it; I have a new car, it cost me $25,000, but how many cars can you buy? It's not real; it's like play money. I save some, but I spend it fast, too. Hell, sometimes I'll fly a broad to Denver or Chicago just for dinner."

While the high status of cocaine adds to its appeal, most people in our studies do not use this drug primarily for its status implications. Most of the heavy users had unquestionable status in the drug community, and some (Tom P., Willie M., and Rufus B.) were rightfully feared by their contemporaries. However, these people were apparently practicing regular, heavy intravenous use of cocaine for something that status cannot buy — that brief sensation of pure pleasure that reportedly accompanies the intravenous high.

Status may be important among low-dose intranasal users, but it is not critical in regular, high-dose cocaine use. Status factors seem to enter most strongly during a person's introduction to cocaine, and are probably more potent in the long run for low-dose than for high-dose users.

Affective-Psychophysical States: Sexuality

Previous reports. Probably no drug has more sexual beliefs associated with it than cocaine. On the street, the drug is called "lady" or "girl" to denote its sensuous, seductive qualities and also to distinguish it from heroin (called "boy"). It is thought by some to enhance sexuality. Others report that cocaine is a "macho" drug that prepares the male to perform prodigious sexual feats (Olden, 1973).

A number of investigators report that cocaine stimulates or enhances sexuality, increases libido, prolongs sexual intercourse, and produces more intense and satisfying orgasms (Ashley, 1975; Gay and Sheppard, 1973; Gourmet Coke Book, 1972; Kolb, 1962; Mayer-Gross, Slater, and Roth, 1960; Waldorf et al., 1977; Wesson and Smith, 1977). However, the cocaine users interviewed by Chopra and Chopra (1930/1931) denied that the sexual act was strengthened or prolonged when using cocaine; they held that, on the contrary, it was markedly weakened. Cocaine users interviewed by Grinspoon and Bakalar (1976) provided mixed reports; although most said cocaine produced sexual stimulation, some said it did not, and at least one reported that the high-dosage user goes beyond sex — "You get beyond most everything except the cocaine" (p. 106). Some early investigators (Anonymous, 1925; Chopra and Chopra; Wolff, 1932) reported that cocaine can induce *sexual inversion* or *homosexuality* in men. Bell and Trethowan (1961) denied this, pointing out that sexual behavior on cocaine is a function of preexisting sexual orientation.

Gay and Shepard (1973) reported that cocaine is a potent aphrodisiac that can "stir the loins of the most sexually jaded." They cited interviews with patients at the Haight-Ashbury Free Clinic in San Francisco which suggest that cocaine can produce multiple orgasms, spontaneous erections, and even priapism (an abnormal persistence of penile erection, usually without sexual desire). On the other hand, a number of workers have reported that in high doses or with heavy, chronic use the sexual effects of the drug are reversed to produce a loss of libido or interest in sex, as well as impotence and frigidity (Ashley; Chopra and Chopra; Wesson and Smith; Wolff). It is thought by some that the "rush" that occurs with heavy intravenous use of the drug can actually serve as a substitute for sexuality (Wesson and Smith, 1977).

Our findings. There was general agreement that cocaine can prolong sexual intercourse if the user has not injected so much that he is unable to attain an erection, or if he had not become so caught up in the cocaine experience that sex became irrelevant. Users' reports as to whether cocaine can produce a more intense or satisfying orgasm were mixed, with some — primarily low-dose users — reporting more sensational climaxes, and others expressing a complete absence of interest in sexuality — "When you're shooting coke you're not interested in sex, just the flash." One heavy user (George B.) expressed doubts that a more spectacular orgasm could occur with high-dose cocaine use — "I don't see how it is possible to have a greater orgasm when you're so numb."

There were some suggestions that chronic use of cocaine produces situational impotence; there were no reports of multiple orgasms, spontaneous erections, or priapism. However, one intravenous user (Rufus B.) reported that on three or four occassions he experienced ejaculation with the cocaine rush.

Only four persons, primarily low-dose users, felt that cocaine was an aphrodisiac. The remainder reported either that cocaine was not the aphrodisiac that it had been touted to be, or else that they were simply not interested in sex when using cocaine. The majority felt that cocaine was a more potent aphrodisiac for women than for men. These observations support earlier investigators (Chopra and Chopra; Ellinwood, 1972) who have suggested that stimulants may produce more intense sexual effects in women than men.

All in all, the findings suggest that sexual effects depend on the amount of dosage. With doses of one gram or less per day, cocaine may enhance sexuality, delay ejaculation, and produce more intense and satisfying orgasms. At doses of more than two grams per day, there is a decrease in interest in sexuality, as suggested by Ashley, Gutierrez-Noreiga (1944), and others. These findings support the hypothesis that cocaine can become a substitute for sex. In fact, when compared with the orgasmic rush that users report accompanies high-dose intravenous use of cocaine, sex may be a pale and lifeless competitor for the user's attention.

There was no evidence that cocaine causes homosexuality. If such claims were true at least some of our men would be actively, indeed, irrepressably homosexual, and that is clearly not the case. That cocaine is taken by some homosexuals cannot be denied, though none served as participants in this research. Several heavy users place such emphasis on being aggresively masculine that an observer might suspect they are running away from unconscious impulses of an opposite sort. But if so, the impulses are buried so deep as to be inaccessible even to such intensive and extensive techniques as those employed in this research. They were not activated even by the high doses that participants in this research customarily took. One or two participants showed some signs of homosexual vectors in their life styles. However, these involvements could easily be explained on grounds other than the activation of homosexuality by cocaine.

Affective-Psychophysical States: Other

Previous reports. In addition to the drug's effects upon sexuality, a number of other adverse affective states have been reported for cocaine. For example, Ashley (1975), and Waldorf et al. (1977) report that increased nervousness, edginess, and hyperirritability are associated with termination of prolonged intranasal use of cocaine. Wesson and Smith, and Siegel (1977), however, report that increased irritability, restlessness, and anxiety occur with recreational use of the drug, while other investigators report these reactions only with heavy or prolonged use (Chopra and Chopra, 1930/1931; Gay et al., 1973b; Kolb, 1925a; Maurer and Vogel, 1967; Wesson and Smith, 1977).

The early literature contained reports suggesting that heavy or prolonged use of cocaine produces depression (Gordon, 1908; Mills, 1905). More recently, Post (1975), in his three-stage theory of the cocaine psychosis, postulated a depressive or dysphoric reaction immediately preceding the paranoid psychosis. In 1977, Wesson and Smith described a case of drug-induced depression in a twenty-four-year-old woman after only a few days of intranasal cocaine use.

While there are some reports of such drug-induced reactions, depression is more commonly associated with withdrawal or abstinence (Brecher and Editors of Consumers' Report, 1972; Cohen, 1975; Eddy et al., 1965; Wesson and Smith). This post-reactive depression state has often been said to be accompanied by an intense craving, indeed an overpowering compulsion, to continue taking the drug (Brecher et al., 1972; Chopra and Chopra; Eiswirth et al., 1972).

Animal research provides some evidence of this craving to continue using cocaine. The drug is a powerful reinforcer. Yanagita (1973) compared the pattern of self-administration of cocaine in monkeys with that of a variety of other drugs — pentobarbital, morphine, meperidine, codeine, amphetamine, methamphetamine, alcohol, and nicotine — and found cocaine to be "very remarkable" both for its total reinforcement power and its toxicity. Similarly, Thompson and Pickens (1970) reported that, in their efforts to self-inject stimulants, rats administered six times as much cocaine as methamphetamine to themselves, and made as many as 2,000 to 4,000 responses per hour for periods of up to six hours.

Woods (1977) noted that when animals are conditioned to self-inject cocaine, investigators must often limit the self-injection to a certain time of day or a specified number. Rhesus monkeys, for example, will go through bouts of severe intoxication if their intake is not restricted (Deneau et al., 1969; Johanson et al., 1976). Such bouts — not unlike the "runs" described by the intravenous users in these studies — may persist unabated for days, and may terminate in convulsions or death, or else in exhaustion and a period of abstinence followed by another bout of self-injection. Similar patterns of cocaine-induced intoxication have been reported with intravenous self-injection in rats (Pickens and Thompson, 1971). Woods stated that when intravenous cocaine was made available to experimental animals in unlimited quantity, the drug killed with amazing speed and reliability, usually within a month and sometimes in less than a week.

Despite such findings, not all investigators agree that depression or compulsion to continue use occurs with abstinence. Ashley (1975) states that abstinence is associated with neither severe depression nor intense craving. "None of the 81 users I interviewed and observed experienced any recognizable discomfort when their cocaine ran out, beyond that feeling we all have when something we like is no longer at hand or readily available" (p. 176–177). Similar observations have been reported by Brecher (1974, cited in Ashley and Waldorf et al. (1977). Grinspoon and Bakalar (1976) found no evidence of severe depression upon termination. They did note, however, that people often want to keep taking cocaine, and this desire can be very intense. They observed that any amount of cocaine set out for use gets used, and it is unheard of for any to be left over.

Another cluster of adverse states reportedly associated with withdrawal are feelings of lethargy, fatigue, lassitude, irritability, and physical exhaustion (Chopra and Chopra, 1930/1931; Gay et al., 1973b; Kolb, 1962; Siegel, 1977; Wesson and Smith, 1977). Ashley reports that with intranasal users this post-reactive lassitude is much like a mild alcoholic hangover; Grinspoon and Bakalar state that these effects are psychophysical reactions to overstimulation of the central nervous system.

Our findings. Our users indicated clearly that heavy use of cocaine is associated with nervousness, tension, and anxiety. The majority of the intravenous users reported that they became nervous, edgy, and anxious whenever they took the drug. While George B. refused to admit that he became more nervous and anxious, his statement that cocaine always made him "restless and hyper as hell" is as close to a definition of tension as one could find. The only two persons who reported no anxiety associated with cocaine (Bill F. and Al G.) were the two lowest users. The feeling of calmness described by Post et al. (1974) in laboratory studies was reported only by Bill F., who anchored the low end of the use-effect curve.

Our findings suggest that cocaine-induced anxiety is dose-related. Low doses (somewhat less than one gram per day) produce a mild euphoria. Although chronic high-dose use (more than one gram per day) continues to produce euphoria, it also produces anxiety. The fears and paranoia that the high-dose users described were of such intensity that these men sharply restricted their contacts with people when using the drug.

Despite the regular experience of anxiety by chronic, high-dose cocaine users, none reported experiencing the drug-induced depression cited by Post (1975) or Wesson and Smith (1977). On the contrary, several high-dose users took cocaine to preclude or temporarily avoid depression and dysphoria.

In our research, both euphoria and anxiety characterized the intravenous cocaine experience, while depression and dysphoria characterized the withdrawal or abstinence reaction. The only user who did not report some kind of depressive reaction upon abstinence was Bill F. He stated, "I don't really feel depressed when I stop using cocaine. I just usually feel tired and wish I hadn't come down so soon." This response is similar to those of intranasal users studied by Ashley (1975) and Grinspoon and Bakalar (1977), but is not characteristic of heavy intravenous users. The reactions of our intravenous users ranged from mild depression and dysphoria among such low-dose users as Arky L., Al G., and Rufus B., to severe depression among some high-dose users —"There is nothing worse than running out of coke!" "I always get anxious on cocaine and get depressed coming off." "I get depressed as hell; I get suicidal thoughts and ideas when I'm coming off. I just try to hang on until its over." While the depressive states following termination contradict the findings from intranasal users, they are consistent with the reports obtained from heavy intravenous users.

There was no way to accurately assess the severity of these depressive states, since intravenous users abruptly terminated these effects with the use of opiates, alcohol, etc. However, some men noted that while the post-cocaine depression can be severe, it is not as intense as that following intravenous use of amphetamine.

Only one man (Tom P.) gave a spontaneous report of hyperirritability upon withdrawal. However, when one considers the insomnia, depression, and physical and mental exhaustion that accompany withdrawal, there seems to be little doubt that many others would have reported such responses had the investigators asked about them directly.

Our findings indicate that most of the men demonstrated psychic dependence upon cocaine and all experienced some craving or compulsion to continue its use. Although this reaction was more striking among heavy users, every man reported regret upon termination. Even Bill F.'s remarks reflect this: "You're going to use it until you run out of cocaine or out of money." Similar observations were reported by heavy users — "After a gram of coke I have this incredible craving for more; it's not a physical thing, but I've traded and sold my TV, tape recorder, or anything to get it." "I always felt I was losing control, because once I got started I *had to* do it." "You don't control cocaine, it controls you." "It's impossible to control cocaine!"

It is a commentary on the powers of cocaine that some men in these studies would sit in a room injecting cocaine every ten or fifteen minutes around the clock (at a rate of ninety-six or more injections per day) until it was gone, even though they were experiencing increasing anxiety, apprehension, and paranoia with each injection. George B.'s description of himself sitting alone on a bathroom stool for two days and nights injecting almost an ounce of pharmaceutical cocaine, or Fred S.'s injecting of the drug, vomiting, and repeating this pattern again and again, vividly portray the intense desire for the effects that intravenous cocaine can produce. These data support the observations of other investigators on the coercive power of cocaine (Burroughs, 1959: Crowley, 1917/1973; Perry, 1972).

Many texts leave the impression that the craving for cocaine is most pronounced upon abstinence or termination. Our findings indicate that craving begins very early in a drug session and continuous throughout episodes of intravenous use. Several men echoed Tom P.'s observation, "After four or five hits you get this crazy compulsion that you have to have more." Another intravenous cocaine user said, "Cocaine is evil. It scares me to death because it's so easy to abuse. If I only do one hit, I can probably walk away from it. If I do two hits I may be able to walk away, but if I get beyond that I can't stop. Beyond that, there is no such thing as saving some of it for a later day; if I have five grams or a half a gram I know I'll do it all at that time." These reports suggest that the rush is a powerful and constant reinforcer that sustains desire for the drug. Reinforcement begins early, and continues even though the user may be becoming more and more toxic with each injection.

Physical and mental exhaustion, fatigue and lassitude, and a "wired" feeling with an inability to relax were common psychophysical states accompanying abstinence. The severity of these symptoms varied from moderate to intense depending upon dosage and the duration of the episode of drug use.

Cognitive Effects

Previous reports. Several reactions which we classify as cognitive have been reported to be associated with use of cocaine. These include users' reports of beliefs in possession of increased physical strength and power (Ashley, 1975; Chopra and Chopra, 1930/1931; Eddy et al., 1965; Lewin, 1931); *hyperphrenia* or feelings of increased mental ability and lucidity (Gay et al., 1973b; 1976; Kolb, 1962; Reinarman, 1977; Waldorf et al., 1977); and a compelling need to put everything in order (Grinspoon and Bakalar, 1976).

Our findings. There was agreement that when using cocaine the participants felt an enhancement of physical strength and a sense of certainty that they could accomplish anything — "You feel like you could gnaw through steel." "You feel like you could do anything, but really all you're interested in is the next hit." "Good girl will make you feel like you can do anything." However, only three men were able to harness these capacities for constructive work: Bill F. felt he could play better when he used cocaine, especially if he took it when he was tired, and George B. was convinced that he outperformed the other salesmen while using the drug — "I not only felt like I could do more work, I did more work! I could do triple what everyone else was doing." Tom P., on the other hand, used cocaine when he was involved in complicated and dangerous cocaine buys — "It keeps me up and keeps me on my toes. I'm sharp and don't miss a thing." These data suggest that cocaine may enhance physical performances. However, separating this effect from related effects such as increased energy and alertness, self-confidence, euphoria, and the absence of fatigue, is impossible within the context of this research.

All the men reported increased mental lucidity and acceleration of mental activity — "I felt my mind was quicker." "I think better and faster on coke." "Your mind runs like crazy, and so does your imagination." "Your mind runs fast, almost like lightening." "Your mind is racing." This acceleration of mental activity was so intense that several reported difficulty maintaining attention while using the drug (Siegel, 1977; Waldorf et al., 1977).

Only two relatively low-dose users (Arky L. and Al G.), reported tendencies or needs to "put things in order." Both reported that on occasion when using cocaine they would launch vigorously into housecleaning activities.

Characterological Effects

Previous reports. In the early twentieth century heavy, habitual use of cocaine was said to be associated with physical emaciation, feebleness and debility, blunting or diminution of intellectual abilities, mental and moral deterioration, loss of will-power, and insanity (Dale, 1903; Gordon, 1908; Mills, 1905). More recently Blejer-Prieto (1965) reported that the psychological and moral deterioration of cocaine users "is obvious." Chopra and Chopra (1930/1931) described the cocaine eaters in India as persons of low morals, habitual liars and pilferers who would resort to anything, however despicable or criminal, to secure their daily dose of cocaine. Wiley and Pierce (1914, cited in Phillips, 1975) pictured "cocaine habituees" at the turn of the century: "When the habit is acquired, the utter undermining of the nervous system is inevitable. There is always the necessity for repeated doses, since the effects soon wear off, and is succeeded by weakness and depression, utter moral degeneration, indulgence in vice and crime in their various forms, followed often by suicide. These are the heritages of the cocaine fiend."

Our findings. Our studies provide no evidence of the characterological effects cited above. As indicated in the discussion of anorexia, none of the men in these studies showed evidence of physical emaciation, feebleness, or debility. Although several recognized that cocaine affects their judgment temporarily, none displayed any overall deficit in intellectual capacity. The distribution of scores on tests of intelligence showed no relation to level of use of the drug.

Only one man, Fred S., could possibly be described as showing "moral deterioration." Fred is downwardly mobile, but this was due largely to his vehement rejection of the hypocrisy and dishonesty he perceived in the values of his parents, not to cocaine per se.

Obviously, when it comes to cocaine, all the persons in these studies have weak willpower. In other areas of life, however, many of them display remarkable powers of will and unusually strong self-discipline. In fact, there seems to be an inverse relationship between level of cocaine use and capacity for self-discipline. Those who take less cocaine seem to be more at the mercy of their environment than those who take more. The latter are characterized by their determination to impose themselves upon their surroundings, to make a mark on their worlds. Most of them will impose rigorous demands upon themselves, and make whatever sacrifices they feel to be necessary.

At some points in their lives, two people in these studies might have fit a turn-of-the-century definition of "insanity." Fred S. was hospitalized for psychiatric problems at age 18, and Tom P. admitted that on some occasions his anger was uncontrollable. In both instances, however, the problems of these men had their origin in conditions existing long before they began taking cocaine.

The Toxic Cocaine Reaction

Previous reports. A diverse collection of physiological reactions has been reported by several investigators to be associated with cocaine poisoning. These include tremors, *ventricular arrhythmia,* convulsions, *mydriasis,* cold perspiration, profuse sweating, deafness, extreme pallor, *tachycardia,* headaches, hypertension, rapid and weak pulse, blindness, vertigo, nausea and vomiting with or without abdominal pain, fainting or unconsciousness, coldness or numbness of the extremities, *anorexia,* muscular rigidity, dry throat, dimness of vision, dizziness, insomnia, *hyperreflexia* or exaggeration of reflexes, lividity of the face, rapid and shallow breathing, cardiac arrest, dyspepsia, *cyanosis,* circulatory collapse, respiratory failure, feelings of heaviness in the limbs, *dysmetria,* stereotyped movements, self-mutilation, and death (Byck and Van Dyke, 1977; Eddy et al., 1965; Isbell and White, 1953; Ritchie et al., 1970; Scheppegrell, 1898; Woods, 1977).

A variety of psychological symptoms are also said to be associated with cocaine poisoning. Heavy or chronic use of cocaine is said to produce an acute paranoid psychosis, similar to that observed in paranoid schizophrenia and the amphetamine psychosis (Ellinwood, 1972; Lewin, 1931; Peterson, 1977; Post, 1975). This psychosis is complete with paranoia and delusions (Chopra and Chopra, 1930/1931; Eisworth et al., 1972; Isbell and White, 1953). Other phenomena associated with this are anxiety and extreme alarm (Eiswirth et al., 1972; Lewin, 1931), a feeling of impending death (Scheppegrell), hyperexcitability and delirium (Mantegazza, 1859/1975; Mills, 1905), agitation and mental confusion (Grinspoon and Bakalar, 1976), fears of imaginary police (Kolb, 1925a; Post, 1975), *bruxism* or teeth-grinding, picking on the face and extremities, and repetitious behavior patterns (Fischman, et al., 1977), visual, auditory, tactile, olfactory hallucinations (Gordon, 1908; Mayer-Gross et al., 1960; Mills, 1905; Siegel, 1977), and even gustatory hallucinations (Siegel, 1977). Visual and auditory hallucinations occur in the cocaine psychosis, but tactile hallucinations — particularly hallucinations of small insects or animals moving in or under the skin, "Magnan's sign" (Magnan and Saury, 1889) — are thought by many to be the hallmarks of the cocaine psychosis.

Not all investigators agree that cocaine produces paranoia or psychosis. Ashley (1975) says that a search of the relevant literature fails to show a single case of a serious toxic reaction to cocaine in the past forty years: "True paranoid reactions and hallucinations are almost never reported by modern users. . . . In the hallucinatory cases, tactile ones — the sensations of insects or tiny animals crawling on or under the skin — are more common than the visual variety — persons or objects appearing smaller than normal" (p. 181). Sabbag (1976) stated, "The country's most reliable experts on cocaine have been unable, either through hospital admittance records or through evidence given by clinical psychiatrists, to uncover any case of psychosis directly attributable to the drug. The best one can gather from the data available is that psychotics who use cocaine will be psychotic" (p. 85). Sabbag states that the notion that cocaine can cause formication (the sensation that insects are crawling on the skin) is also a myth. "That is one of the things they like to tell you will happen if you get on the wrong side of coke — one of the literature's favorite horror stories. It is as untrue as the rest" (p. 86.) Waldorf et al. (1977) also reported that the notion that cocaine causes people to become paranoid is a myth. They observed thirty-two users snort cocaine for a six-month period and did not see a single expression of paranoid ideation.

Our findings. Despite the fact that some persons in these studies were sometimes taking from one to eleven grams of cocaine per day for several days at a time and experienced many symptoms of the toxic reaction, they did not show a wide range of pathological physiological responses. Three were hospitalized for medical problems which they felt were related to the use of cocaine, but none sought emergency medical care; none reported convulsions, fainting, unconsciousness, or vertigo; and none reported rapid and weak pulse, rapid and shallow breathing, respiratory failure, stereotyped movements, self-mutilation, or cardiac arrest. One reported transient respiratory difficulties, and three reported instances of "stabbing" chest pain.

Profuse sweating, mydriasis, gooseflesh, tremors in extremities, headaches (which most attributed to the "cut"), anorexia, dry throat, insomnia, and dizziness (concurrent with or subsequent to injection) were the physiological responses commonly associated with intravenous cocaine use. If tachycardia is defined as heartbeats in excess of 100 beats per minute and if the findings of Fischman et al. (1976) that 32 mg. of cocaine will increase the heartbeat to well over 100 b.p.m., can be generalized, the heavy intravenous users in these studies must have experienced tachycardia. The other most common physiological reactions were nausea — which most men experienced most of the time with the drug — and vomiting. Only four persons reported symptoms which they interpreted as indicating an overdose. Three reported severe chest pain, and John B. cited transient but severe respiratory distress.

The findings of these studies leave little doubt that chronic, high-dose cocaine use can produce both paranoia and temporary psychosis. Most intravenous users experienced intense anxiety, paranoia, hallucinations, delusions, and terror or panic reactions when using the drug. Few low- or intermediate-dose users reported such reactions. In fact, Arky L. and Rufus B. were irritated with the investigators for even suggesting that "their drug" might cause such reactions. However, among men who used more than one gram per day, paranoia and other psychotic symptoms occurred regularly: "You feel you can't trust anyone. You get afraid that something is going to happen. You're afraid people are out to get you. You're afraid people can read your mind. You're afraid the police are going to break in any minute." "Every time I do more than two grams I get paranoid as hell. You're paranoid out of your mind!" "It made me nervous and paranoid 100 percent of the time. I couldn't deal with people; I was afraid of them." Although some participants could be described as generally paranoid individuals, this in no way diminishes the validity of their reports; the fact that they consistently described increased paranoia when they used cocaine and decreased paranoia when they stopped testifies to the drug's effects.

The delusions of these men lacked the systematized and florid qualities — for example, that the FBI, CIA, Mafia, or other organized groups were plotting to harm them — sometimes reported in studies of the amphetamine psychosis. These men all mentioned the same two ideas: the belief that they were being watched, talked about, and followed, and the related belief that the police were about to break in. These findings are consistent with the observations of Kolb (1925a, 1925b), Isbell and White (1953), and others. The selection of the police as the object of their paranoia is striking. One user stated that he had regularly experienced delusions involving the police while practicing heavy intravenous use of cocaine in a foreign country where there were no laws prohibiting its use!

The reactions of heavy, chronic users to drug-induced delusions were primarily defensive in nature. Typically, they did not attack the object of their delusions, but locked and barricaded themselves in a room or, in other instances, fled in panic.

There was no evidence in these studies of the bruxism, picking on the face and extremities, or the compulsive, repetitive behavior patterns reported by Fischman, et al. (1977) to occur with prolonged use of cocaine. Such reactions, however, were easily demonstrated in subsequent research with amphetamine abusers.

Magnan and Saury (1898) reported that tactile hallucinations are the first hallucinatory phenomena to develop with chronic use of cocaine, while visual, auditory, and olfactory hallucinations emerge later. Maier (1926, cited in Grinspoon and Bakalar, 1976) reported that snorters usually suffer only auditory and visual hallucinations, whereas intravenous users more often have tactile hallucinations. This research provides no support for either hypothesis. The hallucinations reported by chronic, high-dose cocaine users were diverse: Only one man (George B.) reported fully formed tactile hallucinations; two (Tom P. and Fred S.) reported visual hallucinations, but all the heavy users reported auditory hallucinations. The men agreed (in retrospect) that the latter emerged in response to normal sounds that they misinterpreted. Two of the men (Arky L. and Willie M.) reported intense itching of their hands, arms, legs, face, or shoulders but interpreted this only as "itching." All men testified that cocaine intensified olfactory sensations, but none reported olfactory hallucinations. The investigators did not question them on the matter of gustatory hallucinations, and none were reported spontaneously.

These results support investigators who have postulated that cocaine can produce a drug-induced psychosis with paranoid delusions and visual, auditory, and tactile hallucinations. However, this research suggests that the immediate physiological consequences of compulsive, high-dose cocaine abuse are less severe and disabling than one might expect. Certainly these men were apparently able to tolerate massive amounts of cocaine without disabling physiological effects. Nevertheless, the paranoia, delusions, agitated and labile anxiety, and hallucinations that accompany heavy, chronic use of the drug can be every bit as real, intense, and disabling as early writers suggested.

Methodological Notes

These findings go far towards reducing some of the confusion in the literature; they provide some of the first facts concerning the effects produced by cocaine with heavy, chronic use. Although this research is based upon retrospective reports in natural, real-life settings, it provides information about the drug's effects that would not be, indeed could not be, obtained in any other way. (That is, no serious investigator would knowingly administer 2,000–3,000 mg. of cocaine to human subjects for long periods of time, out of concern for ethical and moral considerations.)

The effects described by the participants demonstrate both internal and external validity. That is, effects reported by low-dose users differ systematically from those reported by high-dose users, and effects reported at high, low, and intermediate dosage levels are consistent with much of what has been described in the scientific literature. Our conclusions are based upon nine distinctive and separate, but interlocking, investigations. The report of each man is a study in itself and stands alone as such. However, as a carefully constructed collective, the data provide a panoramic picture of the effects of cocaine and the varying, sometimes frightening, social factors associated with its use in the late twentieth century.

These studies also show how important it is to examine the dose-effect relationship at many levels. This is particularly true with a drug like cocaine which has diverse and sometimes even contradictory effects. For example, cocaine's effects upon nervousness, alertness, and anxiety increase with dosage; sociability and sexual interest seem to decrease with increasing dosage; some reactions such as hunger and fatigue are abolished in the low mid-range of the dose-effect curve. Although effects such as restlessness, lucidity, and acceleration of mental activity occur at all levels of usage, other effects — such as paranoia, delusions and hallucinations — emerge suddenly at high dosage levels. Failure to give adequate consideration to the fact that cocaine can produce different or even opposite reactions at different dosage levels has put some investigators in the awkward position of concluding that some drug effects are myths, when in fact they occur at higher or lower levels than those investigated. The situation is a bit like that of a biologist concluding that panda bears do not exist because none are found in Alaska.

Finally, these studies underscore the importance of investigating drug use in real-life situations, among persons who are not members of clinical populations. Effects which appear in laboratories, even with drug-experienced subjects, or in clinical situations are not necessarily universal. For example, these studies show no evidence that stereotyped behavior or an increased proneness to violence are necessary concomitants to cocaine use, though these effects have been claimed by others to result from its use.

Representative Case Method

Our research leaves little doubt that the Representative Case Method is a powerful tool for studying drug abuse. In Chapter 2 we indicated that the method provides a means for testing hypotheses derived from large-scale studies but not validated by research on individuals. This approach reverses the usual strategy of using large-scale studies to validate hypotheses derived from research on individuals. However, the Representative Case Method is a more demanding validational or confirming strategy than large-scale research. If representative case data are collected with sufficient thoroughness, and if fundamental variables (such as dosage level, in the present instance) are adequately taken into account an investigator can speak with confidence about the findings. For example, effects of cocaine which do not occur with George B., Willie M., and Tom P. almost certainly cannot be associated with high-dosage consumption of the drug, even if extrapolations from data collected from low-dosage users suggest otherwise. Furthermore, if people like these all report the same effect, then the effect is genuine, even if no one ever encountered it before in large-scale studies.

Other Representative Case Method investigations are under way with comparable users of amphetamine, opiates, barbiturates and non-users. These are far enough along to show that the method is just as powerful in revealing the differences between the users of opiates, amphetamine, and sedative-hypnotics as in describing users of a single substance. Space does not permit discussion of all the possibilities of the method, but only a little thought is required to realize that it can be a valuable tool in the study of many critical theoretical and practical issues in such fields as psychology, psychiatry, medicine, and sociology.

INTEGRATION

Comprehensive Theories

In general, two models of the psychoactive effects of cocaine have been proposed. One is a direct-relation model, which asserts that the effects of cocaine increase in proportion to dosage level and chronicity. Apparently disparate reactions (such as euphoria and dysphoria) are subsumed under the more general heading of *psychopathology* (dysphoria being more pathological than euphoria) which is postulated to increase with dosage and chronicity. In the case of other effects, a more simple relationship is expected: "A positive correlation of cocaine use and severity of disorganization is suggested. . . . Chronic compared to acute cocaine administration in each case would increase the slope and shift the curve to the left toward greater disorganization at a given dose" (Post, 1975, p. 227). In short, this model assumes that, other things being equal, greater drug use produces greater psychopathology.

The other model can be visualized as being like an inverted U, and is built upon a variable that might be called *arousal*, or *activation*. This model proposes that as dosage increases arousal increases to a maximum and then decreases. Such a model was suggested, though not fully developed, as early as 1924 by Joël and Fränkel (cited in Grinspoon and Bakalar, 1976). They proposed a three-stage process: During the first stage use of cocaine increases sensory acuteness, intensifies attention, speeds up thought-processes, and excites motoric activity; the overall effect of these changes is pleasant. The second stage seems to carry arousal to an extreme, to the point where it is heightened beyond control. Delusions, hallucinations and anxiety develop; the overall effect is no longer pleasurable but becomes aversive. Finally, the third stage produces inhibition — the user comes down the other side of the inverted U. Sensory-motor activity diminishes, thought-processes slow down, and the user feels apathy, indifference, or downright misery.

No single study can produce conclusive evidence regarding comprehensive theories. However, in general both theoretical and empirical considerations lead us to prefer the arousal ("Inverted U") hypothesis. The choice may seem to be merely a matter of whether one prefers to speak of psychopathology or of arousal; however, since the utility of the concept of psychopathology is generally under serious question and since there exists no really objective way to measure it, the issue is not entirely one of preference. Variables like arousal and activation can be indexed in a variety of ways, both physiological and behavioral, and are therefore more useful.

Empirically, the data speak clearly. Low-level users seek mild pleasure and stimulation. Intermediate-level users seek euphoria, excitement, and drive. High-level users sometimes seek arousal (George B., for example), but they invariably wind up in a state of inhibition, isolation, disorganization, and paralysis of adaptive capabilities.

The main weakness of the Inverted U hypothesis is that it fails to account for the immense appeal of the "rush." Although the *average* curve of arousal may rise and then fall off gradually, beyond a certain intermediate level of dosage a moment-by-moment curve of arousal must show sharp increases in arousal (rushes) at each injection, followed by decreases as the rushes diminish. To leave these out would be to ignore the essence of the cocaine experience. In most instances of high-dose usage, the only motivation of the user is to renew the momentary sensations of the rush. Only when numbness, sheer fatigue, or the unavailability of cocaine makes that impossible does drug-taking cease.

The two models, direct and Inverted U, can be reconciled if one assumes that psychological adjustment is a function of the ego-environment relationship, and that optimum adjustment occurs within a range in which this relationship is in balance. In the language of Gestalt psychology, ego is *figure,* while environment is *ground.* At the optimum, exchanges between the two are reciprocal and neither dominates the other. It may be postulated that the effect of cocaine is to enhance or expand the influence of the ego and diminish or shrink the influence of environment. The effect is monotonic; ego enhancement increases as dosage increases (Grinspoon and Bakalar, 1976, pp. 94-95).

For people whose egos are normally weak, small doses of cocaine provide a lift: the pleasurable feeling of increased ego definition and control which occurs on the rising portion of the inverted U. Larger, more chronic doses expand or inflate self-importance still further, making the person feel euphoric, powerful, and almost superhuman, yet totally in command. At this stage, the person is at the top of the inverted U. Still larger doses enhance the figural ego until it destroys the normal ego-environment balance and reaches psychotic proportions. Reality testing becomes impaired; delusions and hallucinations begin; and effectiveness of adjustment suffers because it is dominated by a massively inflated ego. Meanwhile, the influence of environmental factors has diminished below the level that must be maintained if adequate functioning is to continue. In consequence, the ego becomes bloated with impulses that are normally kept under control; the bloating provokes panic and an awareness of vulnerability. The ego responds to the crisis with defensive constriction. The result is isolation, flight, and ultimately implosion of the ego in the face of the tension that accompanies emerging impulses. These defensive maneuvers comprise the cocaine psychosis. It would not be surprising if, as Post (1975) suggests, the dosage level at which these maneuvers appear varies from person to person, depending on the level or type of pre-use adjustment.

Cocaine vs. Amphetamine

A number of investigators have commented on the similarity of the behavioral effects of cocaine and amphetamine (Bejerot, 1970; Fischman, et al., 1977; Jaffe, 1965; Javaid, Dekirmenjian and Davis, 1977; Kramer et al., 1967). While cocaine does not have the phenethylamine skeleton that characterizes amphetamine and its congeners, intravenous use of either drug produces a euphoric rush, feelings of elation, an enhanced sense of physical and mental capacity, increased self-confidence, garrulousness, anorexia, insomnia, and (after heavy or prolonged use) a drug-induced psychosis characterized by paranoia, delusions, and hallucinations.

It is not surprising that two powerful central nervous system stimulants produce similar effects. However, some differences in the behavioral effects of these two drugs emerged during the course of these studies. One difference is in subjective responses. Seven participants had tried amphetamine and all terminated its use once they began using cocaine. Complaints focused on the harsh, driven effects amphetamine produces, the nervous, "wired" and uncomfortable quality associated with it, and the intensity of the "crash" upon abstinence. Such subjective reports leave little question that the amphetamine experience differs from the cocaine experience.

One of the most solidly documented findings has been the discovery that after heavy or prolonged use amphetamine produces rigid, compulsive behaviors or *stereotypy* (Ellinwood, Sudilovsky and Nelson, 1973; Randrup and Munkvad, 1970; Rylander, 1969; Schiørring, 1977; Snyder, 1973). This reaction has been demonstrated with such striking regularity that it has become one of the hallmarks of amphetamine psychosis, for it appears, often accompanied by philosophical concerns about "meanings and essences," immediately prior to the onset of the psychosis (Ellinwood, 1972). We found no evidence of stereotypy or philosophical preoccupations associated with chronic, high-dose cocaine use.

Heavy cocaine users also seem to differ from heavy amphetamine users in their *aggressiveness* and *potential for violence*. The chilling findings reported by Angrist and Gershon (1976), Bell (1973), Carey and Mandell (1968), Noda (1950), Rylander (1969), and R. C. Smith (1972), leave little doubt that heavy use of amphetamine increases violence. Ellinwood (1971) reported on thirteen cases of homicide and a number of other "near misses" that were directly associated with use of amphetamine. He stated that the incidence of amphetamine-induced assaults and homicides might be recognized as much higher if physicians were more fully aware of the problem.

There is no question but that cocaine is associated with violence. Acts of violence were described or alluded to throughout these studies and two men were killed within six months of their completion. However, neither the described acts of violence nor the deaths were induced by cocaine; rather, they were products of the general violence that permeates the drug culture. No one except Fred S. described involvement in any incidents of aggressiveness while under the influence of cocaine. Amphetamine users, on the other hand, seem to be inclined to attack, fight it out, even risk personal harm or injury in their efforts to overwhelm an environment they perceive as hostile. In contrast, cocaine users withdraw, isolate themselves, barricade the doors, and strive to avoid confrontations with the objects of their delusions.

Heavy cocaine users also seem to differ from heavy amphetamine users in terms of *sociability*. High-dosage intravenous amphetamine users tend to congregate in groups and form small, user subcultures (Ellinwood, 1972; Griffith, 1969; Kramer, 1972; R. C. Smith, 1969). In contrast, the heavy cocaine users evidenced solitary use patterns; they withdrew and limited social contacts when using the drug. Amphetamine abusers tend to be more extroverted. Cocaine users lean toward social isolation; they are more thoughtful, introspective, and depressed.

Heavy amphetamine users apparently differ from heavy cocaine users also in *sexual behavior*. Heavy use of amphetamine has been associated with hypersexuality and polymorphous sexual activity (Ellinwood, 1967; Griffith, 1969; Kramer et al., 1967; Lidz, Lidz, and Rubenstein, 1976; Rylander, 1969). In contrast, heavy intravenous use of cocaine in our studies was associated with decreasing sexual interest and activity, and some evidence suggested that cocaine actually can become a substitute for sexuality.

Amphetamine abusers may also differ from cocaine abusers in the *complexity of delusions* which accompany the drug-induced psychosis. Amphetamine abuse is frequently accompanied by complex and systematized delusions involving the family, friends, lovers, gangs, the Mafia, international spy rings, and so on (Chapman, 1954; Connell, 1958; Ellinwood, 1972; Lynn, 1971). In contrast the delusions of cocaine users are simple and straightforward, though no less terrifying.

Heavy cocaine users seem to differ from heavy amphetamine abusers also in *hyperactivity*. A number of investigators have described the frenetic pursuit of activity that accompanies heavy intravenous amphetamine abuse (Davis and Munoz, 1968; Ellinwood, 1972; Kramer et al., 1967; R. C. Smith, 1969, 1972). We ourselves have found clear evidence of intense action-orientation and hyperactivity among amphetamine abusers, but no striking evidence of these effects among heavy cocaine users. On the contrary, heavy cocaine users could be better described as sedentary, seclusive, or even "languishing." Our data suggest that amphetamine is an action-oriented, "locomotor" drug (with subsidiary ideational effects) which mobilizes the user for vigorous activity, while cocaine is an "ideational" drug with subsidiary physical effects. William Burroughs (1959) described cocaine as a cerebral drug: "It hits you right in the brain, activating connections of pure pleasure. The pleasure of morphine is in the viscera. You listen down into yourself after a shot. But coke is electricity through the brain and the C yen is one of the brain alone, a need without body and without feeling. The C-charged brain is a berserk pinball machine, flashing blue and pink lights in electric orgasm. C pleasure could be felt by a thinking machine, the first stirring of hideous insect life" (p. 24).

The intravenous cocaine experience — unlike that of amphetamine, which mobilizes the user for action — is not a means to an end but the end state itself. The user who reaches the "Land of Cockaigne" has found that sought-after place and has no further goal. The only problem is that one cannot stay there forever.

COCAINE USERS

Cocaine Use and Life Themes

The people who participated in this research are unusual in many respects. However, they are not fundamentally different from the rest of us. They are imperfect human beings, pilgrims in life trying to fulfill familiar hopes, dreams, and aspirations in an imperfect world. It is therefore appropriate to consider what, if anything, they have in common.

As a group, our men cannot be described as weak, passive, or ineffectual. On the contrary, the majority are strong, willful, manipulative, and action-oriented; they are counter-dependent individuals who are wary, sensitive to slights, suspicious, and distrustful of others. Though some have illegal occupations, they are nonetheless ambitious, achievement-oriented persons who are willing to fight, struggle, outwit others, and overcome obstacles to make their mark on the world. Of course, there are exceptions: Neither Arky L. nor Al G. are particularly ambitious; both merely get by as best they can. However, Bill F., George B., John B., Willie M., and Rufus B. are trying to fulfill dreams of achievement and success. Even Fred S. has his ambitions, though his life is really devoted to a devious purpose, revenge against his family.

Most of these people took cocaine to gain access to the boundless energy, self-confidence, ebullient optimism, ego-enhancement, and aggressiveness the drug reportedly provides. These characteristics are highly valued in America, where they are touted hourly in commercials and espoused in novels, movies, and dramas on TV. It could therefore be proposed that the men in these studies selected cocaine because it seemed to provide an easy way to fulfill the American Dream. Our participants seem to believe that in cocaine they have found a shortcut to happiness and fulfillment.

A recurring theme in the lives of Arky L., Tom P., George B., Willie M., Rufus B., and even Fred S. has been preoccupation with independence, social isolation, and denial of passivity. These people seem fearful of normal dependency relationships and are intent on making certain that they are self-sufficient enough to need no other human being. They cannot or will not "come in out of the cold."

Fred S. demonstrates a complex and devious variation on this theme. Although his basic pattern is defiance of his father, on occasions Fred would "cave in" and become completely dependent, forcing his father to assume responsibility for him, if only by hospitalizing him or providing expensive psychiatric care. Fred knew well that one can dominate through helplessness as effectively as through direct confrontation.

John B. is also complex. Sometimes he submitted to his needs to be looked after, nurtured, and cared for. However, he just as quickly rejected these and became angry, vindictive, and rebellious, in a cyclic pattern that was confusing for John and drove his wife to distraction.

Bill F. and Al G., the two lowest-dose cocaine users, anchored the other end of the independence-dependence polarity. Both openly expressed needs to be nurtured, looked after, and supported by other people.

None of the men in these studies can allow themselves to get close to anyone, and practically all refuse to allow anyone to get close to them. Indeed, they do not allow themselves to get close to themselves; they do not understand their own motives, needs, and limitations. Consequently, they cut themselves off from the warmth, love, tenderness, and forgiveness everyone needs to be complete. They seem to be trying to live a life of Yang alone, while avoiding the Yin-Yang unity required for wholeness in the human condition. By emphasizing only half of themselves (the animus, in Jungian terms) they have cut themselves off from their darker side (the anima). However, as any Jungian knows, efforts to destroy the unity of psychic life are doomed to fail and ultimately lead to the destruction of those who attempt it.

Given their counter-dependent life orientation and fears of passivity, it is easy to see why these men frequently feel depressed. The conceptualization also suggests why they are drawn to cocaine and how that drug helps them live out their life themes. Use of cocaine — particularly intravenous use — apparently produces a unique high characterized by an experience of bodily warmth, exhilaration and euphoria, enhanced distinctiveness of the ego, feelings of supreme self-confidence, and a remarkable sense of mastery and control. These are reactions that most people get only in glimmering form through interactions with others who love them, care about them, and wish them well, in spite of their faults — and allow them to be themselves.

Cocaine users seem to us to be people unusually sensitive to slights; they have difficulty admitting to themselves that they are frail and need nurture and support, and dare not take those risks of being humiliated, ignored, rejected, or misunderstood that must be taken in the development of trusting interpersonal relationships.

Although these men may have concluded that it is too dangerous to seek intimacy in a hostile and uncaring world, they seem to feel that in cocaine they have found a substitute that fulfills their longing even better. In cocaine they have the friend or ally described by an amphetamine abuser interviewed by Davidson (1964). This woman reported that much of her life had been devoted to avoiding dependence on others: "All of my life I refused to depend on *anybody*. I wouldn't dream of marrying. . . . As a child I fought off all but the essential dependencies on my mother. But the pills allow one to be *secretly* dependent on something inanimate, something that won't desert you or reproach you or ask for something in return" (p. 756).

Earlier we suggested that the main psychological effect of cocaine is to inflate or expand the ego. Each person in these studies seems to have used the drug for the heightened distinctiveness of self-identity, self-confidence, and sense of mastery that it provides. The amount of cocaine needed for that purpose seems to be related to the extent of ego differentiation and the intensity of personal commitment of the user. For example, Bill F., Al G., and Arky L., have uncomplicated ego structures and can apparently be reassured that their identity is intact by fairly low-level stimulation. By contrast, George B., Willie M., Tom P., Fred S., and Rufus B. are intense, ambitious, and committed men who have much to lose if they fail to achieve their goals in life. These people may need greater dosages to reaffirm the integrity and influence of their egos and bring the self into distinct contrast with the environment. In any case, it is apparent that cocaine users seek to inflate and make more salient their own egos, and thus create the illusion of greater control over their personal fate than they actually possess.

Ego expansion must be distinguished from genuine ego growth, for in that distinction lies an important characteristic of cocaine users. Genuine ego growth requires the development of new skills and more complex personality organization as well as the abandonment of older, less effective skills and simplistic views of life. The characteristics of genuine growth are, among other things, greater acceptance of personal responsibility, a sounder appreciation of one's abilities and limitations, and a greater sense of integration of one's internal state with the environment. The growth process is not always happy, involving, as it does, failure as well as success, pain as well as pleasure, and suffering as well as satisfaction. However, in the long run it leaves the person feeling more competent and complete. But the ego-expansion cocaine induces brings no lasting changes; the temporary euphoria is ultimately replaced by the "crash," and the user is left where he was before the drug was taken. Thus, while genuine growth may be visualized as an upward-moving spiral, or heliotrix, ego-inflation is a vicious circle. The illusory paradise of the cocaine experience seems to the user to make genuine growth unnecessary, and the experience itself becomes a substitute for development.

Unfortunately, it is not possible to remain static. The biological maxim is clear and simple: One grows or one dies; and the compulsive cocaine user is a dying organism. Only a few, like George B. and Willie M., are capable of seeing that and trying to do something about it. A few others are more or less aware of it, but feel helpless to alter the course of their lives. Among these are Fred S. and Arky L., both of whom often think of themselves as self-defeating people. Still others simply yield to the inevitable and stop seeking genuine growth (Tom P., Rufus B., Al G.). As for the remaining two, John B. shows evidence of attempts to grow, but seems to be engaged in a prolonged struggle; and Bill F. cannot be identified as a compulsive user at all.

To use a mythological analogy, cocaine is like a False Grail. Though it holds out a promise of fulfillment and everlasting joy, chasing it only leads to a miasma of despair and destruction. Viewed as a totality, the findings of this research have the character of an old-fashioned morality play whose theme is that penalities must be paid if one attempts to take shortcuts to dream, hope, and wish fulfillment.

Considerations for a Theory of Psychological Structure

A complete analysis of the factors contributing to drug use and abuse must account for at least three types of variables. Most attractive to investigators, historically, have been *physiological* factors, which include the influences of drugs on metabolic and neurological processes. Of more recent interest are *social* factors, which include economic, cultural, and political forces affecting drug use. Less thoroughly studied, but increasingly acknowledged, are *personality* factors, which consist of attitudes, traits, and emotions that precede, accompany, and follow drug consumption.

Because our studies have concentrated most heavily on social and personality variables, the following sections survey the related theoretical ideas which guided it and hold promise for future refinement.

Behavioral Adaptation and Life Style

The two concepts organizing our investigations were *behavioral adaptation* and *life style*. A behavioral adaptation is a system of adjustments that take place at the person-environment interface. In our research such aspects of behavioral adaptation as drug of choice, habitual level of use, vocational adjustment, educational achievement, socio-economic background were taken into account during the initial selection of participants.

Behavioral adaptation is the surface expression of a person's life style (second level in figure 13.1). A life style is a network of linkages of overt behavioral adaptations to covert personal dynamics. Through it, incoming stimuli (including the person's own behavior) acquire meanings by being related to past experiences and aspirations. Through it, also, ideas and impulses of internal origin are integrated into outgoing intentional acts. Life styles can be inferred from consistencies in observed behavioral adaptations.

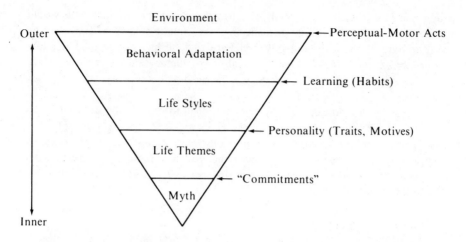

FIGURE 13.1.   Levels of Psychological Structure

Life Themes

As the research progressed it became apparent that each participant's life style was organized around only a few (usually no more than five or six) underlying *life themes* (third level in figure 13.1). Life themes are not to be thought of as traits or motives, for a theme is not an entity or force. Rather, life themes are the organizing principles that make a person's traits and motives understandable. For example, Arky L. has traits of gregariousness and rebelliousness, motives of hostility and revenge, and feelings of rejection and isolation. What gives these coherence is the recurrent theme in Arky's life that he is an alien in a complex and challenging world.

Choice and Inevitability

Several men seem to have made deliberate choices of life themes, and often it seems that their commitments were made very early. For example, Arky L. is aware of his commitment to being a robber and his reasons for making it. George's determination to make himself into a machine or fortress was probably deliberately made, perhaps at a specific moment. In the course of extensive work with business executives, one of the authors (J. V. S.) has noted that many of them can precisely identify the times when they decided to shape their lives in particular ways. Once adopted, a life theme has a fate-like or entelechial quality that makes it seem to have a destiny of its own.

Deliberate choice at the level of ego and life style may help make fate more bearable, but choice has little effect on the ends toward which life themes move. Like the recurrent four-note phrase in Beethoven's Fifth Symphony, life themes are ineluctable. The men in this research sometimes invented variations, slowing down their themes or speeding them up, perhaps changing the key or mode; but sooner or later the themes would play themselves out and the inevitable would come to pass. Bill F. will go on believing that there is a Land of Oz; when he fails to find it, he will probably conclude that he had not wanted it badly enough. Al G. and Tom P. knew the realities of their world and tried to adapt their behavior to assure their safety; yet the inevitable happened, and they lost their lives.

For a while the concept of life themes seemed to provide the key to describing the complexities of the participants. However, the intensive study of more than thirty men (including users of amphetamine, opiates, and barbiturates, as well as our nine cocaine users) showed that this idea required still further development. For one thing, we realized that we had not been concerned sufficiently with the sources of life themes.

Origins of Themes

Life themes are established in childhood and appear to persist into adulthood with little or no modification in basic form. By contrast, behavioral adaptations and life styles can change over time. Essential continuities in life are not always shown in overt behavior — which sometimes alters radically, as in George B.'s cold turkey withdrawal — or in life style — which is subject to developmental change or modification by biological or environmental influences — but in the themes that underlie both.

The same theme may have multiple expressions. For example, John B. sometimes behaves like a naughty adolescent, while at other times he is an aspiring young man trying to make his way into respectable middle-class society. John's theme is not simply that he wants to be a naughty adolescent or a successful middle-class American; it is that he wants to be both! Because that is not possible, John has developed the life style of being sometimes one and sometimes the other; it is the best he can do under the circumstances.

Granted that themes persist, the question remains: Where do they come from? An obvious answer is that they are learned during childhood. This answer has been useful in behavioristic as well as psychoanalytic theories; however, it does not adequately explain why themes are so refractory to change even when behavioral adaptations and life styles are modified. The stout resistance of life themes to external intervention is well-established in clinical practice. Indeed, successful psychotherapy is often described by clients not as a change but as a releasing of one's true self, that is, facilitating the expression of one's life themes.

Explanations in terms of learning also do not account for the intensity of commitment which people make to their themes. These commitments do not have the quality of learned, and therefore alterable, components of a whole. Rather, as Freud himself recognized in his concept of *repetition compulsion,* they have a fate-like quality. This quality makes the men in our studies seem to be living out a destiny over which they have no control and which may cost them their freedom or their lives.

To borrow phraseology from Carl Jung, each of these people is "lived by his myth." A myth is the kernel or core of an "autonomous complex," a numinous, monadic formation that remains subliminal and operates according to its own inherent tendencies, independent of the conscious will. A well-integrated myth may be expressed in creative work; poorly integrated into the rest of the personal structure, it may cause maladjustment (Jung 1971/1922). The myth serves a purpose in human life that is equally important to that served by the ego. In a person who is functioning well, the ego ensures biological survival by adapting to environmental realities, while the myth ensures wholeness through ensuring relatedness to psychic realities.

If Willie M. sees himself as a battered hero subdued by evil powers but whose head, though bloody, remains unbowed, then this is a manifestation of his myth, which he must live to the end. If Fred S. sees himself as the trickster who defeats his enemies by deception and guile but who is doomed to outwit and finally destroy himself, then this is his myth and he will pay the penalty it demands.

Myth, Fate, Destiny

Several theorists have maintained that myths and illusions are necessary in human existence. These ideas have been popularly expressed in Ernest Becker's well-known works, *The Denial of Death* and *Escape from Evil* (1973;1975). On the social level, Joseph Campbell (1973) pointed out that "it has always been on myths that the moral orders of societies have been founded" (p. 10). With the loss of myth and illusions there follows uncertainty, and with uncertainty disequilibrium; the center no longer holds, and there is nothing secure to grasp. The way to health is not through abandoning myth but through establishing a dialogue between perceptions of the outer world and intuitions of the equally vital realities of the inner, psychic world.

Though we have borrowed the idea of myth-determination we have applied it in our own way. This theory is not a theory of predestination, nor does it say anything of the inheritance of ancestral experiences. Up to a point, this theory allows for variation in myth content. It achieves this by three basic propositions:

1. The theory proposes the existence, prior to and independent of the birth of any individual, of an array of myths, fates, destinies, or "potential inevitabilities." (This is no more than saying that the myth of the Savior existed before Christ was born to fulfill it.)
2. The theory proposes the constitutional presence in each individual of a configuration of potentialities suited to some myths but not to others. For example, males are not constitutionally suited to live out easily the myth of the Virgin Mary. In our own studies, it is obvious that a physically frail person with a hunch-back, like Al G., is poorly equipped to live out myths like those that possess Tom P., Willie M., or Rufus B.

3. The theory proposes that, as each individual's constitutional potentialities are modified by early environmentally induced experiences, the range of his or her suitability to available myths is further limited. Conditions are eventually created which invite possession of the individual by a single myth which then determines the themes of that person's life. Possession by myth usually occurs in childhood and involves commitments that exceed the individual's capacity for conscious understanding at the time — sometimes, for the rest of the person's life.

Possession by a myth may be experienced as the making of a deliberate vow, as a religious conversion, or as a sudden insight of a numinous character. But, whether it is so experienced or not, possession is permanent. Apparent changes in mythological content — the frog becoming a prince; the god suffering defeat, destruction, or sacrifice — do not violate this principle; each represents only a stage in the development of the underlying mythical theme.

Consider, for example, the myth that possesses Rufus B. Part I of the myth is obvious; in it he is admired, feared, and envied by everyone — he is the Hero before the Fall. In Part II — the present situation — he is the Hero Descended into Hell, abandoned, friendless, alone, and in danger. It is impossible to imagine that in Part III of Rufus B.'s myth we will see him drifting into peaceful old age, dying in bed surrounded by loved ones; rather, his myth will drive him to renewed efforts at self-assertion, even if — perhaps especially if — they cost him his life. In fact, since his participation in this research it has already driven him to place his life in danger in a daring but nearly fatal escapade.

Future Directions

We have not presented the idea of myth in detail with regard to every participant. Yet we remain convinced that behind every pattern of life themes, a myth, fate, or destiny works itself out. Research in progress will provide more data upon which to base further speculations about the myths that drive people. As more of these are recognized, we may gain sufficient confidence to begin identifying recurrent patterns.

Much remains to be learned about the myths that make peoples' lives: Who are the characters in them? What are the plots? How do the myths of some persons relate to the myths of others? Does the supply of myths change or evolve with the development of culture? Is the "mad scientist" of today fundamentally different from Merlin of the Middle Ages? Is culture itself living out a myth? What is the relation between the myths of individuals, the more inclusive myths of cultures, and the perhaps universal myths that affect humanity as a whole?

At present, it is not possible to say how many universal theme-generating myths there are. The number is probably limited, and in one form or another the most basic myths are probably worldwide and time-independent. In many instances, one can see in drug users thinly veiled allusions to stories of the Holy Grail and to myths of the type that led alchemists to search for the lapis philosophorum. The study and classification of personal myths should have relevance to cultural anthropology and literature as well as psychology and psychiatry for some time to come.

Causal Complexity

In no way do we imply that psychic-mythical factors are the only determinants of drug use or abuse. In some cases and for some drugs — particularly the physically addictive ones — physiological factors can be paramount. In other cases, where distribution, availability, cost, and cultural norms are important, social factors may be critical. In many instances, of course, individual personality may be the overriding cause of drug use or abuse. Combinations of causal factors operate as well, and in clinical or rehabilitation situations the skilled diagnostician must evaluate all possibilities and weigh the contribution of each.

EPILOGUE

As far as could be determined, three months after the last formal assessment none of our nine cocaine users had suffered physical or psychological damage due to their participation in this research. Several seemed more integrated, less apprehensive, and in better control of their lives. Most voluntarily expressed appreciation for the opportunity to participate, stating that they had come to understand themselves better and had learned things that would be helpful. The participants, by and large, are manipulative men; however, they had been paid for their involvement and the investigators could find nothing that would justify their volunteering expressions of appreciation if they were not sincere.

Expressions of appreciation centered around two tasks, the Developmental Life History Interview and the Daily Activities and Experiences Audits. The Developmental Life History Interview, which lasted from six to ten or even more hours was unabashedly a clinical-therapeutic-research tool. The interviewer here made deliberate efforts to confront participants with linkages between their developmental experiences and present behavior. The participants seemed to find these efforts to identify personal continuities helpful.

The Daily Activities and Experiences Audit provided a detailed, hour-by-hour account of the activities, experiences, and feelings of each man from the time he awoke in the morning until he went to sleep that night. (The Audit samples presented in chapters 3–11 were sharply condensed for publication.) When the records of these days had been transcribed, each participant was asked to come in, read the narrative, and make whatever changes, corrections, or deletions he felt were appropriate to guarantee anonymity. The men were fascinated by this look at a blow-by-blow description of their own lives. They made comments such as "Well, I'll be damned!" "That's my life?" "I didn't know that's how I live, but that's it." "Jesus, it's a dull way to live, isn't it?" "I don't like it." "I want my life to be different than that!" and so on.

After continuing this far, the reader may wonder what has happened to these men since the research was completed. Two of them are now dead, one is in prison, and one has been convicted of a felony involving cocaine. These chilling statistics highlight the danger and volatile nature of the world of the heavy cocaine user.

More specifically, Arky L. is now in prison; perhaps he grew tired of the continual struggle for survival or wanted to get away from what he described as "this fucked-up world." Bill F. is in recording school and doing well. Tom P. was shot and killed during the research. He was a violent man in a violent business. Al G. was also killed in a drug-related slaying. One man who knew him well had said that Al "could live forever" in the drug culture because he had no enemies. However, Al was not killed because he had enemies, but because on a given day he was in the company of a man apparently marked for execution. John B. left his job as service-station manager and worked for a while as an apprentice in one of the trades. Both he and George B. suffered accidents that have left them with permanent physical disabilities; their future vocational status is in doubt. Willie M. obtained his divorce and is attending school to become a maitre d'. Fred S. is now a clerk in a large company. The last time we saw him he said there was some "great coke" in town. Rufus B. attempted a spectacular comeback; at last account, he was fighting for survival.

We thank the men who participated in this research. They have shared their lives, their hopes and fears, and their successes and failures with us. They have revealed much about the "Land of Cockaigne" and those who travel there. We wish them well and hope they may find ways to achieve their dreams and aspirations through lawful means.

References

Adriani, J. *The Chemistry and Physics of Anesthesia* (2nd ed.). Springfield, Ill: Charles C Thomas, 1962.

Adriani, J., & Campbell, D. Fatalities following topical application of local anesthetics to mucous membranes. *Journal of the American Medical Association,* 1956, *162,* 1527–1530.

Agrin, A. The great American drug scene. *Journal of Occupational Medicine,* 1972, *2,* 207–220.

Allport, G. The general and the unique in psychological science. *Journal of Personality,* 1962, *30,* 405–442.

Allport, G. *Personality: A Psychological Interpretation.* New York: Henry Holt, 1937.

Angrist, B., & Gershon, S. Clinical effects of amphetamine and L-DOPA on sexuality and aggression. *Comprehensive Psychiatry,* 1976, *17,* 715–722.

Anonymous. Statistical data on cocainism and morphinism in Austria. *Journal of the American Medical Association,* 1924, *83,* 1936.

Anonymous. Cocainism and homosexuality. *Journal of the American Medical Association,* 1925, *85,* 1936.

Ansbacher, H. J., & Ansbacher, R. R. *The Individual Psychology of Alfred Adler.* New York: Harper and Row, 1956.

Ashley, R. *Cocaine: Its History and Effects.* New York: St. Martin's Press, 1975.

Balster, R. L., & Schuster, C. R. Fixed interval schedule of cocaine reinforcement: Effects of dose and infusion duration. *Journal of Experimental Analyses of Behavior,* 1973, *20,* 119–129.

Bakan, D. *On Method.* San Francisco: Jossey-Bass, 1968.

Barker, R. *Ecological Psychology*, Stanford, Calif: Stanford University Press, 1968.

Barash, P. G. Cocaine in clinical medicine. In R. C. Petersen & R. C. Stillman (Eds.), *Cocaine:1977* (NIDA Research Monograph No. 13). Washington, D. C.: U. S. Government Printing Office, 1977, pp. 193–200.

Becker, E. *The Denial of Death.* New York: Free Press, 1973.

Becker, E. *Escape from Evil.* New York: Free Press, 1975.

Becker, H. K. Carl Koller and cocaine. *Psychoanalytic Quarterly,* 1963, *32,* 309–373.

Bell, D. S. The experimental reproduction of amphetamine psychosis. *Archives of General Psychiatry,* 1973, *29,* 35–40.

Bell, D. S., & Trethowan, W. H. Amphetamine addiction and disturbed sexuality. *Archives of General Psychiatry,* 1961, *4,* 74–78.

Bejerot, N. A. A comparison of the effects of cocaine and synthetic central stimulants. *British Journal of Addiction,* 1970, *65,* 35–37. (a)

Bejerot, N. A. *Addiction and Society.* Springfield, Ill.: Charles C Thomas, 1970. (b)

Bender, L. Drug addiction in adolescence. *Comprehensive Psychiatry,* 1963, *4,* 181.

Bentley, W. H. Erythroxylon coca in the opium and alcohol habits. *Detroit Therapeutic Gazette,* September 15, 1880. Reprinted in R. Byck (Ed.), *Cocaine papers: Sigmund Freud.* New York: Stonehill, 1974, pp. 15–19.

Bernfield, S. Freud's studies on cocaine. *Journal of the American Psychoanalytic Association,* 1953, *1,* 516–613.

Bewley, T. Heroin and cocaine addiction. *Lancet,* 1965, *738,* 808–810.

Biggam, A. G., Arafa, M. A., & Ragab, A. F. Heroin addiction in Egypt. *Lancet,* 1932, *21,* 922–927.

Blejer-Prieto, H. Coca leaf and cocaine addiction: Some historical roles. *Canadian Medical Association Journal,* 1965, *93,* 700–704.

Brecher, E. Paragraph Nine of Affidavit Attached to Defendants' Joint Memorandum in Support of Their Motion for Correction or Reduction of Sentence (*United States of America* v. *Foss and Coveney,* U. S. District Court, District of Massachusetts: Criminal No. 73-24-G), 1974.

Brecher, E. M., & Editors of Consumer Reports. *Licit and Illicit Drugs.* Boston: Little, Brown, 1972.

Brown, S. Bibliography on Q-technique and its methodology. *Perceptual and Motor Skills,* 1968, *26,* 587–613.

Buck, A. A., Sasaki, T. T., Hewitt, J., & Macrae, A. A. Coca chewing and health: An epidemiological study among residents of a Peruvian village. *American Journal of Epidemiology,* 1968, *88,* 159–177.

Burroughs, W. *Naked Lunch.* New York: Grove Press, 1959.

Byck, R. (Ed.). *Cocaine Papers: Sigmund Freud.* New York: Stonehill, 1974.

Byck, R., & Van Dyke, C. What are the effects of cocaine in man? In R. C. Petersen & R. C. Stillman (Eds.), *Cocaine: 1977* (NIDA Research Monograph No. 13). Washington, D. C.: U. S. Government Printing Office, 1977, pp. 97–117.

Byck, R., Jatlow, P., Barash, P. and Van Dyke, C. Cocaine: Blood concentration and physiological effect after intranasal application in man. In E. H. Ellinwood, Jr. & M. M. Kilbey (Eds.), *Cocaine and Other Stimulants.* New York: Plenum, 1977, pp. 629–645.

Campbell, J. *Myths to Live By.* 1973. Reprint. New York: Bantam Books, 1977.

Carey, J. T., & Mandel, J. The Bay Area speed scene. *Journal of Health and Social Behavior,* 1968, *9,* 164–174.

Carroll, E. Coca: The plant and its use. In R. C. Petersen & R. C. Stillman (Eds.), *Cocaine: 1977* (NIDA Research Monograph No. 13). Washington, D. C.: U. S. Government Printing Office, 1977, pp. 35–45.

Chambers, C. D., Taylor, W. J. R., & Moffett, A. D. The incidence of cocaine use among methadone maintenance patients. *International Journal of the Addictions,* 1972, *7,* 427–441.

Chapman, A. H. Paranoid psychosis associated with amphetamine usage. *American Journal of Psychiatry,* 1954, *111,* 43–45.

Chassan, J. B. Stochastic models of the single case as the basis of clinical research design. *Behavior Science,* 1961, *6,* 42–50.

Chassan, J. B. *Research Design in Clinical Psychology and Psychiatry,* New York: Appleton-Century-Crofts, 1967.

Chopra, I. C., & Chopra, R. N. The cocaine problem in India. *Bulletin on Narcotics,* 1958, *10,* 12–24.

Chopra, R. N., & Chopra, G. S. Cocaine habit in India. *Indian Journal of Medical Research,* 1930–1931, *18,* 1013–1046.

Clark, R. Cocaine. *Texas Medicine,* 1973, *69,* 74–78.

Cohen, S. Cocaine. *Journal of the American Medical Association,* 1975, *231,* 74–75.

Connell, P. H. *Amphetamine Psychosis.* London: Oxford University Press, 1958.

Connell, P. H. Drug taking in Great Britain: A growing problem. *Royal Society for the Promotion of Health,* 1969, *89,* 92–96.

"Conventional wisdom" on cocaine dangers challenged. *ADAMHA News.* Aug. 24, 1979, pp. 1–2.

Coursey, R. D., & Gaines, L. S. Factor analytic structure of Pearson's Novelty Experiencing Scale. *JSAS Catalog of Selected Documents in Psychology,* 1974, *4,* entire issue.

Crowley, A. *Cocaine.* 1917. Reprint. San Francisco: Level Press, 1973.

Dale, G. M. Morphine and cocaine intoxication. *Journal of the American Medical Association,* 1903, *1,* 1215–1216.

Davidson, H. K. Confessions of a goof ball addict. *American Journal of Psychiatry,* 1964, *120,* 750–756.

Davidson, P. O., & Costello, C. G. *N = 1: Experimental Studies of Single Cases.* New York: Van Nostrand Reinhold, 1969.

Davis, F., & Munoz, L. Heads and freaks: Patterns and meanings of drug use among hippies. *Journal of Health and Social Behavior,* 1968, *9,* 156–163.

Deneau, G. W., Yanigita, T., & Seevers, M. H. Self-administration of psychoactive substances by the monkey: A measure of psychological dependence. *Psychopharmacologia,* 1969, *16,* 30–48.

Dixon, W. E. The drug habit. *British Medical Journal*, 1923, *3*, 543–545.

Downs, A. & Eddy, N. B. The effect of repeated doses of cocaine in the dog. *Journal of Pharmacology and Experimental Therapeutics*, 1932, *46*, 195–198. (a)

Downs, A., & Eddy, N. B. The effects of repeated doses of cocaine in the rat. *Journal of Pharmacology and Experimental Therapeutics*, 1932, *46*, 199–200. (b)

Dukes, W. F. N = 1. *Psychological Bulletin*, 1965, *64*, 74–79.

Eddy, N. B., Halbach, H., Isbell, H., & Seevers, M. H. Drug dependence: Its significance and characteristics. *Bulletin of the World Health Organization*, 1965, *32*, 721–733.

Edison, G. R. Amphetamines: A dangerous illusion. *Annals of Internal Medicine*, 1971, *74*, 604–610.

Edmundson, W. F., Davies, J. E., Acker, J. D., & Myer, B. Patterns of drug abuse epidemiology in prisoners. *Industrial Medicine and Surgery*, 1972, *41*, 15–19.

Eiswirth, N. A., Smith, D. E., & Wesson, D. R. Current perspectives on cocaine use in America. *Journal of Psychedelic Drugs*, 1972, *5*, 153–157.

Ellinwood, E. H., Jr. Amphetamine psychosis: Descriptions of the individuals and process. *Journal of Nervous and Mental Disease*, 1967, *144*, 273–283.

Ellinwood, E. H., Jr. Assault and homicide associated with amphetamine abuse. *American Journal of Psychiatry*, 1971, *127*, 1170–1175.

Ellinwood, E. H., Jr. Amphetamine psychosis: Individuals, settings, and sequences. In E. H. Ellinwood, Jr. & S. Cohen (Eds.), *Current Concepts on Amphetamine Abuse*. Washington, D. C.: U. S. Government Printing Office, 1972, pp. 143–158.

Ellinwood, E. H. Jr. The epidemiology of stimulant abuse. In E. Josephson and Eleanor E. Carroll (Eds.), *Drug Use—Epidemiological and sociological approaches*. Washington, D.C.: Hemisphere Publishing Corporation, 1974, 303–329.

Ellinwood, E. H., Jr., & Kilbey, M. M. (Eds.) *Cocaine and Other Stimulants*, New York: Plenum, 1977.

Ellinwood, E. H., Jr., Sudilovsky, A., & Nelson, M. Evolving behavior in the clinical and experimental amphetamine (model) psychosis. *American Journal of Psychiatry*, 1973, *130*, 1088–1093.

Enforcement can't impede S. American cocaine flow. *U. S. Journal of Drug and Alcohol Dependence*, April, 1978, p. 3.

Erythroxylon coca as an antidote to the opium habit. Editorial. *Detriot Therapeutic Gazette*, June 15, 1880, p. 1.

Evans, M. A., Dwivedi, C., & Harbison, R. D. Enhancement of cocaine-induced lethality by phenobarbital. In E. H. Ellinwood, Jr. and M. Marlyne Kilbey (Eds.), *Cocaine and Other Stimulants*. New York: Plenum, 1977, pp. 253–267.

Finkle, B. S., & McClosky, K. L. The forensic toxicology of cocaine. In R. C. Petersen & R. C. Stillman (Eds.), *Cocaine: 1977* (NIDA Research Monograph No. 13). Washington, D. C.: U. S. Government Printing Office, 1977, pp. 153–192.

Fischman, M. W., Schuster, C. R., & Krasnegor, N. A. Physiological and behavioral effects of intravenous cocaine in man. In E. H. Ellinwood, Jr. & M. Marlyne Kilbey (Eds.), *Cocaine and Other Stimulants.* New York: Plenum, 1977, pp. 646–664.

Fischman, M. W., Schuster, C. R., Resnekov, L., Shick, J. F. E., Krasnegor, N. A., Fennell, W., & Freedman, D. X. Cardiovascular and subjective effects of intravenous cocaine administration in humans. *Archives of General Psychiatry,* 1976, *33,* 983–989.

Fish, R., & Wilson, W. D. C. Excretion of cocaine and its metabolites in man. *Journal of Pharmacy and Pharmacology,* 1969, *21,* supplement, 135–138.

Fog. R. Stereotyped and non-stereotyped behavior in rats induced by various stimulant drugs. *Psychopharmacologia,* 1969, *14,* 299–304.

Freud, S. *Über Coca.* 1884. Reprinted in R. Byck (Ed.), *Cocaine papers: Sigmund Freud.* New York: Stonehill, 1974, pp. 49–73.

Freud, S. Craving for and fear of cocaine. 1887. Reprinted in R. Byck (Ed.), *Cocaine papers: Sigmund Freud.* New York: Stonehill, 1974, pp. 171–176.

Froede, E. Drugs of abuse: Legal and illegal. *Human Pathology,* 1972, *3,* 23–26.

Garlington, W., & Shimota, H. The change seeker index: A measure of the need for variable stimulus input. *Psychological Reports,* 1964, *14,* 919–924.

Gay, G. R., & Sheppard, C. W. Sex crazed dope fiends! Myth or reality? *Drug Forum,* 1973, *2,* 125–140.

Gay, G. R., Sheppard, C. W., Inaba, D. S., & Newmeyer, J. A. An old girl: Flyin' low, dyin' slow, blinded by snow: Cocaine in perspective. *Interational Journal of the Addictions,* 1973, *8,* 1027–1042. (a)

Gay, G. R., Sheppard, C. W., Inaba, D. S., & Newmeyer, J. A. Cocaine perspective: Gift from the sun god to the rich man's drug. *Drug Forum,* 1973, *2,* 409–430. (b)

Goldberg, L. *Narkomani Vanebildning och beroende.* Stockholm: Centralforbundet for nykter hetsundervisning, 1967.

Goode, E. Drug use and grades in college. *Maitre,* 1971, *234,* 225–227.

Gordon, A. Insanities caused by acute and chronic intoxication with opium and cocaine. *Journal of the American Medical Association,* 1908, *2,* 97–101.

Greene, M. H., Nightingale, S., & Dupont, R. Evolving patterns of drug abuse. *Annals of Internal Medicine,* 1975, *83,* 402–411.

Griffith, J. A. A study of illicit amphetamine drug traffic in Oklahoma City. *American Journal of Psychiatry,* 1969, *123,* 560–569.

Grinspoon, L., & Bakalar, J. B. *Cocaine: A Drug and Its Social Evolution.* New York: Basic Books, 1976.

Guilford, J. P. *Fundamental Statistics in Psychology* (3rd ed.). New York: McGraw-Hill, 1956.

Gunne, L. M. & Johnsson, J. Effects of cocaine administration on brain adrenal and urinary adrenaline and noradrenaline in rats. *Psychopharmacologia,* 1964, *6,* 125–129.

498   REFERENCES

Gutierrez-Noriega, C. Accion de la coca sobre la actividad mental de sujetos habituados. *Revista de Medicina Experimental,* 1944, *3,* 1-18.

Gutierrez-Noriega, C. Inhibicion del sistema nervioso central producida por intoxicacion cocainica cronica. *Revista de Farmacologia y Medicina Experimental,* 1949, *224,* 227.

Gutierrez-Noriega, C., & Zapata Ortiz, V. Cocainismo experimental: I. Toxicologia general, acostumbramiento, y sensibilización. *Revista de Medicina Experimental,* 1944, *3,* 303.

Halliday, G. *Influences of Personal Values on Simulated Drug Abuse Research and Rehabilitation,* Unpublished doctoral dissertation, University of Kansas, 1975.

Hammond, W. A. Remarks on cocaine and the so-called cocaine habit. *Journal of Nervous and Mental Diseases,* 1886, *13,* 754-759.

Hammond, W. A. Coca: Its preparations and their therapeutic qualities with some remarks on the so-called cocaine habit. In R. Byck (Ed.), *Cocaine papers: Sigmund Freud.* New York: Stonehill, 1887/1974, pp. 179-193.

Hanna, J. M. Coca leaf use in southern Peru: Some biosocial aspects. *American Anthropologist,* 1974, *76,* 281-296.

Hatch, R. C., & Fischer, R. Cocaine-elicited behavior and toxicity in dogs pretreated with synaptic blocking agents, morphine or diphenylhydantoin. *Pharmacological Communications,* 1972, *4,* 383-392.

Hawks, R. Cocaine: The material. In R. C. Petersen & R. C. Stillman (Eds.), *Cocaine: 1977* (NIDA Research Monograph No. 13). Washington, D. C.: U. S. Government Printing Office, 1977, pp. 47-61.

Ho, B. T., Taylor, D., Estevez, V. S. Englert, L. F., & McKenna, M. L. Behavioral effects of cocaine — metabolic and neurochemical approach. In E. H. Ellinwood, Jr. & M. Marylne Kilbey (Eds.), *Cocaine and Other Stimulants.* New York: Plenum, 1977, pp. 229-240.

Holt, R. R. Individuality and generalization in the psychology of personality. *Journal of Personality,* 1962, *30,* 377-404.

Hrdlicka, A. Trephination among prehistoric people. *Ciba Symposium,* 1969, *1,* No. 6, 1939.

Hutchinson, R. R., Emley, G. S., & Krasnegor, N. A. The effects of cocaine on the aggressive behavior of mice, pigeons, and squirrel monkeys. In E. H. Ellinwood, Jr. & M. M. Kilbey (Eds.), *Cocaine and Other Stimulants.* New York: Plenum, 1977, pp. 457-480.

Isbell, H., & White, W. Characteristics of addictions. *American Journal of Medicine,* 1953, *14,* 558-565.

Jaffe, J. H. Drug addiction and drug abuse. In L. S. Goodman & A. Gilman (Eds.), *The Pharmacological Basis of Therapeutics* (4th ed.). New York: MacMillan, 1970, pp. 276-313.

James, W. *The Varieties of Religious Experience.* 1901. Reprint. New York: New American Library, 1958.

Javaid, J. I., Dekirmenjian, H., & Davis, J. M. Effects of intravenous cocaine on MPG excretion in man. In E. H. Ellinwood, Jr. & M. Marlyne Kilbey (Eds.), *Cocaine and Other Stimulants.* New York: Plenum, 1977, pp. 665-673.

Joël, E., & Fränkel, F. *Der Cocainismus.* Berlin: Springer Verlag, 1924.

Joël, E., & Fränkel, F. Cocainism and homosexuality. Abstracted in the *Journal of the American Medical Association,* 1925, *85,* 1436.

Johanson, C. E., Balster, R. L., & Bonese, K. Self-administration of psycho-motor stimulant drugs: The effects of unlimited access. *Pharmacology, Biochemistry, and Behavior,* 1976, *4,* 45–51.

Johnson, K. G., Abbey, H., Scheble, R., & Weitman, M. Survey of adolescent drug use II: Social and environmental factors. *American Journal of Public Health,* 1972, *62,* 164–166.

Jones, E. *The Life and Work of Sigmund Freud.* New York: Basic Books, 1953.

Jung, C. G. On the relation of analytic psychology to poetry. In J. Campbell (Ed.), *The Portable Jung* (translated by R. F. C. Hall). 1922. Reprint. New York: Viking, 1971, pp. 301–322.

Kaplan, R. *Drug Abuse: Perspectives on Drugs.* Dubuque, Ia: W. C. Brown, 1970.

Kelly, G. A. *The psychology of personal constructs.* Vols. *1* and *2.* New York: Norton, 1955.

Kerlinger, R. Q-methodology in behavioral research. In S. Brown & D. Brenner (Eds.), *Science, Psychology, and Communication.* New York: Teachers College Press, 1972.

Kolb, L. The prevalence and trend of drug addiction in the United States and factors influencing it. *Public Health Reports,* 1924, *39,* 1179–1203.

Kolb, L. Drug addiction in its relation to crime. *Mental Hygiene,* 1925, *9,* 74–89. (a)

Kolb, L. Pleasures and deterioration from narcotic addiction. *Mental Hygiene,* 1925, *9,* 699–724. (b)

Kolb, R. *Drug Addiction: A Medical Problem.* Springfield, Ill.: Charles C Thomas, 1962.

Koller, C. Historical notes on the beginning of local anesthesia. *Journal of the American Medical Association,* 1928, *90,* 1741–1742.

Koller, C. Uber die Verwendung des Cocain zur Anasthesierung am Auge. *Weiner med. Wschr.,* 1884, *34,* Nos. 43 and 44.

Kramer, J. C. Introduction to amphetamine abuse. *Journal of Psychedelic Drugs,* 1969, *2,* 1–16.

Kramer, J. C., Fischman, V. A., & Littlefield, D. C. Amphetamine abuse: Pattern and effects of high doses taken intravenously. *Journal of the American Medical Association,* 1967, *201,* 89–93.

Kramer, J. R. The adolescent addict: The progression of youth through the drug culture. *Clinical Pediatrics,* 1972, *11,* 382–385.

Kuroda, M. On the action of cocaine. *Journal of Pharmacology and Experimental Therapeutics,* 1915, *7,* 423–439.

Lewin, K. *Field Theory in Social Science,* New York: McGraw-Hill, 1953.

Lewin, L. Cocainism. 1924. Reprinted in R. Byck (Ed.), *Cocaine Papers: Sigmund Freud.* New York: Stonehill, 1974, pp. 237–251.

Lewin, L. *Phantastica, Narcotic and Stimulating Drugs, Their Use and Abuse.* New York: E. P. Dutton, 1931.

Lewis, A. Historical perspective. *British Journal of Addiction,* 1968, *63,* 241–245.

Lidz, T., Lidz, R., & Rubenstein, R. An anaclictic syndrome in adolescent amphetamine addicts. *Psychoanalytic Study of the Child,* 1976, *31,* 317–348.

Lindemann, E. The neurophysiological effects of intoxicating drugs. *American Journal of Psychiatry,* 1933/1934, *90,* 1007–1037.

Lindemann, E., & Malamud, W. Experimental analysis of the psychopathological effects of intoxicating drugs. *American Journal of Psychiatry,* 1933/1934, *90,* 853–881.

Louria, D. *Nightmare Drugs.* New York: Pocket Books, 1966.

Ludwig, A. M., & Pyle, R. L. Danger potential of commonly abused drugs. *Wisconsin Medical Journal,* 1969, *68,* 216–218.

Lynn, E. J. Amphetamine abuse: A "speed trap." *Psychiatric Quarterly,* 1971, *45,* 92–101.

Magnan et Saury. Trois cas de cocainisme chronique. *Comptes Rendus des Séances de la Société de Biologie,* 1889, *1,* 60–63.

Maier, H. W. *Der Kokainismus.* Leipzig: Georg Thieme, 1926.

Mair, J. M. M. Experimenting with individuals. *British Journal of Medical Psychology,* 1970, *43* (3), 245–256. (a)

Mair, J. M. M. The person in psychology and psychotherapy: An introduction. *British Journal of Medical Psychology,* 1970, *43* (3), 197–205. (b)

Mantegazza, P. On the hygienic and medicinal virtues of coca. In G. Andrews & D. Solomon (Eds.), *The Coca Leaf and Cocaine Papers.* New York: Harcourt Brace Jovanovich, 1975, pp. 38–42.

Marceil, J. C. Implicit dimensions of idiography and nomothesis: A reformulation. *American Psychologist,* 1977, *32,* 1046–1055.

Martin, R. T. The role of coca and the history, religion, and medicine of South American Indians. *Economic Botany,* 1970, *24,* 438–442.

Matsuzaki, M., Spingler, P. J., Misra, A. L., and Mule, S. J. Cocaine: Tolerance to its convulsant and cardiorespiratory stimulating effects in the monkey. *Life Sciences,* 1976, *19,* 193–204.

Mattison, J. B. Cocaine poisoning. *Medical and Surgical Reporter,* 1891, *65,* 645–650.

Maurer, D., & Vogel, V. H. *Narcotics and Narcotic Addiction,* Springfield, Ill.: Charles C Thomas, 1967.

Mayer, E. The toxic effects following use of local anesthetics. *Journal of the American Medical Association,* 1924, *82,* 876–885.

Mayer-Gross, W., Slater, E., & Roth, M. *Clinical Psychiatry.* Baltimore: Williams and Wilkins, 1960.

McLaughlin, G. T. Cocaine: The history and regulation of a dangerous drug. *Cornell Law Review,* 1973, *57,* 537–573.

McLaughlin, J. J., & Haines, W. H. Drug addiction in Chicago. *Illinois Medical Journal,* 1952, *72,* 27–77.

Mendizabal, F. R. Accion de la coca y de la cocaina in subjectos habituados. *Revista de Medicina Experimental,* 1944, *3,* 317–328.

Mills, C. L. Morphinomania, cocamania and general narcomania and some of their legal consequences. *International Clinics*, 1905, *1*, 159–176.

Minkowski, W. L., Weiss, R. C., & Heidbreder, G. A. A review of the drug problem: A national approach to youthful drug use and abuse. *Clinical Pediatrics*, 1972, *7*, 373.

Mortimer, W. G. 1901. Reprint. *History of Coca: "The Divine Plant" of the Incas.* San Francisco: And/Or Press, 1974.

Musto, D. F. A study in cocaine, Sherlock Holmes and Sigmund Freud. In R. Byck (Ed.), *Cocaine papers of Sigmund Freud.* New York: Stonehill Publishing Co., 1974, 257–270.

Nail, R. L., Gunderson, E. K., & Kolb, D. Motives for drug use among light and heavy users. *Journal of Nervous and Mental Disease*, 1974, *159*, 131–136.

National Clearinghouse for Drug Abuse Information. *Cocaine* (Report Series II: no. 1, January, 1972). Rockville, Md.: Alcohol, Drug Abuse and Mental Health Administration, 1972.

Nie, N., Bent, D. H., & Hull, C. H. *SPSS: Statistical Package for the Social Sciences.* New York: McGraw-Hill, 1970.

Noda, H. Concerning wake-amine intoxication. *Kurume Igakhai Zasshi*, 1950, *13*, 294–298.

Nunnally, J. *Introduction to Psychological Measurement.* New York: McGraw-Hill, 1970.

O'Connor, W. A., & O'Connor, K. S. An ecological approach to treatment: The natural history of institutional change. In D. Berger (Ed.), *Planning for Change in State Hospitals.* Los Angeles: Human Interaction Research Institute, 1978.

O'Connor, W. A. *Problem-resource coordination with target groups* (Final Report, NIMH Grant #R-000004-060), Kansas City, Mo.: Greater Kansas City Mental Health Foundation, 1975.

Offerman, A. Über die Zentrale Wirkung des Cocains und einiger neuen Ersatzpräparate. *Archiv für Psychiatrie*, 1926, *76*, 600–633.

Olden, M. *Cocaine.* New York: Lancer Books, 1973.

Orr, D., & Jones, I. Anaesthesia for laryngoscopy: A comparison of the cardiovascular effects of cocaine and lidocaine. *Anaesthesia*, 1968, *23*, 194–202.

Osgood, E. C., Suci, G., & Tannebaum, H. H. *The Measurement of Meaning.* Urbana: University of Illinois Press, 1957.

Ossenfort, W. F. The treatment of drug addicts at the United States Public Health Service Hospital, Fort Worth, Texas. *Texas State Journal of Medicine*, 1939, *35*, 428–432.

Parke, Davis and Co. Coca Erythroxylon and its derivatives. 1885. Reprint. In R. Byck (Ed.), *Cocaine Papers: Sigmund Freud.* New York: Stonehill, 1974, pp. 127–150.

Partridge, M. Drug addiction – a brief review. *International Journal of the Addictions*, 1967, *2*, 207–220.

Pearson, P. Relationships between global and specific measures of novelty seeking. *Journal of Consulting and Clinical Psychology*, 1970, *34* (2), 199–204.

Penfield, W. Halsted of Johns Hopkins: The man and his problem as described in the secret records of William Osler. *Journal of the American Medical Association*, 1969, *210*, 2214–2218.

Perry, C. The star-spangled powder or through history with coke spoon and nasal spray. *Rolling Stone*, August 18, 1972, no. 115.

Petersen, R. C. Cocaine: An overview. In R. C. Petersen & R. C. Stillman (Eds.), *Cocaine: 1977* (NIDA Research Monograph No. 13). Washington, D. C.: U. S. Government Printing Office, 1977, pp. 5–15. (a)

Petersen, R. C. History of Cocaine. In R. C. Petersen & R. C. Stillman (Eds.), *Cocaine: 1977* (NIDA Research Monograph No. 13). Washington, D. C.: U. S. Government Printing Office, 1977, pp. 17–34. (b)

Petersen, R. C., & Stillman, R. C. (Eds.). *Cocaine: 1977* (NIDA Research Monograph No. 13). Washington, D. C.: U. S. Government Printing Office, 1977.

Phillips, J. L. *Cocaine: The Facts and Myths*. Unpublished manuscript. Washington, D. C.: Wynne Associates, 1975.

Pickens, R., & Thompson, T. Characteristics of stimulant reinforcement. In T. Thompson and R. Pickens (Eds.), *Stimulus Properties of Drugs*. New York: Appleton-Century-Crofts, 1971, pp. 177–192.

Plate, T. Coke: The big new easy entry business. *New York Magazine*, October 1973, pp. 63–75.

Post, R. M. Cocaine psychosis: A continuum model. *American Journal of Psychiatry*, 1975, *132*, 225–231.

Post, R. M. Comparative psychopharmacology of cocaine and amphetamine. *Psychopharmacology Bulletin*, 1976, *12*, 39–41.

Post, R. M. Progressive changes in behavior and seizures following chronic cocaine administration: Relationship to kindling and psychosis. In E. H. Ellinwood, Jr. & M. Marlyne Kilbey (Eds.), *Cocaine and Other Stimulants*. New York: Plenum, 1977, pp. 353–372.

Post, R. M., and Kopanda, R. T. Cocaine, kindling, and reverse tolerance. *Lancet*, 1975, *1*, 409–410.

Post, R. M., Kopanda, R. T., and Black, K. E. Progressive effects of cocaine on behavior and central amine metabolism in rhesus monkeys: Relationship to kindling and psychosis. *Biological Psychiatry*, 1976, II, 403–419.

Post, R. M., & Rose, H. Increasing effects of repetitive cocaine administration in the rat. *Nature*, 1976, *260*, 731–732.

Post, R. M., Kotin, J., & Goodwin, R. The effects of cocaine on depressed patients. *American Journal of Psychiatry*, 1974, *131*, 511–517.

Randrup, A., & Munkvad, I. Biochemical, anatomical, and psychological investigations of stereotyped behavior induced by amphetamines. In E. Costa & S. Garattini (Eds.), *International Symposium on Amphetamines and Related Compounds*. New York: Raven Press, 1970, pp. 695–713.

Reinarman, C. A historical perspective. In D. Waldorf et al., *Doing Coke: and Ethnography of Cocaine Users and Sellers*. Washington, D. C.: Drug Abuse Council, 1977, pp. 1–15.

Resnick, R. B., Kestenbaum, R. S., & Schwartz, L. K. Acute systemic effects of cocaine in man: A controlled study of intranasal and intravenous route of administration. In E. H. Ellinwood, Jr. & M. Marlyne Kilbey (Eds.), *Cocaine and Other Stimulants.* New York: Plenum, 1977, pp. 615–628.

Ritchie, J. M., & Cohen, P. J. Local anesthetics. In L. S. Goodman and A. Gillman (Eds.), *The Pharmacological Basis of Therapeutics* (5th Ed.). New York: Macmillan, 1975, pp. 379–403.

Ritchie, J. M., Cohen, P. J., & Dripps, R. D. Cocaine, procaine and other synthetic local anesthetics. In L. S. Goodman & A. Gilman (Eds.), *The Pharmacological Basis of Therapeutics.* New York: Macmillan, 1970, pp. 371–401.

Rosenberg, C. M. Young drug addicts: Addiction and its consequences. *Medical Journal of Australia,* 1968, *24,* 1031–1033.

Rylander, C. Clinical and medico-criminal aspects of addiction to central stimulants. In F. Sjoqvist & M. Tottie (Eds.), *Abuse of Central Stimulants.* New York: Raven Press, 1969, pp. 251–273.

Sabbag, R. *Snow Blind.* New York: Avon Books, 1976.

Scheel-Kruger, J. Behavioral and biochemical comparison of amphetamine derivatives, cocaine, benzotropine, and tricyclic antidepressant drugs. *European Journal of Pharmacology,* 1972, *18,* 63–73.

Scheel-Kruger, J., Braestrup, C., Nielson, M., Golembiowska, K., & Mogilnicka, E. Cocaine: discussion on the role of dopamine in the biochemical mechanism of action. In E. H. Ellinwood, Jr. & M. Marlyne Kilbey (Eds.), *Cocaine and Other Stimulants.* New York: Plenum, 1977, pp. 373–405.

Scheppegrell, W. The abuse and danger of cocaine. *Medical News,* 1898, *73,* 417–422.

Schiørring, E. Changes in individual and special behavior induced by amphetamine and related compounds in monkeys and man. In E. H. Ellinwood, Jr. & M. Marlyne Kilbey (Eds.), *Cocaine and Other Stimulants.* New York: Plenum, 1977, pp. 481–522.

Schultz, M. G. The "strange case" of Robert Louis Stevenson. *Journal of the American Medical Association,* 1971, *216,* 90–94.

Schultz, P. Ueber die Wirkungswiese der Mydriaca and Miotica. *Arch. Psyiol,* 1898, *23,* 47–74.

Shapiro, M. B. A method of measuring psychological changes specific to the individual psychiatric patient. *British Journal of Medical Psychology,* 1961, *34,* 151–155. (a)

Shapiro, M. B. The single case in fundamental clinical psychological research *British Journal of Medical Psychology,* 1961, *34,* 255–262. (b)

Shontz, F. C. *Research Methods in Personality.* New York: Appleton-Century-Crofts, 1965.

Shontz, F. C. Single organism designs. In P. M. Bentler, D. J. Lettieri, & G. A. Austin (Eds.), *Research Issues 13: Data Analysis Strategies and Designs for Substance Abuse Research.* Washington, D. C.: U. S. Department of Health, Education, and Welfare, National Institute on Drug Abuse, 1976, pp. 25–44.

Siegel, R. K. Cocaine: recreational use and intoxication. In R. C. Petersen & R. C. Stillman (Eds.), *Cocaine: 1977* (NIDA Research Monograph No. 13). Washington, D. C.: U. S. Government Printing Office, 1977, pp. 119–136.

Siguel, E. Characteristics of clients admitted to treatment for cocaine abuse. In

R. C. Petersen & R. C. Stillman (Eds.), *Cocaine: 1977* (NIDA Research Monograph No. 13). Washington, D. C.: U. S. Government Printing Office, 1977, pp. 201–210.

Smith, D. E. The characteristics of dependence in high dose methamphetamine abuse. *The International Journal of Addictions,* 1969, *4,* 453–459.

Smith, D. E., & Fischer, C. M. Acute amphetamine toxicity. *Journal of Psychedelic Drugs,* 1969, *2,* 49–54.

Smith, R. B. Cocaine and catecholamine interaction: A review. *Archives of Otolaryngology,* 1973, *98,* 139–141.

Smith, R. C. The world of the Haight-Ashbury speed freak. *Journal of Psychedelic Drugs,* 1969, *2,* 172–188.

Smith, R. C. Speed and violence: Compulsive methamphetamine abuse and criminality in the Haight-Ashbury District. In C. J. E. Zarafonetis (Ed.), *Drug Abuse: Proceedings of the International Conference.* Philadelphia: Lea and Febinger, 1972, pp. 435–448.

Snyder, S. H. Amphetamine psychosis: A "model" schizophrenia mediated by catecholamines. *American Journal of Psychiatry,* 1973, *103,* 61–67.

Spotts, J. V., & Mackler, B. Relationships of field-dependent and field-independent cognitive styles to creative test performance. *Perceptual and Motor Skills,* 1967, *24,* 239–268.

Spotts, J. V., & Shontz, F. C. The empirical study of the life style and psychosocial correlates of cocaine use and abuse. Remarks given September 16, 1974, for the NIDA Conference, Cocaine Research: State of the Art, Rockville, Md.

Steele, R., Angrest, S., Monroe, S., Brinkley-Rogers, P., & Lesher, S. The cocaine scene. *Newsweek,* May 30, 1977, *89,* no. 22, pp. 20–25.

Stephens, R. C., & Weppner, R. S. Patterns of cheating among methadone maintenance patients. *Drug Forum,* 1973, *2,* 357–366.

Stephenson, W. *The Study of Behavior: Q-Technique and Its Methods.* Chicago: University of Chicago Press, 1953.

Stockwell, G. A. Erythroxylon coca. *Boston Medical and Surgical Journal,* 1877, *96,* 399–404.

Stripling, J. S., & Ellinwood, E. H., Jr. Sensitization to cocaine following chronic administration in the rat. In E. H. Ellinwood, Jr. & M. Marlyne Kilbey (Eds.), *Cocaine and Other Stimulants.* New York: Plenum, 1977, pp. 327–351.

Tatum, A. L., & Seevers, M. H. Experimental cocaine addiction. *Journal of Pharmacology and Experimental Therapeutics,* 1929, *36,* 401–410.

The Gourmet Coke Book. White Mountain Press, 1972.

Thompson, T., & Pickens, R. Stimulating self-administration by animals: Some comparisons with opiate self-administration. *Federation Proceedings,* 1970, *29,* 6–12.

Valliant, G. E. A twelve year follow-up on New York addicts IV: Some characteristics and determinants of abstinence. *American Journal of Psychiatry,* 1966, *123,* 573.

Van Dyke, C., & Byck, R. Cocaine: 1884–1974. In E. H. Ellinwood, Jr. & M.

Marylne Kilbey (Eds.), *Cocaine and Other Stimulants*. New York: Plenum, 1977, pp. 1–30.

Waldorf, D., Murphy, S., Reinerman, C., & Bridget, J. *Doing Coke: An Ethnography of Cocaine Users and Sellers*. Washington, D. C.: Drug Abuse Council, 1977, pp. 16–68.

Wallace, M. B., & Gershon, S. A neuropsychological comparison of d-amphetamine, L-dopa and cocaine. *Neuropharmacology*, 1971, *10*, 743–752.

Wesson, D. R., & Smith, D. E. Cocaine: Its use for central nervous system stimulation including recreational and medical uses. In R. C. Petersen & R. C. Stillman (Eds.), *Cocaine: 1977* (NIDA Research Monograph No. 13). Washington, D. C.: U. S. Government Printing Office, 1977, pp. 137–152.

Wetli, C. V., & Wright, R. K. Death caused by recreational cocaine use. *Journal of the American Medical Association*, 1979, *241*, 2519–2522.

White, R. *Value Analysis*. Glen Garden, N.J.: Society for the Study of Social Issues, 1951.

Wieder, H., & Kaplan, E. H. Drug use in adolescents: Psychodynamic meanings and pharmacogenic effect. *Psychoanalytic Study of the Child*, 1969, *24*, 399–431.

Wiley, H. W., & Pierce, A. L. The cocaine crime. *Good Housekeeping*, 1914, *58*, 393–398.

Williams, E. H. The drug habit in the south. *Medical Record*, 1914, *85*, 247–249.

Wilson, C. W. M. Drugs of dependence. *Practitioner*, 1968, *200*, 102–112.

Wilson, M. C., Bedford, J. A., Buelke, J., & Kibbe, A. H. Acute pharmacological activity of intravenous cocaine in the rhesus monkey. *Psychopharmcological Communications*, 1976, *2*, 251–262.

Wittenborn, J. Contributions and current status of Q-methodology. *Psychological Bulletin*, 1961, *58* (2), 132–142.

Wolff, P. Drug addiction – a worldwide problem. *Journal of the American Medical Association*, 1932, *98*, 175–184.

Woodley, R. A. *Dealer: Portrait of a Cocaine Merchant*. New York: Holt, Rinehart & Winston, 1971.

Woods, J. Behavioral effects of cocaine in animals. In R. C. Petersen & R. C. Stillman (Eds.), *Cocaine: 1977* (NIDA Research Monograph No. 13). Washington, D. C.: U. S. Government Printing Office, 1977, pp. 63–95.

Woods, J. H., & Downs, D. A. The psychopharmacology of cocaine. In National Commission on Marijuana and Drug Abuse, *Drug Use in America: Problem in Perspective. Appendix Volume 1: Patterns and Consequences of Drug Use*. Washington, D. C.: U. S. Government Printing Office, 1973, pp. 116–139.

Woods, L. A., McMahon, F. G., & Seevers, M. H. Distribution and metabolism of cocaine in the dog and rabbit. *Journal of Pharmacology and Experimental Therapeutics*, 1951, *104*, 200–204.

Wurmser, L. Drug addiction and drug abuse. *Maryland State Medical Journal*, 1968, *17*, 68–80.

Wylie, W. D., & Churchill-Davidson, H. C. *A Practice of Anesthesia.* Chicago: Yearbook Medical Publishers, 1966.

Yanagita, T. An experimental framework for the evaluation of dependence liability of various types of drugs in monkeys. *Bulletin on Narcotics,* 1973, *1,* 25–57.

Young, D., & Glauber, J. J. Electrocardiographic changes resulting from acute cocaine intoxication. *American Heart Journal,* 1947, *34,* 272–279.

Zinberg, N. Paragraph three of Affidavit Attached to Defendants' Joint Memorandum in Support of Their Motion for Correction or Reduction of Sentence (*United States of America* v. *Foss and Coveney,* U. S. District Court, District of Massachusetts: Criminal No. 73-24-G), 1974.

Zuckerman, M. Drug usage as a manifestation of a "sensation-seeking" trait. In E. Costa & S. Garratini (Eds.), *International Symposium on Amphetamines and Related Compounds.* New York: Dover, 1970.

Zuckerman, M. Dimensions of sensation-seeking. *Journal of Consulting and Clinical Psychology,* 1971, *36,* 45–52.

Zuckerman, M., & Bone, R. What is the sensation seeker? Personality trait and experience correlates of the sensation-seeking scales. *Journal of Consulting and Clinical Psychology,* 1972, *39,* 308–321.

Zuckerman, M., & Link, K. Construct validity for the sensation-seeking scale. *Journal of Consulting and Clinical Psychology,* 1968, *32,* 420–426.

Index